PRINCIPLES

OF

HUMAN NUTRITION

A STUDY IN PRACTICAL DIETETICS

BY

WHITMAN H. JORDAN

DIRECTOR OF THE NEW YORK AGRICULTURAL EXPERIMENT
STATION ; AUTHOR OF "THE FEEDING OF ANIMALS"

New York

THE MACMILLAN COMPANY

1916

Norwood Press
J. S. Cushing Co. — Berwick & Smith Co.
Norwood, Mass., U.S.A.

PREFACE

An examination of this volume will at once make it evident that it was not prepared for use with students who have specialized in organic and biological chemistry. The object in view was rather such a presentation of the subject-matter related to human nutrition as would be more or less adapted to popular use, but particularly to instruction of students with moderate scientific acquirements, whether in colleges, secondary schools, short courses, schools of domestic science, or correspondence schools. The reliable knowledge bearing on the nutrition of man is mainly to be found in elaborate works on physiology and physiological chemistry, the contents of which are not generally available. Moreover, the highly technical facts are usually not centered around a philosophy of living. The aim here has been to show the adjustment of this knowledge to a rational system of nutrition without insisting upon adherence to technical details that are not feasible in the ordinary administration of the family dietary.

It is needless to state that the author makes no claim to having written on his own authority, but, on the other hand, he has relied upon the conclusions of those authorities and investigators whose sound scholarship in this field of knowledge is unquestioned. The following literature is that which has mainly been considered:

Metabolism and Practical Medicine, Von Noorden; translated by J. Walker Hall.

Textbook of Physiological Chemistry, Abderhalden; translated by William T. Hall.

The Science of Nutrition, Lusk.

A Textbook of Physiological Chemistry, Hammersten; translated by Mendel.

Der Kindes Enahrung, Czerny and Keller.

Chemistry of Food and Nutrition, Sherman.

Foods and their Adulteration, Wiley.

Physiological Economy in Nutrition, Chittenden.

Textbook of Physiology, Howell.

Textbook of Physiological and Pathological Chemistry, Bunge.

The publications on human nutrition of the Office of Experiment Stations.

Papers by Dr. L. B. Mendel.

Generous acknowledgment should be made to Lea & Febiger, Philadelphia, Pa., for permission to use the excellent cuts from Anatomy and Physiology for Nurses by Kimber.

W. H. JORDAN.

New York Agricultural Experiment Station,
Geneva, N.Y., October 27, 1911.

TABLE OF CONTENTS

PART I

THE PRINCIPLES OF HUMAN NUTRITION

CHAPTER I

CHAPTER II

CHAPTER III

CHAPTER IV

CHAPTER V

CHAPTER VI

THE DISTRIBUTION AND TRANSFORMATIONS OF THE DIGESTED FOOD

CHAPTER VIII

PART II

PRACTICAL DIETETICS

CHAPTER IX

CHAPTER XV

The Character and Food Value of Certain Commercial

CHAPTER XVI

CHAPTER XVII

CHAPTER XVIII

PART I

THE PRINCIPLES OF HUMAN NUTRITION

PRINCIPLES OF HUMAN NUTRITION

CHAPTER I

THE PLANT AS THE SOURCE OF HUMAN SUSTENANCE

THE vegetable world sustains a fundamental relation to man's physical being. Plant life is the medium through which the inorganic substances of the soil and air are made available to the uses of the human organism; and so it is with the materials and activities of plants that we must begin a study of the basal facts of human nutrition.

1. The plant stores food substance. — The first step toward supplying man with food is taken when the farmer drops seed into the warm earth. As soon as the young rootlets from a germinating seed come in contact with the soil, and the first leaves reach the air, assimilative growth begins. During the hours of sunlight, matter is constantly gathered in an invisible way, which, after transformation into various compounds, is added to the enlarging tissues of the plant. This continues, perhaps for a season, until the stalk of grain has reached its full height and has attained the ultimate object of its existence in the production of seed. The farmer carries to the field a few pounds of seed, and he returns to his storehouses laden with tons of new material, perhaps hay, perhaps grain. From somewhere, in some way, the plant has gathered various substances, often no less than ten thousand pound per acre in a single year, and has manufactured them into forms that are nutritively useful to man.

2. The plant stores energy. — Plant life not only builds tissue : it stores energy, as we may easily discover. The farmer's boy learns this when he feels the hot glow of the fire that is fed by forest wood. The wood disappears, but he is warmed by the radiant heat. It has occurred that when fuel was scarce and costly and grain was abundant and cheap, the Western farmer has burned his corn. As with the wood, the materials which were collected from the soil and air were dispersed in invisible forms during the combustion which liberated the heat energy, except a small heap of ashes on the hearth.

3. Relation of plant substance to animal life. — But ordinarily, the substance of farm crops is produced, not for fuel but for food purposes, and in this use of vegetable matter we come in contact with a set of phenomena equally complex and equally important and interesting to those of its growth. The child gradually attains a man's stature. What is the source of this added tissue? It is plant substance which in other combinations was collected from soil and air. The child eats his daily food and makes his daily gain of tissue. If his food were withdrawn, his body would waste, and in time death would ensue. We, therefore, cannot resist the conclusion that the bones, blood, and flesh of the human body are derived from food.

The plant does more than to supply building material for the animal[1] body, for the living organism is kept warm. No matter how cold the surrounding atmosphere, we find

[1] Man is an animal, and the nutritive processes of his body are similar to those in all other higher animal organisms, the mechanism being different.

by the use of a thermometer that in health man's temperature remains at about 98.4° F. with not over one degree normal variation. Just as the Western farmer obtained heat by burning corn in the fireplace, so do human beings maintain their body temperature at the necessary degree by consuming food to be burned. The combustion is not so rapid as occurs in the fireplace, but the chemical changes are the same, only more slowly carried on.

Food not only builds man's body and warms it, — it furnishes it with motive power. The energy which the plant acquires during its time of growth through vital processes is transformed in part into motion. Man is a living mechanism, a combination of muscles and levers which are moved, not by means of a spontaneous internal generation of energy, but through a supply from without, the energy stored in the plant.

If we use the plant for fuel, we get heat alone; if it is consumed as food, we get heat, motion, and the production of body tissue. In the first instance, the plant substance, except the mineral portion, is wholly broken up into simpler compounds which escape in unseen gaseous forms, the liberated energy becoming manifest as heat. If the plant is used by man as food, a greatly varying proportion of its dry matter is retained to form his body substance, and the remaining part suffers oxidation, largely into the same compounds that are carried away by the draft from the fire on the hearth, with an accompanying liberation of energy that manifests itself in motion and heat. As a result, there is built a living organism that is warmed to a temperature generally much above that of the surrounding air, and which is the seat of complex internal activities and is capable of performing external work.

CHAPTER II

THE CHEMICAL ELEMENTS INVOLVED IN THE NUTRITION OF THE HUMAN BODY

THE facts which are fundamentally necessary to a broad understanding of human nutrition pertain, first of all, to the materials out of which vegetable and animal tissues are constructed. It is important to know both what these are and what are their sources.

4. Number of elements involved. — About seventy substances are now believed to be chemical elements, *i.e.*, substances that cannot be resolved into two or more simpler ones, and of which, so far as known, all forms of matter are composed, the variety of their combinations being almost infinite. It is remarkable that comparatively few of these fundamental substances — about one-fifth — are intimately related to the growth of plants; and those that occupy a prominent place in human nutrition are even less in number. It is necessary to mention only fifteen elements in this connection, some of which are of minor importance: carbon, oxygen, hydrogen, nitrogen, sulfur, phosphorus, chlorine, silicon, fluorine, potassium, sodium, calcium, magnesium, iron, and manganese.

5. Sources of elements. — At ordinary temperatures, four of these, oxygen, hydrogen, nitrogen, and chlorine, are gases, and the remaining ones are solids. Four are constant and important ingredients of the atmosphere;

6

viz., carbon, oxygen, hydrogen, and nitrogen, and they also exist in the soil in gases, as well as in combination in liquids and solids; the other eleven, though sometimes present in the air in minute quantities, are found to no appreciable extent except as fixed compounds in water and in the crust of the earth, or in plants and animals. Nearly all of these elementary substances are absolutely essential to man's existence. From the standpoint of necessity, they are, therefore, nearly all of equal value; but if we take into consideration the relative ease and abundance of the supply, certain ones rise to a position of supreme importance.

A. THE ELEMENTS AND THEIR SOURCES

6. Carbon. — This is a familiar substance in common life. Anthracite coal and charcoal are examples of impure carbon. Graphite in lead pencils is also carbon, and so are diamonds. When wood chars or food is burned in an overheated oven, the partially decomposed materials become black, revealing the presence of carbon, the other elements with which it was associated being driven out.

An immense quantity of carbon exists in the air, combined with oxygen as carbon dioxid or carbonic acid gas. The average proportion by weight of this compound in the atmosphere is stated to be .06 per cent, and as the weight of a column of air one inch square is fifteen pounds, it follows that over every acre of land there is 26.2 tons of carbon dioxid, or 7.7 tons of carbon. As we know that plants draw their supply of this element from the atmosphere, and as vegetable tissue is its only source to animal life, we are able to assert, with confidence, that the carbon in the tissues of the human body was once floating in space.

A long time` ago, Boussingault determined the average yearly amount of carbon which was withdrawn from the air by the crops grown on a particular field during a period of five years, and found it to be 4615 pounds. This is no more than is acquired by a large crop of maize. As a matter of fact, plants, as well as animals, contain a larger proportion of this element than of any other, and the amount of this substance which enters into the processes of growth and decay in the vegetable and animal kingdoms is almost beyond comprehension. It is natural to wonder whether the atmospheric supply is equal to the demand. Any anxieties we may have concerning this should be removed by learning that during many years the percentage of atmospheric carbon has not changed appreciably. The processes of decay on the earth's surface, the combustion of wood and coal as fuel and of carbon compounds by animal life, are returning carbon to the air as rapidly as it is being withdrawn. This is the round traveled, — from the air to the plant, from the plant to the animal, and from the animal back to the air, — a cycle in which this element has been moving since life began, and in which it will continue to move so long as life exists.

7. Oxygen. — This element is, next to carbon, the most abundant component of vegetable and animal tissues, and it stands second to none in its relation to the vital processes of nearly all forms of life. It is not a substance with which we are familiar by sight, because we ordinarily come in contact with it as a transparent, colorless gas. We live and move in it, for it is an important and uniformly abundant constituent of the atmosphere. The air is over one-fifth oxygen by volume, the proportion by weight being slightly larger. More than twenty-one million pounds of this element are contained in the air above a single acre of land, a quantity which remains remarkably constant, and which is surprisingly uniform over the entire surface of the globe. While it is being continuously withdrawn from the air for the uses of life and to maintain fuel combustion and processes of decay, it is, like carbon, continuously returned.

Vast quantities of oxygen are also contained in water, as this compound, which fills the ocean and lakes, and is abundant in the crust of the earth, is nearly 89 per cent oxygen. It is estimated also that the solids in the crust of the earth are one-half oxygen. That which enters directly into the uses of animal life is, however, chiefly that which is derived from the atmosphere and water.

Not a plant grows or animal lives excepting through the circulation of oxygen, during which it passes into fixed combinations and back again to the free form. Man uses the free oxygen in breathing and returns it to the air in part combined with carbon as carbon dioxid. This compound the plant appropriates, retaining the carbon for its tissues and giving back the uncombined oxygen to the atmosphere to be again used by animal life. All decay and many other chemical changes require the presence of this element. What we speak of as fire is due to its union with the elements of the fuel.

Oxygen bears an indispensable relation to the mechanical forces that man now employs, for it is the agent which maintains combustion in the furnaces of our industries.

All the activities of life are intimately related to it.   When a plant grows, oxygen is torn from its union with other elements by the dominating power of the sun's rays, and energy is stored in vegetable tissue.   When this tissue is used as food, the oxygen returns to its former combinations through the opportunities offered by the vital processes of the animal, and the hidden forces of the plant compounds are thus manifested in a variety of ways. Human toil is sustained by the energy thus stored and liberated.

8. Hydrogen. — This element, which, in a free state, is the lightest known gas, is found abundantly in nature only in combination with other elements.   The minute quantities which exist in the air are due to volcanic action and possibly to decay under certain conditions.   As a manufactured product, it has an important use in producing intense heat and in filling balloons.   Hydrogen constitutes about one-ninth of water by weight, and is found in a large number of soil compounds.   It is an essential constituent of vegetable and animal tissues, although it exists in the compounds of living organisms in a much smaller proportion than carbon or oxygen.   Plants obtain it largely from water, and it is furnished to the animal body in water and in other compounds.

9. Nitrogen. — Probably no element has been given more attention in its relations to human nutrition than has nitrogen as such and in its compounds.   Like oxygen, it is an invisible, tasteless, and odorless gas which forms in the free state a large part of the earth's atmosphere. The air has been considered to be approximately 77 per cent free nitrogen by weight, but the discovery of the new element, argon, which has heretofore passed as nitrogen, will slightly modify previous determinations.

Nowhere outside of the air, in the tissues of living organisms, and in certain mineral deposits, does nitrogen exist in any form in comparatively large quantities. The soil spaces contain it, and it is taken into solution in small proportions by all natural waters. It is found in the mineral, as well as organic, compounds of the soil, but in quantities which seem insignificant as compared with other elements, such as oxygen and silicon. Few agricultural soils contain over one-half of one per cent of combined nitrogen. Minute quantities of its compounds exist in the atmosphere, which are being constantly carried to the soil in rain-water and as constantly replaced by the ammonia from decomposing animal and vegetable matter and by the products of the oxidation of nitrogen through electrical action and combustion. Notwithstanding this comparatively small supply of nitrogen compounds, they play a prominent part in human nutrition both commercially and physiologically.

Nitrogen compounds are especially important because the available supply is often dangerously near the demand, or even below it. The nitrogen found in the air is inert for animal uses, and is ignored by a large majority of plants. Much of that in the soil is also unavailable. Moreover, its immediately useful compounds on the farm are constantly subject to loss, — first by processes of fermentation, such as those in manures, which the farmer cannot wholly prevent, and second by soil losses which are to some extent beyond control. Many of the commercial products of the farm also carry away much nitrogen. The sources of supply to balance this outgo are the nitric acid and ammonia of the rainfall, the free nitrogen captured by legumes, and whatever comes from purchased fertilizers and foods. These facts relate primarily to plant production, but they also sustain an essential relation to the maintenance of human life, and cannot be ignored in a discussion of the physical problems that relate to human welfare.

Physiologically, the nitrogen compounds stand in the front rank. They are necessary building material for the fundamental tissues of the animal, and are intimately related to the prominent chemical changes that are involved in growth and in the maintenance of life. It is safe to assert, too, that variations of these compounds in the food may have an important influence on health and the character of the body structure.

As a result of these conditions which relate to the supply of useful nitrogen and to its important rôle, we find that it has assumed a prominent place in commerce. For these reasons, the control, even though only partial, which the farmer may now assume over the income and outgo of the nitrogen compounds valuable to agriculture is a triumph of modern science and an important feature of national economics.

10. Sulfur is a common and familiar substance. As an element it is not widely distributed in nature, but its compounds are found in all soils and natural waters, and in all the higher forms of animal and vegetable life. We know it as " brimstone " when fused in sticks, and as " flowers of sulfur" when sublimed in a finely divided form. Its most common commercial compounds are sulfuric acid and the sulfates of potash, soda, lime, and magnesia. This element is an essential part of some of the most important animal tissues, and is supplied in food in the form of the sulfates and in its protein combinations.

11. Phosphorus occupies an important place among the elements of nutrition. In the uncombined form it does not exist in nature, as that found in laboratories is produced only by chemical means. Its compounds are found everywhere. The phosphates of calcium and magnesium are widely distributed in soils, and large deposits of calcium phosphate are known, from which is obtained the crude phosphatic rock that serves as a basis for the manufacture of commercial fertilizers. All foods in their natural forms contain phosphorus, combined in certain fats and nitrogen compounds which stand in close relation to the vital processes. It is distributed in the flesh of man and, combined with calcium and oxygen, constitutes a large part of bone.

12. Chlorine, which is a constituent of common salt, is essential to human nutrition. At ordinary temperatures it is, in the free state, a greenish-colored, disagreeable gas. When combined with hydrogen, it forms hydrochloric acid, a compound which is necessary to the digestion of food.

13. Potassium, combined with oxygen and hydrogen, gives us the caustic potash of the market. The ashes of all plants contain this element, a familiar illustration of this fact being the potassium carbonate leached from wood ashes by hot water in the old-fashioned way of making soft soap. The saleratus formerly used in bread-making was a potassium compound. This element is found in the flesh of animals, mostly in the form of the phosphate, and is abundantly supplied for the purposes of nutrition by dietaries that are not too largely made up of artificially treated foods.

14. Sodium is the basal element of common salt (sodium chloride); and this is about the only sodium compound we need to mention, for this is the one that serves almost wholly as a source of this element to human food.   Sodium plays an important part in the digestion of food, because it is the basis of certain bile salts and is concerned in other ways in the digestive processes.

15. Calcium, when united with oxygen, forms lime, which is one of our commonest commercial articles.   Large masses of lime rock, or calcium carbonate, exist in many parts of the earth's surface, and every soil contains more or less of lime compounds.   As compounds of this element are always found in plants and in the milk of all animals, a mixed diet of unmodified vegetable and animal foods nearly always furnishes a supply sufficient to meet the demands of animal life.   The growing child makes a generous use of lime, because in union with phosphoric acid it is the chief building material of the bony frame-work.   A deficiency of food lime is sure to cause abnormal development of the bony structures.

16. Iron, one of the elements of living organisms, needs no description, because its common properties are familiar to every one.   Iron rust and iron ore are oxides of this element, and when the oxygen is removed from these, we have the bright gray metal of commerce.   Though taken up by plants and animals in small quantities only, iron is absolutely essential to their growth and welfare, but because of its abundance the imperative character of the demand is never realized in ordinary experience. It is intimately related to the life processes of the human organism.

B. Proportions of the Elements in Plants and Animals

The facts which have been reviewed concerning the elements out of which the tissues of plants and animals are built are properly supplemented by a statement of the proportions in which these are found in living organisms. This information is necessary to an understanding of the relations of supply and demand which exist between the vegetable and animal kingdoms and the raw materials of the inorganic world.

17. In plants. — It is estimated by a German scientist, Knop, that if all the species of the vegetable kingdom, exclusive of the fungi, were fused into one mass, the ultimate composition of the dry matter of this mixture would be the following: —

TABLE I

	%
Carbon	45.0
Oxygen	42.0
Hydrogen	6.5
Nitrogen	1.5
Mineral compounds (ash)	5.0

The composition of various plant substances used as human food shows considerable variations from these average figures.

Carbon constitutes a larger proportion of the dry substance of plants than any other element, and there is certainly no species that is an exception to this rule. Oxygen stands next in order, followed by hydrogen, and then nitrogen. It is an important fact in the economy of nature that those elements which, on the average, make up 93.5 per cent of the dry matter of plants have as their main source either the atmosphere or water. Only a small percentage of the dry matter of food plants is drawn from the dry matter of the soil, and it is this part of plant substance which is economically important to those engaged in the production of human food.

The elements of the ash vary somewhat in different plants or parts of plants. For illustration, their proportions in the dry matter of several kinds of plant substance that enters into the human diet are given in this connection : —

TABLE II

Ash Elements in Cereal Grains and Vegetables[1]

	Wheat	Maize	Oats	Beans	Potatoes	Carrots	Radishes	Spinach	Parsnips
	Per Cent	Per Cent	Per Cent	Per Cent	Per Cent	Per Cent	Per Cent	Per Cent	Per Cent
Potassium .	.51	.36	.46	1.25	1.89	1.68	1.93	2.27	2.18
Sodium . .	.029	.012	.039	.029	.08	.86	1.14	4.32	.053
Calcium . .	.043	.023	.08	.129	.07	.44	.77	1.40	.39
Magnesium .	.14	.135	.134	.16	.112	.14	.13	.63	.163
Iron . . .	.017	.008	.026	.012	.029	.038	.144	.38	.038
Phosphorus .	.41	.29	.35	.62	.28	.31	.343	.74	.412
Sulfur . .	.0032	.0044	.022	.049	.099	.14	.19	.45	.101
Silicon . .	.018	.014	.57	.011	.036	.06	.031	.35	.036
Chlorine . .	.006	.013	.029	.065	.131	.25	.66	1.02	.183

[1] Calculated from Wolff's " Aschen Analysen."

18. In animals. — We are not ignorant of the proportions of the chemical elements in the bodies of our larger animals, including man. Lawes and Gilbert, of England, and the Maine Experiment Station, in this country, have made analyses of the entire bodies, or nearly so, of steers and other domestic animals. These results, combined with our knowledge of the constitution of the compounds of the animal tissues, enable us to calculate very closely the proportions of carbon and other elements in the entire body of man and bovines : —

TABLE III

	Man	Fat Ox. Lawes and Gilbert	Two Steers, 2-yr. Old. Maine Station
	Per Cent	Per Cent	Per Cent
Carbon	63.1	63.0	60.0
Oxygen	20.2	13.8	14.1
Hydrogen	9.9	9.4	9.0
Nitrogen	2.5	5.0	5.8
Mineral compounds (ash)	4.3	8.8	11.1

As the proportion of carbon is much larger in the fats than in the other compounds of the animal body, it is easy to see that the ultimate composition of the ox would vary with his condition, whether lean or very fat. The figures given suffice to show, however, that animals, like plants, contain much more of carbon than of any other element, and that the quantities of the remaining elements stand in the same order in the plant and in the animal, the striking differences being the greater proportion of oxygen in

c

the former and of carbon and nitrogen in the latter. The plant and animal are alike, therefore, in consisting chiefly of those elements which are derived from air and water. Carbon, oxygen, and hydrogen constitute from 83 to 86 per cent of the bodies of fat oxen and steers, raw materials which nature supplies without cost, leaving less than one-sixth of the animal body to be built from elements derived from the soil that have, in part, a commercial value for crop production, which is the fundamental consideration in the production of human food.

19. Ash elements in animal body. — In order to compare the plant and animal, it is desirable to consider the elements found in the ash or mineral portion of the animal body. We will return for this information to the analysis of a fat ox made by Lawes and Gilbert. These investigators found that the ash, constituting 8.8 per cent of the dry substance of the entire body, was made up as follows, the mineral or inorganic constituents of the human body being given for comparison : —

TABLE IV

	Ox	HUMAN BODY
	Per Cent	Per Cent
Phosphorus	1.53	1.13
Calcium	2.80	2.50
Potassium	0.26	0.12
Sodium	0.20	0.10
Magnesium	0.07	0.07
Oxygen, combined with the above	3.29	
Silicon, sulfur	0.65	0.14
	8.80	

Of the elements other than oxygen which appear in the ash, phosphorus and calcium take a leading place as to quantity, although sulfur, potassium, and sodium are essential, even if present in relatively small amounts.

CHAPTER III

THE COMPOUNDS OF HUMAN NUTRI-TION

THE human body consists primarily of elements, but we ordinarily regard it as made up of compounds. These are groups of elements united in such fixed and constant proportions that they have as uniform properties, under given conditions, as the elements themselves. In discussing the composition and uses of human foods and their relation to the structure, composition, and activities of man as an organism, we refer chiefly to the compounds of carbon rather than to carbon itself. To be sure, the investigator of the problems of nutrition often conducts his researches and formulates his conclusions with reference to the elements, but when the information he secures reaches the language of practice, we speak of proteins, carbohydrates, and fats. Commerce recognizes these compounds, also. It is necessary, therefore, for the student of human nutrition, whether as a scientist or as one who would thoroughly understand dietetics, to become well informed about those substances that in various proportions form the organized structure of plants, and that furnish not only the energies that are manifested by animal life, but all the materials out of which animal tissues are built.

A. CLASSES OF MATTER

Before passing to a consideration in detail of the proximate constitutions of plants and animals, it is desirable

20

to reach a clear understanding of certain broad divisions into which we classify all matter, either living or dead, which has been organized by the vital forces of the various forms of life.

20. Combustible and non-combustible. — One of the most common and familiar phenomena of the physical world is the destruction of vegetable or animal matter by combustion, with the result that only a small portion of the original material is left behind in visible and solid forms. Fuel, such as wood or coal, is largely consumed when ignited, and we have as a residue the ashes. If we incinerate hay, corn, or wheat, we get the same result. The gradual decomposition of exposed dead vegetable or animal matter that occurs in warm weather is a process essentially similar to the combustion of fuel, only more prolonged. In view of these facts, it is customary to classify all the tissues of plants and animals into the combustible and incombustible portions, the former being that part of the ignited or decayed substance which disappears in the air as gases, and the latter the residue or ash. It should be well understood that combustion does not involve a loss of matter; only a change into other forms. If we were to collect the gases which pass off from a stick of wood that is burned, consisting mostly of carbon dioxid, vapor of water, ammonia, and, perhaps, certain other compounds of nitrogen, we would find that their total weight, plus that of the ash residue, is even greater than that of the dry wood, because the carbon and the hydrogen of the wood have taken to themselves from the air, during the combustion, an increased amount of oxygen. The carbon, oxygen, hydrogen, and nitrogen of the plant or animal tissue belong mainly to the combustible portion, although two of these elements are found in the ash compounds. The remainder of the fifteen elements previously named are supposed to appear wholly in the ash.

The relation in quantity of the combustible and incombustible parts of vegetable and animal dry matter and the wide variations in the proportions are illustrated below : —

TABLE V

	Combusti-ble	Non-combustible (Ash)
	Per Cent	Per Cent
Potato tubers	95.5	4.5
Maize kernel	98.3	1.7
Wheat kernel	98.0	2.0
Oat kernel	96.9	3.1
Field bean	96.4	3.6
Cucumber	86.8	13.2
Spinach	83.6	16.4
Rhubarb	85.6	14.4
Body of fat ox	91.2	8.8

The significance of these facts is, that the chemical change which we call combustion is one of the phenomena of human nutrition. Substances which may suffer either slow or rapid oxidation outside the human organism may undergo complete or partial combustion within this organism; or, stated in another way, the part of the plant which " burns up " in the fireplace or crucible is the part which in general undergoes the same change within the human organism in so far as the food is digested.

21. Organic and inorganic. — The terms *combustible* and *incombustible* are less used, perhaps, than two others, which represent practically the same divisions of plant or animal substance; viz., organic and inorganic. In chemical literature, the portion of a plant or animal which suffers combustion is called the organic, and the ash is known as the inorganic or mineral part. These terms are evidently based upon the erroneous assumption that the compounds which burn and break up into simpler ones are peculiarly those which sustain necessary and vital relations to life, and are formed only through the functions of living organisms. As a matter of fact, many of these so-called organic compounds have been synthesized (built up) artificially, and while the dry substance of the plant is organized chiefly by building up compounds of carbon, oxygen, hydrogen, and nitrogen, which suffer combustion, compounds of sulfur, phosphorus, chlorine, potassium, sodium, and calcium are also constant and essential constituents of the juices and tissues of the plant and animal; and, although the latter elements may finally wholly appear in the incombustible part or ash, they have, nevertheless, sustained in other combinations important relations to nutrition and growth. It is true, however, that the portion of a food material which is commonly spoken of as organic embraces those compounds that furnish practically all the energy which is utilized by animal life and much the larger part of the building material.

B. THE GROUPS OR CLASSES INTO WHICH THE COMPOUNDS IN PLANTS AND ANIMAL LIFE ARE DIVIDED

The known compounds that belong to life in all its forms are of great number and variety, and doubtless many are yet to be discovered. These sustain important relations to human needs, some serving as food, some as medicine, and some in the arts. It is fortunate that comparatively few must be considered in discussing the science of human nutrition. Moreover, it is convenient that the compounds which play a leading part in human nutrition are designated, especially for practical purposes, in classes rather than singly, even though this custom tends to more or less looseness of expression and definition.

The same classification is used for the compounds of both the vegetable and animal kingdoms, and they are now divided into the following general groups : —

> Water
> Ash (mineral compounds)
> Proteins (nitrogenous compounds)
> Carbohydrates
> Fats (or oils)

In this instance, accuracy is sacrificed to convenience. The class names have come to be regarded, more or less, as representing entities having fixed properties and functions, whereas each class contains numerous compounds differing widely in their characteristics and in their nutritive value and office. Moreover, these terms have a variable significance as used under different conditions. No one of them except water uniformly represents just the same mixture of compounds when applied to foods of unlike source.

22. Distribution of elements in the classes of compounds. — Before passing to a detailed description of these compounds, singly or in groups, it will be well to gain a clear understanding of the relation which the fifteen elements previously mentioned sustain to these classes of substances. This can be seen most readily by a tabular display.

All vegetable or animal matter	Incombustible or inorganic matter	Water	Oxygen, Hydrogen
		Ash	Oxygen, Sulfur, Chlorine, Phosphorus, Silicon, Fluorine, Calcium, Magnesium, Iron, Manganese, Potassium, Sodium
	Combustible or organic matter	Proteins and non-proteins	Carbon, Oxygen, Hydrogen, Nitrogen, Sulfur (generally), Phosphorus (sometimes), Iron (in a few cases)
		Carbohydrates, fats, acids	Carbon, Oxygen, Hydrogen

The ash, which, on the average, constitutes about one-twentieth of the plant, and never more than one-tenth of the animal, may contain thirteen of the fifteen elements, while the larger proportion of living matter consists mostly of the compounds of three or four elements, in no case of more than six or seven. From this point of view, it becomes strikingly evident that the dominant elements of life, quantity alone considered, are those derived from the air and water.

Water

Water fills a very important place in human nutrition. It is everywhere present, generally in some useful way. All plant substance, all animal tissue, foods, and nearly all the material things with which man comes in contact in his daily life are made up of more or less water, or are associated with it. Sometimes this is very evident, as with green plants or juicy fruits. It is not so evident with wheat, flour, and corn meal. If, however, we submit almost any substance, no matter how dry it may appear, except, perhaps, glass and metals, to the heat of an oven at 100° C., we find that a material loss of weight occurs; and if we so arrange that whatever is driven off is first drawn through some substance that entirely absorbs the water which has been vaporized, we learn that the decrease in weight is nearly all accounted for by the water thus collected.

23. Determination of water. — This fact suggests to us the chemist's way of determining the proportion of water which any particular material contains. He weighs out a certain amount of the substance and then keeps it in an oven at 212° F. for five hours, perhaps, after which it is reweighed. The difference in the two weights, or the loss, is assumed to be all water, and the percentage in the original substance is easily calculated. That portion of the material which is left behind after the water is evaporated we call the *dry substance,* or *water-free substance.*

24. Hygroscopic water. — Water is associated with plant and animal tissues in two ways, hygroscopically and physiologically. It is easy to illustrate the former way by an object lesson. If an ounce of corn meal were to be dried in an oven as described, it would, as stated, lose in weight. If it were subsequently allowed to remain exposed in the open air, it would return quite or nearly to its original weight. The loss would be due to water driven out, and the gain to water absorbed from the atmosphere, which we call *hygroscopic moisture.*

All solids attract moisture up to a certain proportion, which varies with the substance and with the atmospheric conditions that prevail. The surfaces of the particles of matter are ordinarily covered with a thin film of water which is thicker on a cold, wet day than on a warm, dry day; and so certain foods, when exposed to the air, weigh less at one time than at another, because the percentage of hygroscopic water varies. An equilibrium will always be established between the attraction of a substance for moisture and the tension of the vapor of water in the surrounding air, which accounts for the effect of temperature and of the degree to which the air is saturated with water vapor. As all substances do not have the same attraction for moisture, therefore, under similar atmospheric conditions, one food may retain more water than another.

25. Physiological water. — Water that is held physiologically is that which is a constant and essential part of

living organisms, in which relation it is necessary to life
and performs certain important functions. These functions are of three kinds: (1) The presence of water in the
tissues of plants and animals gives them more or less
firmness or rigidity combined with elasticity; (2) water
acts as a food solvent; (3) water is the great carrier of
food materials and of waste products from one part to
another of the vegetable or animal organism.

26. Water in living plants. — Water constitutes a large
proportion of the weight of all living plants, especially
during the period of active growth. The cured hay, as
any farmer's boy knows, weighs much less than did the
green grass when it was cut, and this loss in weight is due
almost wholly to evaporation of water from the tissues of
the plant under the influence of the sun and wind. This
water, which is contained in the tubes and inter-cellular
spaces of the stalk or leaf, is exactly the same chemical compound as pure water found anywhere else, and has no
more value for food, excepting that it is pure and is not
subject to the contamination which sometimes occurs in
streams and wells. There is no such thing as the so-called
" natural " water of plants which has a peculiar nutritive
value or function. Vegetation water should be distinguished from sap or plant juice. Sap is more than water;
it is water holding in solution certain substances such as
sugars and mineral salts. When the plant is dried, these
soluble compounds do not pass off, but remain behind as
part of the dry matter.

27. Proportion of water varies. — The proportion of
water in plants varies greatly in different species, and in
some species according to the stage of growth or the sur-

rounding conditions. These facts have more importance than is generally recognized, because the food value of vegetable substances is influenced by the proportion of dry matter. It is always necessary to know the percentage of water in vegetables and fruits before we can estimate their worth as food.

The variations in water content of the living tissues of different species of plants or parts of plants, as well as its large proportion, is well illustrated by the following average figures : —

TABLE VI

WATER IN GREEN VEGETABLES

	PER CENT
Asparagus	94.0
Cabbage	90.5
Green peas	78.1
Lima beans	68.5
Onions	87.6
Pumpkin	93.4
Potatoes (tuber)	78.9
String beans	87.2
Sweet-potatoes	71.1
Tomatoes	96.0
Turnips	89.4

28. Much water in immature plants. — Immature plants contain more water than older or mature ones. Young pasture grass is more largely water than the same plants would be after the seed is formed. This fact is consistent with the very rapid transference of building material during the active stages of growth. Analyses of samples of timothy grass cut at the Maine State College in 1879, and at the Pennsylvania State College in 1881, show the marked influence of the stage of growth upon the water content of the living plant: —

TABLE VII

	MAINE STATE COLLEGE Percentage of Water
Nearly headed out	78.7
In full blossom	71.9
Out of blossom	65.2
Nearly ripe	63.3

	PENNSYLVANIA STATE COLLEGE Percentage of Water	
	Highly Manured	No Manure
Cut June 6, heads just appearing . .	79.7	76.5
Cut June 23, just beginning to bloom	69.7	69.1
Cut July 5, somewhat past full bloom	61.4	60.0

What is true of timothy is probably true of all vegetables in the perfectly fresh state.

29. Effect of soil moisture. — The proportion of water in plants is influenced by the lack or excess of soil moisture. The soil, and not the atmosphere, is the source of supply of vegetation water, which, taken up by the roots, traverses the plant and passes into the atmosphere through the leaves. If the supply is abundant, the tissues are constantly fully charged, but if, by reason of drought, the soil becomes very dry, the outgo of water by evaporation may exceed the income. What farmer has not seen his corn with rolled leaves during an August drought! The vegetation water had fallen below the normal, or below what was necessary to maintain the tissues in their usual condition of rigidity.

30. Water in dry foods. — The proportion of moisture in flour, meal, and other food materials has much to do with their preservation in a sound condition. New grains when packed in large masses are subject to fermentations, which injure their quality and diminish their food value. This is due to the fact that sufficient moisture is present to allow the growth of low forms of life with certain attendant chemical changes. Food materials containing 20 per cent or more of water, when stored in large quantities or in closed vessels, are almost certain to heat and become musty or moldy, always involving a loss of nutritive value. It is well if the moisture in flour and other stored cereal preparations does not exceed 10 or 12 per cent.

31. Water in the animal. — Water is an important and abundant constituent of animal organisms, from the lowest to the highest forms. The blood, which is one-twentieth or more of the weight of the human body is approximately four-fifths water. The soft tissues of farm animals have been found to contain from 44 per cent to 75 per cent, according to the species and conditions of the animal. The most extensive and complete analysis so far made of the entire bodies of animals were performed by Lawes and Gilbert at Rothamsted, England. In this country four steers were analyzed at the Maine Experiment Station, and in the study of human nutrition problems many determinations of water have been made of parts of the carcasses of bovines, swine, sheep, poultry, and game. The figures are as follows : —

TABLE VIII

WATER IN ENTIRE BODY

	PER CENT
Ox, well-fed, Lawes and Gilbert	66.2
Ox, half fat, Lawes and Gilbert	59.0
Ox, fat, Lawes and Gilbert	49.5
Steer, 17 months old, medium fat, M.E.S.	59.0
Steer, 17 months old, medium fat, M.E.S.	56.3
Steer, 27 months old, fat, M.E.S.	51.9
Steer, 27 months old, fat, M.E.S.	52.2
Calf, fat, Lawes and Gilbert	64.6
Sheep, lean, Lawes and Gilbert	67.5
Sheep, well-fed, Lawes and Gilbert	63.2
Sheep, half fat, Lawes and Gilbert	58.9
Sheep, fat, Lawes and Gilbert	50.9
Sheep, very fat, Lawes and Gilbert	43.3
Swine, well-fed, Lawes and Gilbert	57.9
Swine, fat, Lawes and Gilbert	43.9
Chicken, flesh	74.2
Fowl, flesh	65.2
Goose, flesh	42.3
Turkey, flesh	55.5

It is very evident that, in general, considerably more than half of the weight of the bodies of our domestic animals consists of water, the range in all species and conditions here mentioned being from 42.3 per cent to 67.5 per cent.

32. Effect of age and condition. — The percentage of water varies with the species, age, and condition. Swine carry a notably small proportion. The calf's body, even though fat, is comparatively watery. It is very noticeable that with oxen, sheep, and swine the lean animals contain a much larger proportion of water than do the fat. This does not mean that in the process of fattening the fat is substituted for water, and so expels it from the organism, but that the increase in fattening has a much smaller percentage of water than the body in its original lean condition. This is well illustrated by the data from two independent investigations at Rothamsted and at the Maine Experiment Station. The former investigation showed that when swine, sheep, and oxen are fattened, the increase contained from 20 per cent to 24 per cent of water, this being half the proportion found in the entire bodies of the lean animals. The Maine Station results established the fact that in the increase of two steers from the age of 17 months to 27 months, during which time a fattening ration was fed, there was 42 per cent of water, the bodies of the younger steers having 58.2 per cent. It is well understood that beef from mature animals " spends " better than that from young, the same observation being made in comparing lean and fat beef. Modern investigation shows clearly that the reason for this lies partly in the difference in water content. Dry matter, and not water, is the measure of food value.

Ash

The ash or mineral part of plants or animals has occupied a minor place in the discussions pertaining to the principles and problems of animal nutrition. Much is said and written about the carbon compounds of living organisms, but the compounds of the mineral world, in their relation to foods and to the processes of growth, are generally passed by with brief comment, much less than would

D

be profitable. It is certainly desirable to gain a clear understanding of the combinations, distribution, and functions of these bodies. Their importance as necessary constituents of foods and animals is no less than pertains to the carbon compounds, although their scientific and commercial prominence as related to animal nutrition is much less.

As previously stated, the mineral portion of a plant or animal is measured by the ash or residue after combustion, the principal ingredients of which are the following : —

ACIDS			ACIDS		
Hydrochloric acid .	.	HCl	Potash		K_2O
Sulfuric acid	. . .	H_2SO_4	Soda		Na_2O
Phosphoric acid	. .	$H_6P_2O_8$	Lime		CaO
Silicic acid .	. . .	SiO_2	Magnesia		MgO
Carbonic acid .	. .	CO_2	Iron oxid		Fe_2O_3

Other mineral compounds are found in the ash from various forms of vegetable life, but those mentioned are all that we need to discuss at length.

33. Combination of ash elements. — The acids and bases do not exist in the ash as shown, but they are united to form salts, and so we have the chlorides, sulfates, phosphates, and carbonates of potassium, sodium, calcium, and magnesium. These are nearly all familiar objects in common life, as, for instance, sodium chloride (common salt), potassium chloride (the muriate of potash of the market), potassium sulfate (the sulfate of potash of the market), calcium sulfate (of which gypsum or land plaster is composed), calcium phosphate (burned bone is chiefly this compound), potassium phosphate (a compound of phosphoric acid and potash found chiefly at the druggist's), and calcium carbonate (limestone).

It should be remembered that the compounds in the ash are not necessarily those of the plant or animal. During the process of ignition, organic compounds are broken up, the acid and basic elements of which enter into other combinations in the salts of the ash. Much of the lime in the ash is in union with carbonic acid, which in the plant may have been associated with vegetable acids, such as oxalic and tartaric, and part of the sulfur and phosphorus of the ash comes from the nitrogen (protein) compounds.

These salts differ greatly in their properties. Some are soluble in water, others are not. To the former class belong all the chlorides, and the potassium and sodium sulfates and phosphates. The normal phosphates of calcium and magnesium are insoluble in water, but soluble in various acids. These facts are important in showing what salts may be found in the plant and animal juices, and what effect leaching with water or other solvents might have upon the inorganic portion of human foods.

34. Ash elements in plants. — The ash elements of plants are important in this connection because they are the main source of the same elements of the human body. These may be held in plant tissue in three ways: in organic combinations, as the inorganic salts of the sap, and in crystals and incrustations. Outside of phosphorus and sulfur, comparatively little is known of the relations of the important ash elements to plant structure. The ash from different plants and parts of plants is by no means uniform in composition and quantity, even in the same species or class of materials, although with the grains there is some degree of uniformity in this respect. Certain factors cause variations, such as species, stage of growth, fertility, the part of the plant, and changes due to manufacturing processes, and the variations which occur pertain not only to the amount of ash, but also to its composition.

Different species of plants, and consequently different foods, are greatly unlike in their content of mineral matter. The figures below illustrate this fact, further confirmation of which may be had by consulting more extended tables : —

TABLE IX

THE MINERAL COMPOUNDS IN CERTAIN VEGETABLES AND GRAINS [1]

(Per cent in the dry matter)

	POTASH	SODA	LIME	MAGNESIA	IRON OXID	PHOSPHORIC ACID	SULFURIC ACID	SILICA	CHLORINE
Potatoes . . .	2.27	0.11	0.10	0.19	.04	0.64	0.25	0.08	0.13
Turnips . . .	3.64	0.79	0.85	0.30	.06	1.02	0.90	0.15	0.41
Carrots . . .	2.02	1.16	0.62	0.24	.05	0.70	0.35	0.13	0.25
Radishes . . .	2.32	1.53	1.08	0.22	.21	0.78	0.47	0.07	0.66
Spinach . . .	2.73	5.81	1.96	1.05	.55	1.69	1.13	0.74	1.02
Parsnips . . .	2.63	0.07	0.55	0.27	.05	0.94	0.25	0.08	0.18
Winter wheat .	0.61	0.04	0.06	0.24	.03	0.93	0.01	0.04	?
Oats (with hulls)	0.56	0.05	0.11	0.22	.04	0.80	0.06	1.22	0.03
Barley	0.56	0.06	0.07	0.23	.03	0.92	0.05	0.68	0.03
Maize kernel . .	0.43	0.02	0.03	0.22	.01	0.66	0.01	0.03	0.01
Peas	1.18	0.03	0.13	0.22	.02	0.98	0.09	0.02	0.04
Field beans . .	1.51	0.04	0.18	0.26	.02	1.41	0.12	0.02	0.06

[1] Wolff's "Aschen Analysen."

We observe as we study the previous figures that phosphoric acid, potash, lime, and magnesia are the more prominent mineral compounds in plants, and it is with these that we find the most marked variations. The dry matter of vegetables and of peas and beans is much richer in potash and lime than is that of the cereal grains, and radishes and spinach have a relatively large amount of iron. Other differences occur. The amount and kind of mineral matter ingested in the food may be varied greatly by the selection of food materials.

35. Influence of manufacturing process and cooking on the ash constituents of plant substance. — Many substances utilized as human food, especially grain products, have an ash content that is determined more or less by certain processes of manufacture, especially milling. For instance, wheat flour is only a part of the kernel, the bran being removed. This bran, which is the outside of the kernel, is especially rich in mineral ingredients, much richer than the inner part of the kernel.

TABLE X

ASH CONTENT OF WHEAT AND ITS MILLING PRODUCTS

	WATER	ASH
	Per Cent	Per Cent
Wheat kernel	10.2	1.8
Wheat flour	10.6	0.4
Wheat germ	10.4	2.7
Wheat shorts	10.1	3.1
Wheat bran	10.4	5.9

The whole kernel contains about 2 per cent of ash, the bran about 6 per cent, and wheat flour less than .5 per cent. When vegetables and meats are cooked in water or are steamed, the soluble salts are leached out, in part at least.

36. The mineral compounds of animal bodies. — The mineral compounds of animals are nearly similar in kind to those of plants, but are very different in relative proportions. This is made plain by a comparison of the figures given below : —

TABLE XI

ASH IN PLANTS AND ANIMALS (PER CENT)

	Total	Potash	Soda	Lime	Magnesia	Phosphoric Acid	Sulfuric Acid	Silicic Acid	Chlorine
Dry substance .									
Maize kernel . .	1.4	.43	.02	0.03	.22	0.66	.01	.03	.01
Wheat kernel . .	2.0	.61	.04	0.06	.24	0.93	.01	.04	
Fresh bodies									
Fat ox	3.9	.14	.12	1.74	.05	1.56		.01	
Fat sheep . . .	2.9	.14	.13	1.19	.04	1.13		.02	
Fat swine . . .	1.8	.10	.07	0.77	.03	0.73			

Potash is much less prominent in the composition of the animal than is the case with plants, and phosphoric acid and lime are much more so. In general, more than 80 per cent of the ash of the animal body consists of phosphoric acid and lime in combination largely as calcium phosphate, whereas these two compounds constitute less than one-half of the ash of maize and wheat kernels.

37. The distribution of ash compounds in the animal body. — The bones contain a very large proportion of the ash constituents found in the animal body, the soft parts being poor in mineral salts. Usually the ash makes up between 60 and 70 per cent of bone, and the bony framework is from 6 to 9 per cent of the entire bodies of domestic animals. More than 80 per cent of the ash of bone is calcium phosphate, which is associated with calcium carbonate, calcium fluoride, calcium chloride, and magnesium phosphate.

The bones of all species of animals, including man, show a remarkable similarity of composition, the average of which would not be far from the following : —

TABLE XII

In 100 Parts of the Ash of Bone (Average)

Calcium phosphate	83.9
Calcium carbonate	13.0
Calcium in other combinations	0.35
Fluorine	0.23
Chlorine	0.18
	97.66

The muscular tissue and other soft parts of the animal body contain less than 1 per cent of incombustible bodies. The ash from flesh is mostly phosphoric acid and potash, accompanied by comparatively small amounts of soda, lime, and magnesia and minute quantities of chlorine and iron. Unquestionably, potassium phosphate is the predominating salt in flesh, as calcium phosphate is in bone.

The blood contains a variety of mineral substances, the

chief of which is sodium chloride, or common salt, although a small amount of iron is present, having a most important function. In the bile, soda is abundant, combined mostly with the peculiar organic acids of this secretion. Chlorine is a constant constituent of the gastric juice, its presence as chlorhydric acid being essential to digestion.

38. Forms in which the ash elements exist in the plant or animal. — As has already been suggested, the mineral elements are combined differently in the ash from what they were in the plant or animal substance before ignition. Because calcium or potassium phosphate is found in plant ash or the ash of animal tissue, it does not follow that such a compound existed in the unburned substance. For instance, the phosphorus in a grain of wheat is combined in certain organic compounds such as nucleo-proteins and phytin. Sulfur exists in certain proteins. When ignition occurs, there is a rearrangement of the elements, and we find the phosphorus and sulfur present in the ash of the wheat kernel in inorganic salts. It is a mistake, in most cases, to speak of any food material containing the compounds that are found in its ash. Recent investigations have demonstrated the absence of inorganic phosphorus in the cereal grains, unless these have been subjected to fermentation, when inorganic salts of phosphorus may be present.

The Nitrogen Compounds

The nitrogen compounds of the vegetable and animal kingdoms have received much attention from scientific investigators and writers during the past fifty years. It is quite the custom to declare that certain members of this class of substances are the ones most important in the domain of animal nutrition, and many writers have given to them so prominent a place in discussing nutrition problems as to almost ignore the other nutrients. Certain investigators claim, on the other hand, that from the economic point of view the function and relative value of protein have been unduly magnified. Whatever may be the correct opinion, it is very evident that the present tendency is towards a fuller discussion of the office and value of the other classes of nutrients.

There can scarcely be any disagreement, however, concerning the general proposition that the compounds of nitrogen play a leading part in the processes and economy of human nutrition. This is true for several reasons : —

(1) The nitrogen compounds are those fundamental to the energies of the living cells which make up the tissues of plants and animals. The basic substance of the active cell is protoplasm, a complex nitrogenous body, which Huxley called " the physical basis of life." Around this primal substance seem to center all vital activities, especially the transformation of the raw materials of the inorganic world into the organized structures of plant life and the transformations of food compounds into the tissue substance of the human body.

(2) These compounds are structurally essential to the growth of living tissues and to the formation of milk.

(3) Foods rich in nitrogen have reached a position of great commercial importance, and they bear relatively high market prices.

Protein

For the sake of brevity and convenience, certain nitrogen compounds of human foods, both vegetable and animal, are designated as a class by the single term *protein*. This term includes such compounds as albumins, globulins, and similar or related organic nitrogen bodies found in human foods. When, therefore, it is stated that a food stuff contains a certain percentage of protein, reference is made to the total mass of nitrogen compounds present, which may be many in number and of greatly differing characteristics.

39. Determination of protein. — It should be stated, by way of preliminary explanation, that, in the past, the proportion of protein (total nitrogen compounds) in foods has been ascertained by determining the total amount of nitrogen and then multiplying its percentage number by the factor 6.25. This method is based on the assumption that the average percentage of nitrogen in the proteins is 16, which is not true to so close a degree of approximation as was formerly believed to be the case. It may happen in some instances that a determination made in this way is sufficiently accurate, while in other cases the margin of error is large. Recent investigations with perfected methods show percentages of nitrogen in the numerous single proteins found in the grains ranging from 15.25 to 18.78. These are largest in certain oil seeds and lupines and smallest in some of the winter grains. Prominent authorities concede that the factor 6.25 should be discarded, and suggest the use of 5.7 for the majority of cereal grains and leguminous seeds, 5.5 for the oil and lupine seeds, and 6 for barley, maize, buckwheat, soja bean, and white bean (*Phaseolus*), rape, and other brassicas. Nothing short of inability to secure greater accuracy justifies the longer continuance of a method of calculation which is apparently so greatly erroneous.

40. Various proteins unlike. — As previously stated, protein is the accepted name for a class of compounds. Just how there came about such a grouping of a large number of substances under a single head it is not necessary to consider in this connection, but it should be made clear that the individual compounds which are included under this term are in part so unlike in chemical and physical properties as to warrant the assertion that they have but little in common except that they contain nitrogen; and we may believe that their unlikeness in composition is no greater than the differences in their nutritive functions. Moreover, the total protein of any particular foodstuff may be a mixture of several individual proteins. These mixtures differ greatly in the individual cereal grains.

It is very evident that it is not only convenient, but necessary, to classify such a heterogeneous group of bodies into subdivisions more nearly alike in their characteristics. When we come to consider doing this, we find there has existed a most unfortunate confusion of terms.

41. Classification of proteins. — Some years ago a system of classification was reported by a committee on nomenclature, representing the Association of Agricultural Colleges and Experiment Stations.[1]

The first classification given is essentially this one, although there are included in it certain distinctions very

[1] Report 1898, pp. 117–123.

clearly set forth by Professor Atwater in a paper associated with the above-mentioned report.

In the arrangement adopted it was recognized that certain nitrogen bodies included under protein are so unlike the main and important members of this group as to be properly styled non-protein. It is also conceded that there are simple or native proteins which seem to stand in the relation of " mother " substances to a large number of protein bodies that have been modified either by various external agencies, or are the result of a union of proteins with compounds of another class.

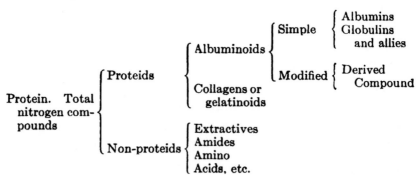

Other nitrogen compounds are included with the protein by the present methods of chemical analysis, such as alkaloids and nitrates, but these are so uncommon in foods, or are present in such small quantities, that they may be safely ignored.

Quite recently committees representing certain scientific bodies [1] have recommended quite a different classification from the foregoing. The terms used in this classification are explained in the text which follows: —

[1] *Am. Jour. Phys.*, Vol. XXI.

Proteins . .	Simple	Albumins Globulins Glutelins Alcohol solubles Albuminoids Histones Protamines	
	Conjugated	Nucleoproteins Glycoproteins Phosphoproteins Hæmoglobins Lecithoproteins	
	Derived	Primary derivatives	Proteans Metaproteins Coagulated proteins
		Secondary derivatives	Proteoses Peptones Peptides
Non-proteins	Extractives Amides Amino acids		

The two classifications are given in this connection because much literature on nutrition recognizes the former, and the latter is now more or less in use. Certain differences should be noted. In the latter the term *proteid* is abandoned, and the term *albuminoid* is made to refer to the bodies classed as collagens or gelatinoids in the former grouping. Besides, the newer classification makes a more minute division of the proteins on the basis of constitution and characteristic properties.

42. The true proteins. — The proteins are the main and important nitrogen compounds either in the plant or in the animal. The nitrogenous bodies of seeds are little else than proteins, while young plants, and especially roots, such as beets and turnips, contain more nitrogen in the non-protein form. Proteins are the chief constituents of muscular tissue. Their chemical constitution is not definitely known. No investigator has yet been able to search out their manner of combination, but it is generally considered to be very complex, even to the extent of several thousand atoms. These bodies are constructed from the simpler ones of the inorganic world through the vital energies of plants, and they apparently must come to the animal fully organized.

43. Ultimate composition of proteins. — The ultimate composition of the proteins, that is, the proportions of the elements which they contain, has been carefully studied, and while there are material differences among them in this respect, the limits of variation are not especially wide, as can be seen from the following figures taken from Neumeister : —

TABLE XIII

ELEMENTARY COMPOSITION OF THE PROTEINS

	PER CENT	AVERAGE
Carbon	50.0 to 55.0	52.0
Hydrogen	6.5 to 7.3	7.0
Nitrogen	15.0 to 17.6	16.0
Oxygen	19.0 to 24.0	23.0
Sulfur	0.3 to 2.4	2.0

We see that the number of elements ordinarily found in the proteins is five, nitrogen and sulfur being those that chiefly distinguish these bodies from all others which make up the mass of combustible matter. Two other elements are found in certain of these bodies, as, for instance, phosphorus in casein and iron in a constituent of blood.

44. Familiar examples of proteins. — Proteins are familiar objects in the home, and their properties are matters of common observation. When the farmer's boy secures the tenacious cud of gum from the fresh wheat gluten, or when the housewife watches the strings of coagulated albumin separate from the cold water extract of fresh lean beef that is brought to the boiling point, or observes the white of an egg harden into a tough, white mass as it is dropped into boiling water; when we note the stiffening of the muscular tissue of the slaughtered animal or the rapid formation of strings of fibrin in the cooling blood, — in all these instances there are manifested certain chemical or physical properties which pertain to these most important and useful compounds.

Simple Proteins

45. The albumins. — There are several albumins. They are found in the juice of plants, in certain liquids of the animal body such as the serous fluids, in muscle, blood, and milk, and abundantly in eggs. Unlike other proteins, these compounds are soluble in pure cold water, and when such a solution is heated to the boiling point, they separate from the liquid by coagulation and become insoluble unless acted upon by some strong chemical.

When macerated beef is treated with cold water the albumin in it goes into solution, and if this extract is boiled to make beef tea, it is a matter of common observation that the albumin separates in clotted masses. None remains in the tea. It is well for the housewife to know that all lean meat contains this substance, which by prolonged treatment with cold water may be removed to the detriment of the residue.

The clear serous fluid which is left after removing the clot from blood contains albumin, which may also be coagulated by heat. After the casein is removed from milk by acid or rennet, the albumin of the milk remains in the whey. It is this which in part causes milk to clot if brought to the boiling point. One of the most familiar examples of this class of proteins is the white of an egg, which, when cooking in boiling water, becomes a hard, white, coagulated mass. Albumin in the serous fluids and in blood is called serum-albumin; in milk, lact-albumin; and in eggs, ova-albumin.

A small proportion of the proteins of plants is found to be albumin; for instance, Osborne found .3 to .4 per cent in wheat, .43 per cent in rye, .3 per cent in barley, .5 per cent in soja beans, and some in most seeds. This possesses essentially the same characters as the animal albumin described previously. Whenever a vegetable substance is leached with water, it is probably this protein which would be the first to suffer removal or destructive fermentation.

46. The globulins. — It is fully recognized that when plant and animal tissues are treated with water, but a small part of the proteins dissolve. If, however, we add to the water a mineral salt, especially common salt (sodium chloride), sufficient to secure a 10 per cent solution, an additional and considerable amount of protein may be extracted. These compounds are called globulins, and differ from the albumins in being insoluble in pure water and in a *saturated* solution of certain mineral salts, such as sodium chloride. The globulins form an important part of the protein content of plants and of animal tissues, both in quantity and in having a maximum nutritive usefulness.

47. Plant globulins. — In plants these proteins seem to be especially abundant and widespread. Our most recent and most reliable knowledge of plant proteins comes from investigations conducted in the laboratory of the Connecticut Agricultural Experiment Station, chiefly by Osborne. In these researches the seeds of many species of agricultural plants were studied, all of which were found to contain globulins. In some the proteins consisted largely of these compounds. The percentage content in certain seeds was determined approximately : —

TABLE XIV

GLOBULINS IN CERTAIN SEEDS

	PER CENT		PER CENT
Kidney bean	20.0	Wheat	0.6
Cottonseed meal	15.8	Lentil	13.0
Peas	10.0	Horse bean	17.0
Lupin	26.2	Maize	0.4
		Soy bean	Chiefly globulin

The seeds of the legumes, as a rule, contain the largest proportion of these proteins, the cereal grains having only a very small part of their protein in this form.

From present knowledge, many seeds appear to have characteristic globulins which differ among themselves

E

in their chemical properties. These have been given names derived from the general names of the species in which they are found. Thus we have amandin in almonds, avenalin in oats, corylin in walnuts, excelsin from the Brazil-nut, phaseolin in several species of beans, glycin in the soy bean, maysin in maize, vicilin in horse beans, lentils, and peas, vignin in the cow-pea, and tuberin in the potato. One globulin called edestin appears to be quite generally distributed in the seeds of agricultural plants, having been found in a larger number than any other protein yet discovered, including all the cereals, castor bean, cottonseed, flaxseed, hemp, squash, and sunflower, though it is not abundant in any of these.

48. Animal globulins. — The animal globulins of which we have definite knowledge are those that exist in the muscle and in the blood. The names which some of them bear are myosin, fibrinogen, and paraglobulin. If finely divided, well-washed muscle (lean meat) is treated with a 10 per cent salt solution, first by rubbing it in a mortar with fine salt, and then adding enough water to secure the proper strength of solution, a globulin is dissolved to which the name *myosin* has been given. The view has been generally accepted that this compound does not exist as such in living muscle, but forms there by coagulation upon the death of the animal. This change has been looked upon as similar to the coagulation of blood through the formation of fibrin, and is regarded as the explanation of the stiffening of dead muscles (rigor mortis). The theory has been broached that a " mother " substance exists in the living muscle, from which myosin is formed in much the same way as fibrin is developed in clotting blood from a preëxisting body, but no single view as to exactly what occurs is fully accepted. There is, nevertheless, a general agreement that rigor mortis is due to a clotting of the muscle, accompanied by marked chemical transformations, one final product being myosin. The theory is advanced that ferments are present in the muscle, to the influence of which these changes are due, and without which they do not occur.

Another prominent and remarkable globulin is the fibrinogen found in the blood. It is common knowledge that when blood is drawn from the veins and cools, it clots, — a phenomenon which is nothing more than the formation of strings of fibrin. Fibrin as such is not found in living blood, but is one of the products into which fibrinogen splits when exposed blood cools, probably because of the influence of a ferment. Stranger than all is the fact that so long as the blood is retained in the arteries and veins, even if the animal dies and grows cold, this clotting does not appear.

Serum-globulin is a collective name for several globulins, which exist in blood serum and in the other fluids of the animal body, such as lymph and its allies, including those exudations which pertain to diseased conditions, especially dropsical.

One more protein has been generally classified as a globulin, although differing in some respects from the other members of this class, and more recently is classed as a phosphoprotein. Reference is made to vitellin, which is the principal protein in the yolk of eggs. It is there intimately mixed with certain peculiar phosphorized bodies, which we shall notice later.

49. Glutenins. — These form a large part of nitrogen compounds of the cereal grains and possibly of other seeds. They are insoluble in water, alcohol, and neutral salt solutions, but readily dissolve in very dilute acids and alkalies. The glutenin of the wheat, found in the tenacious substance that is left after washing the starch out of wheat flour, is the best-known protein of this class and is an important constituent of wheat flour, existing there to over 40 per cent of the total protein.

50. Alcohol-soluble proteins.[1] — Alcohol-soluble proteins have been found in all the cereal grains so far examined. The principal ones to be mentioned are gliadin from wheat, zein from corn, and hordein from barley. Gliadin is practically as abundant in the wheat kernel as is the glutenin with which it is associated, the two together constituting over 80 per cent of the total proteins of that cereal. The proportion of gliadin in wheat flour has much to do with its quality for bread-making purposes. It appears that the best bread flour contains about twice as much gliadin as glutenin.

51. Albuminoids. — This term, according to the classification in common use in the United States, has been understood as including various proteins such as the albumins, and globulins. The latter classification recommended confines the term to the proteins found chiefly in the animal body in such parts as the cartilages, bones, feathers, hair, hoofs, horns, and nails. These proteins are also obtained from the threads of silkworms and from sponges. The albuminoids have group names, such as *collagen* in carti-

[1] Osburn proposes the name *prolamins*. *Science*, Vol. XXVI, pp. 417–427.

lage and bone, *keratins* in feathers, hair, hoofs, horns, nails, and similar exterior tissues, *fibroin* in the threads of silkworm, and *spongin* in the framework of sponges.

Gelatin, so well known to the housewife, is derived from collagen. It is a matter of common observation that when meat containing tendons (cartilage) is submitted to the action of boiling water, there is obtained in the extract a gelatinous substance which becomes evident when the extract is cooled. This gelatin is insoluble in cold water, but dissolves in hot. As a dry commercial article, it is a tenacious substance, which, when prepared in thin layers, is transparent. When collagen and gelatin are acted upon by tannic acid, as, for instance, when the skin of an animal is treated with an extract from hemlock or oak bark, the result is a substance which does not putrefy and which gives to the tanned hide the properties of leather. Gelatin is much used in various food preparations.

It is characteristic of the keratins such as hair and horn that they contain a relatively large proportion of sulfur, the analysis of horn and hair showing as high as 5 per cent, the average amount in horn being 3.3 per cent. The keratin bodies serve to give rigidity and wearing qualities to certain exterior animal tissues.

52. Histones, protamines. — The proteins in these two groups do not occur as such in nature, and are only obtained by separating them from some combination. The two groups are alike in being basic in character and in being found in the spermatozoa of fishes. Histones have also been obtained from the blood corpuscles of a goose and from the white blood corpuscles of thymus glands.

Conjugated Proteins

53. Nucleoproteins. — These are complex, phosphorus-bearing proteins that sustain an important nutritive function. They are regarded as a combination of *nuclein* with an albumin, the nucleins being compounds of *nucleic acid* and albumin, and nucleic acid yielding on cleavage phosphoric acid, certain nitrogenous bases known as *purins*, and in all cases a carbohydrate.

The nucleoproteins are associated with the nuclei of the cells that make up both plant and animal tissues, and consequently are found in the flesh of animals that is used for food. They are relatively abundant in glandular tissues such as the spleen, pancreas, thymus gland, and liver. The spermatozoa masses of fishes are especially rich in these bodies. Because certain bases known as purins which arise from the cleavage of nucleoproteins are regarded as the progenitors of uric acid, persons with uric acid tendency are advised to avoid eating certain animal foods such as beef and liver, or any others known to contain these compounds. Experiments show that the feeding of certain tissues rich in nucleoproteins increases the output of uric acid, while adding to the diet a large amount of purin-free proteins such as albumin does not have this effect.

54. Glycoproteins (Glucoalbumins). — These are bodies that upon cleavage are decomposed into a protein and a carbohydrate. The best-known glycoproteins are the mucins that are secreted, for instance, by the mucous membranes of the air passages and of the alimentary canal and by certain glands such as the salivary. Certain of these compounds contain phosphorus, and others do not.

55. Phosphoproteins (Nucleoalbumins). — Like the nucleoproteins, these compounds contain phosphorus, but on cleavage do not yield the purin bases that under certain conditions are to be avoided. The best-known phosphoprotein is the casein of milk, a compound exceedingly important in human nutrition, especially with the young.

This compound is a secretion of the mammary gland of many species of animals, and doubtless originates in the contents of the gland cells. As will be seen later, the casein from different species of mammals differs somewhat in chemical and physical properties. Casein is insoluble in water, but exists in milk in suspension. It is not coagulated by heat, but curdles when a weak acid is added to milk, as, for instance, vinegar. The same result is produced by a generous quantity of common salt. When milk is ingested into the human stomach, the casein coagulates (the milk curdles) through the action of a ferment in the gastric juice (see p. 90), and this coagulation is unlike with milk from different species. The action of this ferment on casein is utilized in cheese making in the development of a curd which, with its inclosed fat, is separated from the whey and pressed into compact masses and later allowed to undergo certain changes due to other ferments.

Other phosphoproteins exist, one being the vitellin in the yolk of eggs, which, as prepared, contains lecithin. (See p. 82.)

56. Hæmoglobins. — Blood contains a peculiar compound known as *hæmoglobin*. When decomposed, it

separates into a protein, globin, and a coloring matter
(pigment), which, when charged with oxygen, is called
hæmatin. This hæmoglobin in the blood of mammals
contains, besides carbon, nitrogen, oxygen, and hydrogen,
sulfur and iron. The latter varies in per cent from .34
to .48, and sustains an essential relation to the functions
of the blood. The blood pigment has the property of
taking up and releasing oxygen with great readiness, carrying its load of oxygen out of the lungs, giving it up to oxidation processes in various parts of the body, and bringing
to the lungs in its place the resulting carbon dioxid to be
discharged into the air. The blood changes color with the
acquisition and loss of the oxygen.

57. Lecithoproteins. — From the yolk of eggs, the
mucous membranes, and the kidneys, and doubtless from
other sources, are obtained a conjugated protein containing lecithin. The constitution and special function of this
body are not well understood.

Derived Proteins

These are divided into *primary* and *secondary* protein
derivatives. Primary protein derivatives are those that
have been slightly modified by the incipient action of water,
very dilute acids, or enzyms, or are the result of the action
of acids and alkalies whereby products soluble in weak
acids and alkalies are formed. Coagulated proteins resulting from the action of heat and alcohol are classed in
this division.

Secondary protein derivatives are those in which the
modifying changes (hydrolytic or the taking up of water),
through the action of acids or enzyms, have proceeded

beyond the incipient stage with the formation of bodies that are soluble in water. In this division, the most important compounds are the proteoses and the peptones, the latter having suffered a greater change by hydrolysis than the former.

Primary Protein Derivatives

58. Proteans and metaproteins. — When proteins are acted upon by acids or alkalies, they are modified in proportion to the strength of the reacting acid or alkali and the length of time that the action continues. With acid or alkalies of sufficient strength, there are formed products soluble in weak acids and alkalies.

59. Coagulated proteins. — There are several agents which convert albumins and other proteins into a coagulated mass, such as a boiling heat, alcohol, and certain neutral salts and the action of an enzym. For instance, with albumin from flesh or the white of an egg, boiling water converts it into a coagulum that is insoluble in water and is only rendered soluble by such agents as acids and alkalies upon heating.

Dropping a soluble protein into alcohol has the same effect. Globulins are, as a rule, affected in the same way. The nature of this modification is not known.

Secondary Protein Derivatives

60. Proteoses, peptones. — When various proteins, such as an albumin or globulin, are subjected to the action of a weak acid or of certain enzyms, they undergo what is known as hydrolysis. This change involves a cleavage (splitting) of the protein body, accompanied by the taking

up of the elements of water. In this way are formed
proteoses and peptones, the latter being proteins that are
soluble in water. A proteose is an intermediate stage
between the original protein and a peptone, and it receives
a name according to its source, as albumose, globulose,
and caseose, according as an albumin, a globulin, or casein
is its source.

Peptone was formerly regarded as the final product of
enzym action in digestion, but we now know that the
digestion of the proteins proceeds much farther. These
hydrolyzed bodies are found abundantly in the digestive
tract during digestion, the proteoses as stated being an
intermediate stage of digestion between the original proteins and the peptones. This means that the formation
of the final products of protein digestion is a progressive
step. Proteoses and peptones may also be obtained by
laboratory methods. It should be noted that commercial
peptones are largely proteoses.

61. Important properties of the proteins. — The previous description of the various groups of proteins cannot
be understood to its fullest extent excepting by those who
have a good knowledge of the fundamentals of organic
chemistry. Nevertheless, the facts given serve to impress
the important chemical and physical properties which
these bodies possess, and point to the necessity of studying
them individually in their relation to foods and nutrition.
It is not rational to speak of protein as if the term represents
an individual entity; but the members of this general class
of compounds must be considered by sub-classes at least,
in discussing the use of raw material in cookery and in
meeting dietary conditions.

There are several points that the dietician should keep in mind. One is the solubilities of the different proteins, another the effect produced upon them by heat, and another their relations to acids and ferments, — facts that will develop more fully as we proceed. A fact still more important is the varying constitution of the protein molecule, and consequently the possible variation in the nutritive function of the individual proteins.

62. The unlike constitution of proteins from different sources. — We have already seen that certain proteins are particularized in part by containing phosphorus, others sulfur, and others iron. The significance of these differences will become evident as we discuss nutritive processes. A phosphorus-bearing protein may have, and undoubtedly does have, a nutritive function that cannot be exercised by an albumin not carrying phosphorus.

It is well known that when proteins are submitted to the action of acids, alkalies, and certain ferments (enzyms), they break up into simpler compounds, which we speak of as cleavage products. It is very significant that the kind, and especially the proportions, of these products differ greatly with different proteins. For instance, the purin bases, which certainly sustain important physiological relations, are present in beef and certain glands used as food, but absent in milk and eggs. The variations in the decomposition products of certain vegetable proteins are striking, as also are the differences in this respect between vegetable and animal proteins. These cleavage products are sometimes spoken of as the "building stones" of the proteins. The following table is worthy of attention : —

TABLE XV

COMPOUNDS[1] INTO WHICH VARIOUS PROTEINS ARE BROKEN BY CLEAVAGE

	Gliadin Wheat	Gliadin Rye	Hordein Barley	Corn	Glutenin Wheat	Egg Albuminin	Ox Muscle	Chicken Muscle	Fish Muscle	Fibrin
	%	%	%	%	%	%	%	%	%	%
Glycocoll . . .	0.02	0.13	0.00	0.00	0.89	0.00	2.06	0.68	0.00	——
Alanine . . .	2.0	1.33	0.43	2.23	4.65	2.22	3.72	2.28	——	3.00
Leucine . . .	5.61	6.30	5.67	18.60	5.95	10.70	11.65	11.19	10.33	——
Proline . . .	7.06	9.82	13.73	6.53	4.23	3.56	5.82	4.74	3.17	2.40
Phenylalanine .	2.35	2.70	5.03	4.87	1.97	5.07	3.15	3.53	3.04	1.20
Glutaminic acid	37.33	33.81	36.35	18.28	23.42	9.10	15.49	16.48	10.13	3.50
Tyrosine . . .	1.20	1.19	1.67	3.55	4.25	1.77	2.20	2.16	2.39	1.00
Arginine .	3.16	2.22	2.16	1.16	4.72	4.91	7.47	6.50	6.34	——
Lysine	0.00	0.00	0.00	0.00	1.92	3.76	7.59	7.24	7.45	0.30
Histidine . . .	0.61	0.39	1.28	0.43	1.76	1.71	1.76	2.47	2.55	——
Ammonia .	5.11	5.11	4.87	3.61	4.01	1.34	1.07	1.67	1.33	——

As these compounds into which the several proteins are split may be regarded as the building stones out of which the animal proteins are constructed, the foregoing figures are significant.

In this connection it should be noted that a comparison of vegetable and animal proteins shows a close resemblance in the kind of building stones out of which they are constructed, although the proportions are unlike.

[1] There is no popular terminology with which to describe these compounds, that are known only to the chemist. They are distinguished from one another by their structure and chemical relations, and are stated in this connection simply to show that important structural differences exist between the proteins named.

Nitrogen Compounds that are Non-Proteins

In the usual method for determining the proteins of a food by multiplying the total nitrogen present by a factor, there is included in the calculation nitrogen that does not come from true proteins, but from compounds that possess physical and chemical properties greatly removed from those which characterize albumin and other true proteins. Their office as nutrients is also less comprehensive than that of the proteins.

63. Amides.— Certain non-proteins which are spoken of under the term *amides* are found chiefly in plants. Asparagine, first found in young asparagus shoots, and glutamine, found in germinating pumpkin seeds, are amides. They are soluble in water, and consequently are diffusible throughout the plant tissues. It is believed that they are the forms in which the nitrogen compounds of the plant are transferred from one part to another, as, for instance, from the stem to the seed. It has generally been held that these bodies are more abundant in young plants than in mature. A larger part of the nitrogen of roots and tubers is found in these compounds than in other foods, the proportion in grains being the least, and is very small indeed. Such investigations as have been conducted point to the conclusion that amides are not muscle-formers, as is the case with proteins. This is a reason for regarding the protein of certain vegetable foods as of less value than that of the grains and grain products.

64. Extractives. — These are bodies found in the extract obtained from beef with cold water. After the albumin has been removed from such an extract by boiling, these compounds, known as *creatin* and *creatinin*, chiefly constitute the nitrogenous solids that remain. The food value is small, if anything, for they appear to be eliminated from the body in the urine without change.

CHAPTER IV

THE COMPOUNDS OF HUMAN NUTRITION, CONCLUDED

CARBOHYDRATES, ACIDS, FATS, AND OILS

MUCH the larger proportion of the dry matter of human foods consists of non-nitrogenous material. This is especially true of the cereal grains. While these nitrogen-free compounds are not regarded by many as fundamentally so important as are the proteins, in quantity they unquestionably occupy the first rank. The activities of plant life are largely devoted to their production, and their use by animal life is correspondingly extensive. They may properly be called the main fuel supply of the animal world. Other nutrients aid in maintaining muscular force and animal heat, to be sure, but these compounds are the principal storehouse of that sun-derived energy which furnishes the motive power exhibited in all animal life. They are also important in other ways, for they fill a necessary office in the formation of milk and in the fattening of animals.

65. Elementary composition. — The compounds of this class contain only three elements, — carbon, hydrogen, and oxygen. They may be derived, therefore, wholly from air and water, and they constitute that portion of

human foods which is drawn from never failing and
costless sources of supply.

The elementary composition of typical nitrogen-free
bodies is given in this connection: —

TABLE XVI

	CELLU-LOSE	STARCH	GLUCOSE	SACCHA-ROSE	STEARIN	OLEIN
	Per Cent	Per Cent	Per Cent	Per Cent	Per Cent	Per Cent
Carbon	44.4	44.4	40.0	42.1	76.7	77.4
Hydrogen	6.2	6.2	6.7	6.4	12.4	11.8
Oxygen	49.4	49.4	53.3	51.5	11.0	10.8

66. Classification. — The non-nitrogenous compounds
of foods are usually divided into two main classes, viz.
carbohydrates and similar bodies and fats and oils. The
first class often bears the name *nitrogen-free extract*, but
the carbohydrates are its principal members. The second
is known by the chemist as *ether-extract*, because ether is
used to extract the fats or oils from the vegetable substances in which they are contained. The actual fat
obtained from vegetable foods is always less, however,
than the ether-extract, because the ether takes into solution other compounds than the fats. It should be noted
that the last two compounds of the above table, which are
fats, are relatively richer in carbon and hydrogen and
poorer in oxygen than the other compounds mentioned,
which are carbohydrates. This fact has an important
relation to nutritive values.

The Carbohydrates

The carbohydrates as a class make up a large proportion of plant substance and constitute a generous share of human food. While the compounds of this class are not structurally important to the animal organism, they fill a large place in the animal economy in maintaining the vital processes. They are among the longest known and most familiar substances that are now used as food by the human family.

In order to understand the carbohydrates as individual compounds and in their relations to each other and to the processes of nutrition, it is necessary to consider them, in general outlines at least, from the standpoint of the chemist.

The term *carbohydrates*, like the term *protein*, is collective, and includes a great variety of compounds. By their common names we know them as celluloses, starches, sugars, gums, vegetable mucilages, and so on. Chemically we distinguish them by their structure and by their relation to one another.

The Sugars

When considered from the standpoint of efficiency, the sugars are among the most valuable of all the carbohydrates, although in quantity they are less important than the starches, at least in raw food materials.

Unlike starch, they are found in solution in the sap of growing plants. It is probable that these are the forms in which carbohydrate material is transferred from one part of the plant to another. It is easy to see that some such medium of exchange is necessary. The actual pro-

F

duction of new vegetable substance takes place in the leaves. When, therefore, cell-walls and starch grains are to be constructed in the stem and fruit, the building material must be carried from the leaves to these parts in forms which will readily pass through intervening membranes. Excepting certain soluble compounds, closely related to starch, the sugars appear to be the only available bodies fitted for this office.

It is very seldom that a plant contains only a single sugar. Generally two or more sugars are found together. This is especially the case in the corn plant, sorghum, and the fruits; and the proportions of each depend somewhat upon the stage of growth of the plant.

67. Classification of sugars according to structure. — The structure of certain sugars is such that their molecules cannot be divided into simpler compounds that retain the carbohydrate character, and these are known as monosaccharides. To this class belong glucose (grape sugar) and fructose (fruit sugar). On the other hand, there are a large number of carbohydrates, one molecule of which by treatment in certain ways may be converted into two or more molecules of a mono- (simple) sugar. For instance, one molecule of starch, when submitted to the action of an acid or of certain ferments, breaks up into several molecules of glucose, and we call starch a poly-saccharide; and to this class belong sucrose (cane sugar), maltose (malt sugar), lactose (milk sugar), cellulose, the starches and gums, all of which may be split up into mono- or simple sugars. The *poly-sugars* are subdivided into di-, tri-, and so on, according as they break up into two, three, or more molecules of a simple sugar.

There are subdivisions of the mono-sugars also, on the basis of the number of carbon atoms in their molecules, and thus we have the names *diose, triose, tetrose, pentose, hexose, heptose,* etc., for sugars having two, three, four, five, six, seven, or more carbon atoms in the molecule. It may be remarked here that it is among the hexose (six carbon) sugars or their multiples that we find the carbohydrates most important to human nutrition.

A. The Mono-saccharides or Simple Sugars

The simple sugars that are most important in human nutrition are dextrose (grape sugar), levulose (fruit sugar), and galactose (from milk sugar). These are hexose (six carbon) sugars. The pentoses are also simple sugars; but, as we shall see, they scarcely occur in nature, being obtained chiefly by splitting up certain gums.

68. Dextrose. — An important simple sugar is *dextrose* or *grape sugar*, or what is known in the market as glucose. Excepting in the hands of the chemist, it is seldom seen as crystals, although these appear in the " candying " of honey and raisins. Its commercial forms are as a constituent of molasses and the sirups. Dextrose is found in practically the same plants that contain saccharose, such as sorghum, maize, and the fruits. So far as known, it is always associated with some other sugar. On account of its difficult crystallization and a lower degree of sweetness, it is less valuable for commercial purposes than cane sugar. That which appears in the market is largely made from starch by the use of an acid, and it is often utilized for adulterating the more costly saccharose. Many seem to regard glucose as a substance deleterious to health, but in consideration of the fact that, in digestion, starch and most other sugars are reduced to this compound before entering the circulation of the animal, this view does not seem to be sustained. In fact, there is a lack of evidence to show the ill effect of glucose either upon man or animals.

69. Levulose. — Another simple sugar is *levulose* or *fruit sugar*, the composition of which is identical with dextrose, but which has a different chemical constitution. It accompanies dextrose, and is found in some fruits in considerable quantities, and especially in honey. It is as sweet as cane sugar, but does not form crystals with the same readiness.

70. Galactose. — This is obtained by a cleavage of milk sugar (see later) into this sugar and dextrose. It may also be obtained from certain gums.

71. The pentoses. — There are several pentoses, none of which occur in nature, but which are prepared by chemical methods from the gums. Thus, from gum arabic containing arabin, arabinose may be obtained, and from zylin (wood gum) zylose may be prepared. Certain of these sugars have been isolated from animal compounds. They also have been found to appear in human urine. They are of great importance in the nutrition of herbivorous animals, but appear in human food only to a limited extent.

B. The Di-saccharides

These carbohydrates are all sugars which may be decomposed into two molecules of a simple sugar, or one molecule of each of two simple sugars. They are only three in number, — saccharose or sucrose (cane sugar), maltose (malt sugar), and lactose (milk sugar).   When acted upon by weak acids or certain ferments, they break by cleavage (hydrolysis) as follows : —

Saccharose + water = dextrose + levulose
Maltose   + water = dextrose + dextrose
Lactose   + water = dextrose + galactose

These are the changes that occur during the digestion of food.

72. Saccharose. — The most important of these, commercially considered, is *saccharose*, which is the ordinary crystallized sugar of the markets.   As a human food it is widely used, is especially valuable, and its manufacture and sale constitute a prominent industry.   This sugar is obtained mostly from two plants, sugar cane and the sugar beet.   It also exists abundantly in sorghum, pineapples, carrots, and in considerable proportions in the stalk of ordinary field corn.   The first spring flow of sap in one species of maple tree is richly charged with it, and in a few states large quantities of maple sirup and sugar are manufactured.

Saccharose is not a prominent constituent of unmodified human foods.   While it occurs in sweet-potatoes and in roots, and perhaps in minute proportions in certain seeds, it is only in the fresh corn plant, sorghum, pineapples, and sugar beets that it constitutes a material part of the food substance.

The fruits generally contain saccharose, mixed with other sugars and organic acids, and upon the relative proportions of these compounds depends the character of the fruit as to acidity or sweetness.

73. Maltose. — A sugar that is intimately related to the first growth which occurs in the germination of seeds is *maltose*, for it stands as an intermediate product between the store of starch in the seed and the new tissues of the sprout. The solution that the brewer extracts from the malted grains contains this compound as the principal ingredient, and through succeeding fermentations in the beer vats it is broken up into alcohol and other compounds. It sustains an important relation, therefore, to the production of beers and other alcoholic liquors. The glucose sirups found in the markets sometimes contain small quantities of this sugar. It is also found abundantly in the intestinal canal during the digestion of food, being derived from starch and other carbohydrates through the action of ferments. Maltose is similar to cane sugar in ultimate composition, but not in constitution, though as a nutrient it evidently has an equivalent value. So far as known, however, it does not appear to occur in material quantities in foods.

74. Lactose. — The only sugar of animal origin which is abundant in farm life is the lactose that is found in milk and which is known in commerce as milk sugar. The milk of all mammals contains sugar, which appears to be the same compound with every species so far investigated. When they are fed wholly from the mother, this is the only carbohydrate which young mammals receive in their food. The average proportion of sugar in the milk of domestic animals varies from three to six parts in a hundred, cow's milk containing about five parts. When the cream is removed, much the larger part of sugar remains in the skimmed milk, and in cheese-making it is nearly all found in the whey, from which the milk sugar of commerce is obtained. Very soon after milk is drawn, unless it is heated to the point of sterilization, or is treated with some antiseptic, the lactose begins to diminish in quantity, being converted into lactic acid through the action of what is known as lactic acid organisms (bacteria). Sour milk, therefore, is different from sweet in at least one compound, and this change causes at least a slight modification of food value.

C. The Poly-saccharides

This group includes a large number of carbohydrates that may be considered as complexes of the simple sugars already described. Indeed, they make up the principal bulk of the carbohydrate content of the raw materials from which human food is prepared. The poly-saccharides may be divided into three sub-groups, the starch group, the gum and vegetable mucilage group, and the cellulose group, the first being the one of greatest importance in human nutrition.

76. The Starches. — Starch is a widely distributed and abundant constituent of vegetable tissue. Food plants, especially those most used by the human family, contain it in generous proportions, in some seeds as much as 60 or 70 per cent being present. Probably only water and cellulose are more abundant in the vegetable world.

Starch does not exist in solution in the sap, but is found in the interior of plant cells in the form of minute grains which have a shape, size, and structure characteristic of the seed in which they are found. Potato starch grains are large, about $\frac{1}{300}$ of an inch in diameter, and are kidney-shaped, while those of the wheat are smaller, about $\frac{1}{1000}$

of an inch in diameter, and resemble in outline a thick burning-glass. Corn starch grains are angular, being somewhat six-sided, and those of other seeds show marked and specific characteristics. These differences in size and shape furnish the most important means of detecting adulterations of one ground grain with another, as, for instance, when corn flour is mixed with wheat flour.

Unless modified by some chemical change, starch is not dissolved by water. The starch grains are not affected at all by cold water, and, in hot water, at first only swell and burst. Prolonged treatment with hot water causes chemical changes to more soluble substances. For this reason the simple leaching of a food material removes no starch by solution. At the same time the cooking of a ground grain so breaks up and liberates the starch grains that they are probably acted upon more promptly by ferments in the digestive fluids.

The proportion of starch in plant substances used for human food varies greatly. The dry matter of many seeds, such as rice and the cereal grains, wheat, maize, barley, or oats, is largely made up of starch. The same is true of potatoes and other tubers. Johnson quotes the following figures from Dragendorff : [1] —

TABLE XVII
Amount of Starch in Dry Matter

	Per Cent		Per Cent
Wheat kernel	68.5	Peas	39.2
Rye kernel	67.0	Beans	39.6
Oat kernel	52.9	Flaxseed	28.4
Barley kernel	65.0	Potato tubers	62.5

[1] "How Crops Grow," p. 52.

It appears that in grain plants starch forms most abundantly during the later development of the seed. At the Maine Station none could be found in very immature field corn cut August 15, while on September 21 the dry matter of the whole plant on which the kernels had matured to the hardening stage contained 15.4 per cent. In general, the stem and leaves of forage plants are poor in starch.

The distribution of starch in seeds is worthy of note. The grain of wheat has been carefully studied in this particular, and it is found that this body does not normally exist in the seed coatings, this tissue consisting largely of mineral matters, proteins, cellulose, and gums. On the contrary, the germ and the interior material deposited around it are rich in starch. To be sure, wheat bran, which is now very largely the outer seed coats of the grain, has more or less, but this is due to imperfect milling.

Starch is an important commercial article, and for this purpose is mainly obtained from corn and potatoes. Special forms of starch used in cookery are sago, tapioca, and arrowroot. It is used as human food, as a source of dextrin and in other ways. By treatment with an acid, corn starch is converted into the glucose of our markets, dextrin and maltose being intermediate products.

76. Glycogen. — This is the only uncombined carbohydrate found in the animal body in appreciable quantity outside the forms that are in the blood circulation. It is sometimes called animal starch. It is a white powder, soluble in water, and may be extracted in small amounts from the muscles and liver. (See p. 139.) It is formed out of the sugars that are taken into the circulation from the digestive tract, and, as we shall see, is a reserve store of fuel for the maintenance of muscular energy, and in this way it performs a very important office in nourishing the animal body. It was formerly believed that another carbohydrate exists in muscle called *inosite*, but it is now known that this substance belongs to a different class of compounds.

77. The pentosans. — These bodies are very widely distributed in nature, being found in the leaves, stem, roots, and seeds of a great variety of plants, in algæ and in beets and turnips. Some pentosans are known as gums, such as gum arabic, gum tragacanth, and cherry gum. Pentosans, on hydrolysis, yield pentose sugars, among which are arabinose and zylose. These gum-like substances exist in such human foods as beets and turnips, spinach, cabbage, and other vegetables that serve more or less as human food.

78. Galactans, mannans, levulans, dextrans. — These are compounds of little importance in human nutrition that are more or less associated in the framework of a great variety of plants or parts of plants, including seeds, beets, and turnips, tubers and bulbs, algæ, lichens, molds, and the wood and bark of many species of trees. On hydrolysis they yield galactose, mannose, levulose, and dextrose, respectively.

Together with the pentosans these compounds make up the least valuable part of certain vegetable foods.

79. The pectin bodies. — Another class of compounds much like the gums, and perhaps related to them chemically, is the pectin bodies. Some of these substances are gelatinous in appearance. The jellying of fruits, such as apples and currants, is made possible by their presence. They exist in greater abundance in unripe fruit than in the ripe, consequently the former is selected for jelly-making. When such fruits are cooked, the pectin which they contain takes up water chemically and is transformed into a gelatinous substance, and the secret of jelly-making is in stopping the cooking process before the chemical transformations have passed beyond a certain point. Mucilages not greatly unlike the gums and pectins exist in certain seeds and roots, the most notable instance being flaxseed.

80. Dextrin, which is sometimes spoken of as a gum, is made by heating starch to about 200° C. It may also be produced by treating starch with a dilute acid. Dextrin is undoubtedly formed on the outer part of the loaf when wheat bread is baked. It is soluble in water.

81. Cellulose. — This is found in the tough or woody portion of plant tissue. In tables of food analyses we find the term *crude fiber*, which consists largely of cellulose, a familiar example of which in a nearly pure form is the cotton fiber used in making cloth. Crude fiber is separated from associated compounds by the successive treatment of vegetable substance with weak acids and alkalies, and as so determined is sometimes improperly taken to represent the amount of cellulose in a plant. While crude fiber is mainly cellulose, it contains a small proportion of other compounds, and, besides, more or less cellulose is dissolved by the acid and alkali treatment, so that the percentages of crude fiber given in food tables only approximately measure the cellulose present.

All plant tissue is made up of cells, the walls of which

are chiefly or wholly cellulose.   It is this substance out of which is built the framework of the plant, and which gives toughness and rigidity to certain of its parts.   The more of this plant tissue contains, the more tenacious it is, other things being equal, and the more difficult of mastication.

The proportions of cellulose in the different parts of a plant are greatly unlike.   It is usually most abundant in the stem, with less in the foliage and least in the fruit. With vegetables like potatoes and turnips, the leaves are much richer in fiber than the tubers or roots, which contain a comparatively small proportion.   Of the grains or seeds considerable is present in the outer coatings, while but little is found in the interior.   Considering human foods of plant origin, we find that vegetables such as celery, lettuce, beets, and turnips are relatively rich in crude fiber, while tubers, flours, and meals contain only small amounts.   In certain by-products from the grains, like bran, which is made up mostly of the seed coatings, fiber is present in fairly large proportions, while in flour derived from the inner parts of the grain the percentage is almost negligible.

The stage of growth at which a plant is used for food purposes has a marked influence upon the proportion of crude fiber.   In young, actively growing vegetable tissue, the cell-walls are thin, but, as the plant increases in age, these thicken chiefly through the deposition of cellulose. In general, the toughness and hardness of mature plants, as compared with young, is due to the increased proportion of woody fiber, although the decrease in the relative amount of water in the tissues and the deposition of other substances have more or less effect.   The rapid toughening of young asparagus tips and the tenderness of young beets as compared with old ones are cases in point.

The Acids

Other substances besides those of a carbohydrate character are included in the nitrogen-free extract. Chief among these are the organic acids, compounds which are found mostly in the fruits, although they appear in certain fermented products, such as sauerkraut and sour milk. The most important and well known of these are acetic acid, found in vinegar, citric acid in lemons, lactic acid in sour milk, malic acid in many fruits, such as currants and apples, and oxalic acid in rhubarb. Probably these acids are sometimes free, but the trend of opinion is that generally they are united with potassium or some other base, forming an acid salt. Excepting the fruits, only fermented foods contain acids to an appreciable extent. When milk sours, the sugar in it is changed to lactic acid under the influence of a ferment. In sauerkraut, various acids are formed at the expense of the carbohydrates that are in the material which is subjected to fermentation.

Fats and Oils

The fats or oils are compounds greatly important in the nutrition of man. There are many individual fats, those known in common life as tallow, lard, butter, and oils, such as linseed and cottonseed oils, being mixtures of three or more of these.

When any finely ground foodstuff, either vegetable or animal, is submitted to the leaching action of ether, chloroform, or certain other liquids, several compounds are taken into solution, the main and important ones being fats or oils. These bodies make up the chief portion of such an extract from seeds, while material so derived from other vegetable materials also contains a considerable amount of wax, chlorophyll, and other substances. Tables that show the composition of foods have a column which is sometimes designated " ether-extract," and sometimes " fats or oils." The former is the more accurate term, because the compounds which it is the intention to describe are often no more than half fats or oils. The real value of the " ether-extract " from different foods is partly determined, therefore, by its source. When it is all oil, or nearly so, it is worth much more for use by the animal than when it is made up to quite an extent of other bodies.

82. Fats in grains and seeds. — The proportions of fat or oil in foods vary within wide limits. In general, seeds and their by-products contain more than the stem and leaves, the differences in the percentages of actual oil being greater than is indicated by the ether-extract. But little is found in the dry matter of roots and tubers. Among the cereal grains and other more common farm seeds, corn and oats show the largest amounts, the proportion in dry matter being from five to six in one hundred, while wheat, barley, rye, peas, and rice contain much smaller percentages, wheat having about 2 per cent, and rice sometimes not over one-fifth of 1 per cent. Agricultural seeds that are especially oleaginous are cottonseed, flaxseed, sunflower seeds, and the seeds of many species belonging to the mustard family, such as rape. Peanuts, coconuts, and palm nuts are also very rich in oil. The average percentages in these seeds and nuts are approximately as given below : —

TABLE XVIII

OIL IN CERTAIN SEEDS

	PER CENT		PER CENT
Linseed	34	Peanuts	46
Cottonseed	30	Coconuts	67
Sunflower seed	32	Palm nuts	49
Rape seed	42	Poppy seed	41
Mustard seed	32		

The oils from all the above are important commercial products, being used in a great variety of ways in human foods and in the arts. In many cases, the refuse from this extraction goes back to the farm as food for cattle. This is especially true of linseed and cottonseed.

83. Fat-rich foods. — Certain of the raw materials used in the human dietary are practically all fat or oil, such as lard, butter, and the salad oils. Meats such as pork, beef, and mutton are rich in fats, the proportion depending greatly on the condition of the animal from which the meat comes.

84. Nature and kinds of fats. — The vegetable and animal fats and oils may, for convenience' sake, be discussed in two divisions, the neutral fats or glycerides and the fatty acids. The neutral fats are combinations of the fatty acids with glycerin. When, for instance, lard is treated at a high temperature with the alkalies, potash, and soda, glycerin is set free, and an alkali takes its place in a union with the fatty acids. This is the chemical change which occurs in soap-making. There are several of these neutral fats, the ones most prominent and important in agriculture

being those abundant in butter and in the body fats of
animals; viz. butyrin, caproin, caprylin, caprin, laurin,
myristin, olein, palmatin, and stearin, the last three being
the most abundant and important in human foods. Butyrin is a combination of butyric acid and glycerin, stearin
of stearic acid and glycerin, and so on. Because these
are combinations of three molecules of a fatty acid radical
with one of glycerin, they are sometimes named tri-
stearin, tri-palmatin, and tri-olein, and so on. Some
single fats (glycerides) are compounds of two or three
fatty acid radicles united with glycerin in the same
molecule. As glycerin is an alcohol, and as combinations
of an alcohol and acids are ethers, the neutral fats are
really ethers (esters), although they differ greatly from our
conceptions of an ether, which is gained from ethyl ether
or the ether of drug stores.

85. Physical properties. — These individual fats possess
greatly unlike physical properties. They are all soluble
in benzine, chloroform, and ether, and insoluble in water.
At the ordinary temperature of a room, some are liquid
and some are solid, olein belonging to the former class, and
palmatin and stearin to the latter. It is a matter of common observation that butter, lard, and tallow differ in
hardness at a given temperature, and by the use of a thermometer it may easily be discovered that their melting
points are not the same. As these animal fats are in all
cases chiefly mixtures of olein, palmatin, and stearin, stearin
and palmatin being a solid at ordinary temperatures, and
olein a liquid at anything above the freezing point, it is
evident that the relative proportions of these compounds
will affect the ease of melting and the hardness of the mix-

tures of which they are a part. Stearin melts at 71.7° C. and palmatin at 62° C. Tallow, having more stearin than lard and butter, and less olein, is consequently much more solid on a hot day.

The composition and physical properties of the fat from a beef animal seem to vary according to the age of the animal and the locality of the body from which the fat is taken. Fat from an old animal melts at a lower temperature than that from a young animal, and the same is true of fat taken from the outside of the body as compared with that taken from the inside. Fat from herbivora is in general harder than that from carnivora.

86. Milk fat. — Milk fat contains not only the three principal fats, but also the others mentioned, butyrin, caproin, caprylin, caprin, laurin, and myristin, in small proportions, and these latter tend to give butter certain properties that distinguish it from the other animal fats, which are almost wholly palmatin, olein, and stearin. These special butter fats are liquid at ordinary temperatures. Doubtless the flavor, texture, and resistance of butter to the effects of heat are much influenced by the proportions of the numerous fats it contains, but there is much connected with this subject of which we are still ignorant.

87. Fatty acids. — Free, fatty acids exist in nature. They are not found in butter, lard, and tallow unless these substances have undergone fermentations, or, as we say, have become rancid. The characteristic flavor of strong butter is due to free butyric acid, which, because of fermentations, has parted from the glycerin with which it was originally combined in the milk. In plant oils, on the other hand, are found considerable proportions of the free

G

fatty acids, some of which have not been discovered so far in animal fats, either free or uncombined.

88. Ether-extracts. — Perhaps no one has studied plant oils more thoroughly than Stellwaag, who investigated the ingredients of the ether- and benzine-extracts from plants. His results show that not only do these extracts include substances which are not fats, but that a considerable proportion of free, fatty acids is always present, sometimes in quantities exceeding the neutral fats: —

TABLE XVIII *a*

COMPOSITION OF ETHER-EXTRACTS (PER CENT)

	NEUTRAL FATS	FREE FATTY ACIDS	MATERIAL NOT SAPONIFIABLE
Potatoes	16.3	56.9	10.9
Beets	23.0	35.3	10.7
Maize, kernel	88.7	6.7	3.7
Barley	73.0	14.0	6.1
Oats	61.6	27.6	2.4

It appears, as before stated, that ether-extract, especially that from vegetables, may consist, to some extent, of materials which should not be classed among the fats. The extracts from the grains proved to be nearly all oil. Moreover, the grain oils were made up principally of glycerides, and those from potatoes and beets consisted largely of free, fatty acids.

89. Lecithins. — There is a group of bodies closely related to the fats, which are often called the phosphorized fats. Reference is made to the *lecithins*. It has previously been stated that neutral fats are combinations of fatty acids and glycerin (glycerol). Lecithins are compounds in which one of the radicals of a fatty acid is replaced by a compound of phosphoric acid. They are widely distributed in nature. They appear to be an active component of every cell, both of vegetable and animal tissue, and they are especially abundant in seeds, in the nerve system, in fish, eggs, and in the yolk of eggs. These bodies evidently fill an important place in plant and animal nutrition. These are good theoretical reasons for suggesting that lecithins serve as a stepping stone to the synthesis of the nucleoproteins. In digestion they behave like the true fats.

CHAPTER V

THE DIGESTION OF FOOD

WE have accepted so far without discussion the almost self-evident fact that the food is the immediate source of the substance and energy of the animal body. It now remains for us to consider the way in which nutrition is accomplished. The first step in this direction is the digestion of food. It is necessary for food ingredients to be placed in such relations to the animal organism that they are available for use. This involves both condition and location. The various nutrients in the exercise of their several functions must be generally distributed to all the interior parts of the animal body. It is obvious that bread and meat as such cannot be so distributed, and so their compounds must, in part at least, be brought into soluble and diffusible condition, in order that they may pass through the membranous lining which separates the blood vessels and other vascular bodies from the cavity of the alimentary canal.

90. Digestion and assimilation. — In discussing physiological relations of food, two terms are employed : viz., digestion and assimilation. Digestion refers to the preparation of food compounds for use, by rendering them soluble and diffusible, — changes which are accomplished in what we call the alimentary canal, a passage that begins with the mouth, includes the stomach and intestines, and ends with the anus. Assimilation signifies the appropriation of nutrients, after digestion, to the maintenance of the vital processes and to the building of flesh and bone, — processes taking place in the tissues, to which the nutritive substances are conveyed by the blood. The two terms are entirely distinct in meaning, although they are confused in popular speech.

91. General changes in food through digestion. — In digestion, food undergoes both mechanical and chemical changes. It is masticated, that is, ground into finer particles, after which, in its passage along the alimentary canal, it comes in contact with several juices which profoundly modify it chemically. That portion of it which is rendered diffusible is absorbed by certain vessels that are embedded in the walls of the stomach and intestines, and is conveyed into the blood. The insoluble part passes on and is rejected by the animal as worthless material, and constitutes the solid excrement or feces. The forms in which the nutrients are conveyed into the circulation are believed to be the following: The proteins, previous to absorption into the blood, are converted into soluble bodies, proteoses and peptones, or mainly into simpler nitrogen compounds resulting from a more extensive cleavage, or more probably into all these forms; the carbohydrates enter the blood as sugars, chiefly as dextrose. The fats are changed into a finely divided form either as such or as fatty acids and soaps. The function of digestion is to transform the various nutrients into these forms. A study of digestion includes, then, a knowledge of mastication, of the sources, nature, and functions of the several digestive juices, and a consideration of the various conditions affecting the extent and rapidity of digestive action.

A. FERMENTS

The changes involved in rendering food compounds soluble are intimately connected with a class of bodies known as ferments, to which brief reference has already been made, and it seems necessary before proceeding to a consideration of digestion as a process to learn something of the nature and functions of these agents, which are actively and essentially present in the digestive tract.

A ferment may be defined in a general way as something which causes fermentation; in other words, the decomposition of certain vegetable or animal compounds with which it comes in contact under favorable conditions. Ferments have been classified into two kinds, organized and unorganized. The so-called organized ferments are low, microscopic forms of vegetable life, generally single-celled plants. Those known as unorganized ferments are not living organisms, but are simply chemical compounds.

92. Organized ferments. — When milk is allowed to remain in a warm room for several hours, it becomes sour. An examination of it chemically shows that its sugar has largely or wholly disappeared and has been replaced by an acid. A study of the milk with the microscope, before and after souring, reveals the fact that there has been a marvelous increase in it of single-celled organisms or plants. The presence of this form of life is regarded as the cause of the change of the sugar into lactic acid. We have here a so-called lactic acid ferment, which may typify the organized ferments known as bacteria. Numerous other fermentations of the same general kind are common to everyday experience. The changes in the cider barrel and the wine cask, the spoiling of canned fruits and vegetables, and the heating of hay and grain are illustrations of what is accomplished by these minute organisms.

Bacteria that cause disease and which multiply in the organs, and other tissues of the animal body, may also be properly called ferments, because in their growth new compounds, *toxins*[1] perhaps, are formed which are as truly fermentative by-products as the carbonic acid and alcohol of cider and beer making. As this subject viewed on its pathogenic side is not important in this connection, we need to study organized ferments only so far as they relate to the preservation of foods and to changes in the alimentary canal. We shall be best equipped for controlling ferments and preventing their destructive action if we know what they are, and understand the general conditions under which they thrive. We should also know how, and to what extent, their action occasions harm.

93. Structure. Distribution. — The organized ferments are classed in the vegetable kingdom. As a rule, each individual plant is a single cell, varying in shape and so minute as to be invisible to the unaided sight. It corresponds in its general structure to the cells which make up the tissues of the higher vegetable species, *i.e.*, it consists of a cell-wall inside of which are protoplasm and other forms of living matter. These organisms are distributed everywhere, — in the air, in the soil, on surfaces of plants, and in the bodies of animals.

---

[1] Poisonous albuminous bodies, produced by bacterial action; as, for instance, in typhoid fever, diphtheria, tetanus, and other diseases.

Whenever the right opportunity offers itself, they multiply and bring about all the results attendant upon their growth.

94. Conditions of growth. — The conditions essential to their development are the proper degree of moisture and temperature and the necessary food materials. Thoroughly dry animal and vegetable substances do not ferment. Flour and meal that have been dried to a water content of 10 per cent will keep a long time without loss from fermentative changes. The heat in a bin of new grain, with its subsequent musty condition, is due to the fermentations that are made possible through the presence of considerable moisture. Thorough drying is a preventive of destructive fermentations.

There is a temperature at which each vegetable ferment thrives best, and there are limits of temperature outside of which the growth of these forms of life does not occur, or is very slight. Numerous species thrive between 75° and 100° F. Fermentable materials like fruit and meat at the freezing point or below are not subject to fermentations. The boiling point of water kills most bacteria, and temperatures above 150° F. retard or entirely prevent their growth.

95. Results of fermentations. — Like all life, these organisms must have food. Many species find this in acceptable forms in vegetable and animal products. Because these products generally contain the sugar, proteins, and mineral compounds which nourish bacteria, many of them are the prey of ferments under proper conditions of moisture and heat. The prevention of fermentation in foods is desirable because it occasions a loss of nutritive value and often produces undesirable flavors. The loss becomes evident when we consider the nature of the chemical changes that occur. For instance, when sugar of cider is broken up through the influence of a bacterium, the carbon dioxid and alcohol are formed through the appropriation of free oxygen. This means that combustion occurs, causing the liberation of energy which otherwise would have been available if the sugar had been taken as food. Many fermentations involve oxidation, all of which are destructive of food value.

96. Manner of action. — Several theories have been advanced to account for the action of the organized ferments. One is that these little plants use sugar and other compounds as food, deriving energy and growth therefrom, the carbonic acid, alcohol, and other new bodies being the by-products of this use. Another is that these organisms produce an unorganized ferment which brings about the fermentative changes, and their action is therefore indirect. Indeed, it seems to be definitely proved that it is possible to separate from the cells of the yeast plant a ferment that, in the absence of the yeast plant itself, converts sugar into carbon dioxid and alcohol. This shows that the effective agent in bacterial fermentations is, after all, a chemical substance, or an unorganized ferment. These later discoveries tend to remove the distinction that has been made between organized and unorganized ferments. Whatever may be the real explanation of the changes that occur, fermentations due to plant growth are among the most useful agencies with which we deal, and may be the most harmful. The yeast plant is an organized ferment, and in bread-making it is useful, but the putrefaction of meats under the influence of another ferment causes loss.

The digestive tract of man is inhabited by countless numbers of bacteria. These are found to some extent in the stomach, but most abundantly in the intestines, especially in the colon. The two main types in which we are interested in their relation to digestion are the *fermentative* or those that attack the carbohydrates, especially the sugars, and the *putrefactive*, or those that cause decomposition of the proteins. The former are most active in the stomach and when carbohydrate-bearing foods, especially sweets, *are eaten in excess*, or for any reason the food remains an abnormally long time in the stomach, as when the organ is weak muscularly, an uncomfortable, and sometimes dangerous, evolution of acids and gases occurs. As the presence of hydrochloric acid tends to inhibit the growth of these organisms, an insufficient secretion of gastric juice gives an opportunity for stomach fermentations that would not occur under normal conditions.

The putrefactive fermentations, which are favored by a heavy meat diet, begin in the lower part of the small intestine and reach their maximum in the colon. In excessive meat eating, particularly when the food residues remain for an unusually long time in the intestines, putrefactive products may be evolved to a harmful extent, sometimes causing serious results. But with healthy individuals under proper conditions of diet the bacteria present in the digestive tract are at least not harmful, and according to older views, now more or less discredited, are useful adjuncts of digestion.

97. Unorganized ferments. — There is another class of ferments which is termed unorganized, and to which the general name *enzym* is given. These are the ferments especially important in digestion. They are merely chemical compounds which produce a peculiar effect upon certain bodies with which they come in contact. If a thin piece of lean beef be suspended in an extract from the mucous lining of a pig's stomach, to which has been added a small proportion of hydrochloric acid, the liquid being kept at about 98° F., the beef will soon begin to soften, afterwards swell to a more or less jelly-like condition, and finally dissolve. The same general result would occur with fish, blood fibrin, or the coagulated white of an egg. When starch, which is not affected by pure, warm water, is placed in a warm water solution of crushed malt, it soon dissolves, leaving a comparatively clear liquid. A chemical examination of these preparations will reveal the fact that the compounds of the meat are present in solution in somewhat modified forms, and that the starch has been changed to a sugar or other soluble bodies. In both cases substances insoluble in water have become soluble and diffusible.

The cause of these changes is the presence of typical bodies, one in the pig's stomach and one in the malt, ferments of the enzym class, the former of which renders proteins soluble, the latter acting to produce a similar result with the insoluble carbohydrates. This action is different from that of the organized ferments, where oxidation occurs in many cases. The enzyms simply induce the proteins and starch to take up the elements of water, which apparently does not greatly diminish their energy value. How this is done cannot be explained in simple terms, if at all. Our knowledge of the manner of the change rests entirely upon theoretical grounds. The digestion of food is largely accomplished through the specific effect of enzym bodies, of which every digestive fluid contains one or more. Examples of these are the pepsin and pancreatin of the drug store that contain enzyms mixed with more or less of impurities. The various enzyms are often given names according to their function : *invertase*, which inverts or splits sucrose ; *glucase*, that changes any carbohydrate into glucose ; *lactase*, that splits lactose into simpler sugars. In general, the ferments acting on starch are called *diastases*. Those acting on proteins to produce hydrolysis and cleavage are designated as *proteolytic*.

B. The Mouth

98. Mastication. — The first step in the digestion of food is to reduce it to a much finer condition. This is done in the mouth, the teeth being the grinding tools. This comminution is essential for two reasons: (1) it puts the food in condition to be swallowed, and (2) fits it for the prompt and efficient action of the several digestive fluids. It is necessary for all food materials to be broken down and moistened in order that they may be swallowed. Even if they could be conveyed to the stomach in a coarse form, the process of rendering their constituents soluble would proceed very slowly. Common experience teaches us how much more quickly finely powdered sugar or salt will dissolve than will the large crystals or lumps. The more finely any solid is ground, the larger is the surface exposed to the attack of the dissolving liquid.

Prompt and rapid solution of food is essential, because, if it is too long delayed, uncomfortable and injurious fermentations are likely to set in, and, because of imperfect digestion, the final nutritive effect of a meal may be diminished, and health may be impaired. For these

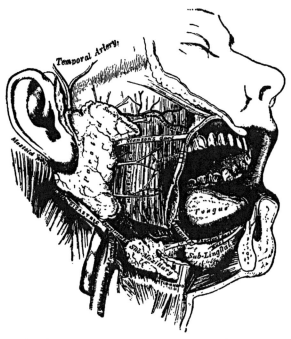

FIG. 1. — Glands secreting the saliva, — parotid, sublingual, submaxillary.

reasons, persons with diseased teeth, or those who have lost teeth, may not properly prepare their food for digestion.

99. The saliva. — During mastication there is poured into the mouth a liquid called the saliva, which has two important functions : (1) it moistens the food, and (2) it causes a chemical change in certain of the constituents of the food.

The saliva has its origin in several secretory glands known as the salivary glands that are adjacent to the mouth cavity, and from these this liquid is poured into the mouth through ducts that open in the cheek and under the tongue. The chief of these glands are located in the side of the face just in front of the ear, and between the lower jaw and the floor of the mouth, and are called the parotid, the submaxillary, and the sublingual. Other glands of this character are scattered in the cheeks and at the base of the tongue. The anatomy and arrangement of these organs are not essential to our subject. We are chiefly interested in the liquid which they secrete.

100. The saliva and its action. — The saliva is a transparent and somewhat slimy liquid, and contains generally not less than 99 parts in 100 of water, and one part or less of solid matter. It is alkaline in reaction, because of the presence of compounds of the alkalies. The specific chemical effect exerted by this liquid on the food constituents is shown by subjecting starch to its action. When this is done, the starch gradually disappears as such and is replaced by a solution of maltose, the same sugar that we find in barley malt. The agent which is active in causing this change is a ferment, *ptyalin*, which is always present in the saliva of man and of some animals. It is classed among the diastatic ferments, because it has an office similar to that of a diastase in the germination of seeds; viz., the transformation of starch into a sugar. This transformation proceeds through successive stages from starch to dextrins, and from dextrins to maltose. Cooked starch is readily susceptible to the action of saliva, while raw starch is more slowly attacked by it. This does not mean that raw starch may not be finally digested by the human subject. This change begins in the mouth, and probably continues in the stomach, until the food becomes so acid that the ferment ceases to act, for ptyalin is inactive in an acid medium.

The action of saliva in the stomach does not cease suddenly, however, but proceeds until the masticated food is rendered wholly acid by mixing with the gastric juice. There is a not inconsiderable absorption of sugar from the stomach, notwithstanding the fact that the stomach secretes no agent that acts on starch. A certain proportion of the starch of foods is acted on by the saliva, partly in the stomach, but the main transformation to sugar occurs farther on in the digestive tract. The saliva also moistens the food, which is a most important office, for it is a necessary preparation to the act of swallowing. It is estimated that an adult secretes not far from one quart of saliva in 24 hours.

C. The Stomach

101. The gastric juice. — When the food leaves the mouth, it passes down the esophagus into the stomach. The only modifications it has suffered up to this point are its reduction to a finer condition and a slight action of the mouth ferment upon the starch. After the food is swallowed, changes of another kind begin, affecting the protein compounds especially. There is at once poured upon the food the gastric juice, a liquid that is secreted in large quantity by glands located in the inner or mucous membrane of the stomach. This juice, like all the diges-

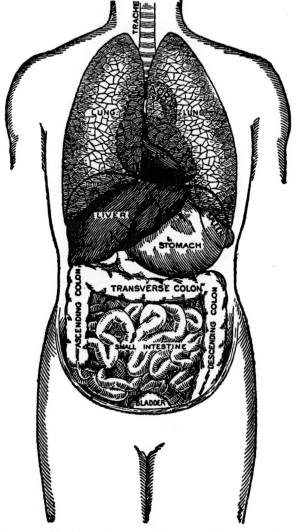

tive fluids, is mostly water, the proportion being between 98 and 99 parts of water to less than two parts of solids. The latter consist of ferments, a certain amount of free or uncombined hydrochloric acid, and a variety of mineral compounds, prominent among which are calcium and magnesium phosphates and the chlorides of the alkalies, common salt being especially abundant.

Fig. 2.—Position of organs of thorax and abdomen that are related to digestion and excretion. (Morrow.)

102. Gastric enzyms. — Especial interest pertains to the ferments of the gastric juice, one of which, in connection with free hydrochloric acid, causes a most important change in the proteins of the food, such as egg albumin and the gliadin and glutenin of the wheat kernel by reducing them to soluble forms. We know quite definitely about this action, because it can be very successfully produced in an artificially prepared liquid. If the mucous lining of a pig's stomach, after carefully cleaning without washing with water, is warmed for some hours in a very dilute solution of hydrochloric acid, an extract is obtained which has the power of dissolving lean meat, wheat gluten, and other protein substances. The active agent in causing this solution is *pepsin*, an unorganized ferment or enzym which is present in the gastric fluid of all animals. It changes proteins to peptones, bodies that are soluble and diffusible. This change is not a single step, for the protein passes through successive stages in the form of proteoses before it reaches the peptone form. Another ferment present in the gastric juice is the one which gives to rennet its value as a means of coagulating the casein of milk in cheese-making, and is called *rennin*. The action of this latter body is especially prominent in the stomach of the calf when fed exclusively on milk, and it is the calf's active stomach, the fourth in the mature animal, which is the source of commercial rennet. A similar coagulation of casein takes place in the human stomach, especially no-ticeable in the milk that is rejected from the stomachs of infants, this being a normal result in digestion. Some investigators do not distinguish between rennin and pepsin. Still another ferment which food meets in the stomach is lipase (steapsin), that has the property of decomposing fats. This ferment, or similar ones, plays a prominent

H

part in intestinal digestion, but there is no proof that the
fats are acted on in the stomach to any appreciable extent
when they enter the stomach in meat or other solid or
liquid forms.   Emulsified fats appear to be quite extensively acted on in the stomach, especially in milk, a
fact important in the feeding of infants.   Recent investigations, particularly those of Cannon, have brought
out some very interesting facts concerning the way in
which the stomach manages the food during its retention in that organ.   The following diagrams[1] show

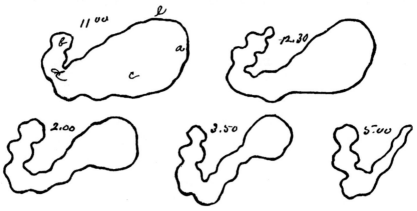

Fig. 3. — Changes in the form of the stomach during digestion.
a. fundus.   *b.* pylorus.   *c.* middle portion.   *d.* duodenal region.

the general arrangement of the parts of the stomach
and its changes in form during digestion.   The food
is introduced into the stomach through the esophagus
and is lodged first in the fundus or cardiac end.
From there it is moved by degrees toward the pylorus from which it enters the small intestine.   It

[1] Originally appearing in *American Journal of Physiology*, 1898. Vol.
1, p. 370.

has been taught that this movement is brought about by the churning of the stomach throughout its entire length. Cannon showed the error of this conclusion. From his observations it appears that the fundus end of the stomach is quiet at first. The waves of peristaltic constriction begin at the duodenal and middle portions and move the food. toward the pylorus. In this way the constrictions that begin near the pyloric end gradually extend toward the cardiac end. The latter part of the stomach is distended after a full meal, but gradually diminishes in size during digestion. Moreover, the character of the gastric juice is not the same from the different areas of the stomach, that from the middle portion being rich in acid, and that from the cardiac and pyloric ends being neutral or nearly so. These facts show that the food remains for some time in the fundus and meets there a neutral liquid, consequently the alkalinity of the mass is maintained for a time, and the saliva acts on the starch for a much longer period than has been supposed. It is believed, too, that the length of time the food remains in the stomach varies with its kind. The digesting mass is not forced into the intestine, until it becomes well saturated with free acid at the pylorus, a result that will be reached later with a meat, than with a vegetable, diet; for it is plain that much more acid will be required to combine with the proteins of the meat than with the smaller amounts in carbohydrate foods and so free acid is longer in accumulating.

103. Gastric stimuli. — The gastric juice is not constantly poured into the stomach to accumulate there, but is secreted as it is needed under the influence of certain stimuli. These stimuli may be classed as psychic and chemical. Appetizing odors when there is a strong desire to eat, and the agreeable taste of food in the mouth of a hungry person are important psychic or "nervous" influences that promote gastric digestion through an adequate supply of the digesting fluid. Other stimuli that may be called chemical, are the direct or indirect reaction of certain substances such as meat extracts, proteoses, sugars, alcohol, and condiments, upon the secretory activity of the stomach. This stimulus comes later than the psychic, but is more prolonged. The more recent researches indicate that the first products of digestion, reacting on the stomach inner membranes, cause the formation of a substance, a *secretin*, which, carried by the blood stream to the cells of the stomach glands, excites gastric secretion. It now seems possible that sometime we shall have a definite dietetic method of influencing gastric secretion rather than a medicinal, for it appears that certain food compounds may stimulate, and others, such as fats, retard, stomach activity. The psychic (nervous) factor is no less important. If this is so, it is seen how necessary it is that one shall eat with pleasure rather than through compulsion. Satisfaction with one's diet is a determinative element in good digestion. Moreover, condimental stimulation is a poor makeshift for the effect of a healthy liking for food.

Digestion is aided by movement of the ingested food mass through contractions of the walls of the stomach. It is easy to see how bad digestion occurs in a stomach that is weak muscularly or that fails to secrete gastric juice sufficient in quantity or normal in constitution, and how difficult it is to remedy such conditions.

D. DIGESTION IN THE INTESTINES

The chemical changes which the food undergoes in the large and small intestines are exceedingly complex and concerning which we have greatly insufficient knowledge. When the partly digested food from the stomach (chyme)

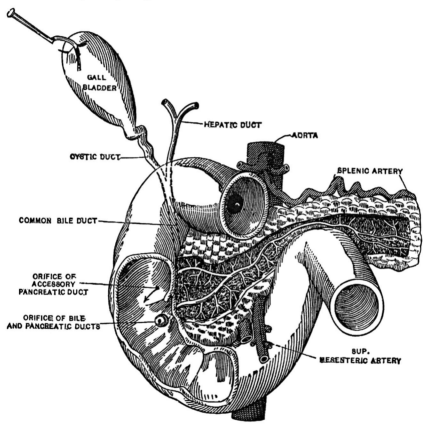

FIG. 4. — Ducts introducing the bile and pancreatic juice into small intestine. (GERRISH.)

reaches the intestines, it meets several liquids secreted by such special glands as the liver, pancreas (sweet bread), and certain smaller glands that are distributed in the membranes of the intestinal walls. The liver secretes the bile, pancreatic juice comes from the pancreas, and various intestinal juices flow from the small glands along the intestinal walls.

104. The bile. — This is a secretion of the cells of the liver and from the inner wall of the gall bladder, that from the former source being thinner, less ropy, and poorer in solid matter than that secreted by the gall bladder. After elaboration, bile is stored in part, at least, in the gall bladder. Human bile is a golden yellow liquid, alkaline, and bitter in taste. That from the gall bladder has been found to contain from 82 per cent to 90 per cent of water or from 10 per cent to 18 per cent of solid matter. The liver bile is poorer in solids, analyses showing the proportion of water to be from 96.5 per cent to 97.5 per cent. The solids of bile include a great variety of compounds, the chiefest of which are certain bile salts and pigments.

Numerous other compounds are present, such as fats, soaps, cholesterin, urea, and mineral salts.

105. Bile salts. — The bile salts are mainly sodium compounds of *glycocholic, taurocholic,* and related acids and the best-known pigments which occur under normal conditions are *bilirubin,* which is reddish yellow, and *biliverdin,* which is green. Several other pigments occur in the concretions which form in the gall bladder, known as gallstones. No ferment (enzym) has been found in the bile, at least in more than traces.

106. Secretion of bile. — The secretion of the bile is irregular in quantity, and, as is the case with gastric juice, appears to be induced by chemical excitants of which acids, especially hydrochloric, seem to be especially effective. Of the nutrients, the proteins exert the most influence in this respect. The acceleration of secretion occurs at a greatly varying time after food ingestion, the maximum flow being determined by the kind of food.

The bile compounds are in evidence in certain pathological conditions. When for any reason the discharge of bile into the intestine is retarded and the organism attempts to eliminate it through the kidneys, the tissues become charged with its compounds and take on a yellowish coloration, and the subject is said to have jaundice, — a condition sometimes attended with serious results. Concretions are formed in the gall bladder that in man are characterized by the presence of cholesterin, a bile compound.

107. The pancreatic juice. — This secretion has the most comprehensive action on the food nutrients of any one of the intestinal liquids. It originates in the pancreas (sweet bread). Its flow is intermittent, being induced by the reaction especially of the acids in the partially digested foods from the stomach. The amount secreted and its composition appear to change with the kind of food. It contains about 87.5 per cent of water and 12.5 per cent of solid matter. This secretion acts upon all classes of nutrients, as it contains a variety of ferments greatly unlike in function.

108. Protein-splitting enzyms.—Among these are at least two, and possibly several, which act on proteins, including trypsin (possibly not a single body), as the main one, and one that, like erepsin (see p. 105), splits peptones into simpler compounds and seems to supplement the action of trypsin. Trypsin acts in neutral or in alkaline solutions, a free mineral acid like hydrochloric completely stopping its operation. Organic acids, like lactic, do not seem to have this effect. In conjunction with other enzyms, it splits food proteins into simpler compounds, viz., monamino and diamino acids, tryptophane and other bodies, all of which may be regarded as the building stones of the original proteins. As we have seen, these simpler bodies are not the same in kind or proportions for all proteins.

109. Steapsin. — The pancreatic secretion acts vigorously on fats, not only splitting them into fatty acids and glycerin, but, in conjunction with the bile, also effects their emulsification, this latter result being aided, doubtless, by the soaps which are formed from a union of the fatty acids and the alkaline bases (mostly sodium) in the bile. This is a true saponification. The cleavage of the fats is due to an enzym to which the name of *steapsin* is given, also called *lipase*.

110. Amylopsin. — We have seen that starch is acted upon to a small extent by the saliva, and that this action is not prolonged in the stomach beyond the time when the stomach contents become fully acidified. Starch digestion is therefore carried on mainly in the intestines, chiefly, if not wholly, by a diastatic ferment in the pancreatic juice which has the power of hydrolyzing the starch mostly into maltose. This pancreatic diastase, called *amylopsin* by some authors, is not found in the digestive tract of infants until more than one month after birth. The **presence** of bile is very favorable to its action.

111. Intestinal juices. — Mention has been made of juices that are secreted by small glands distributed in the walls of the intestines. These appear to be quite important factors in digestion, as they supplement the action of the ferments of the pancreatic juice. It appears to be shown that an enzym *erepsin* is found in these juices, that is unable to act upon any of the native proteins except casein, but has the power of decomposing proteoses and peptones into simpler compounds, particularly the amino acids. These secretions seem to contain, also, a ferment that converts maltose into dextrose, and in infants and young animals they also contain a lactose- (milk sugar) splitting enzym. It is held that trypsin does not exist as such in the pancreatic juice when poured into the small intestine, but that this enzym is formed from a mother substance (trypsinogen) in the pancreatic juice after it comes in contact with the intestinal juice, this result being accomplished through the action of a body, probably secreted from the intestinal walls and called by Pawlow *enterokinase*.

112. Intestinal bacteria. — So far, in presenting the relation of ferments to digestion, only the unorganized ferments or enzyms have been considered. While these are chiefly concerned in normal digestion, organized ferments are present throughout the entire intestinal canal and play a part in food changes. They are most abundant and active in the lower part of the small intestine and the upper part of the large. They act upon the proteins, causing putrefaction, dissolve cellulose, and cause a decomposition of the carbohydrates. The products of these fermentations may be in part the same as those produced in pancreatic digestion, but these include also indol and skatol, which have the characteristic fecal odor, volatile fatty acids, and gases, some of which are carbon dioxid, hydrogen, marsh gas, and hydrogen sulfide.

Under certain conditions fermentations of this character, which up to a certain extent are normal and may be beneficial, proceed so far as to be deleterious to health. Anything which retards digestion, such as imperfect mastication, excessive eating, abnormal amounts of meat in the diet, and failure of the organs secreting the digestive fluids to supply these fluids in sufficient abundance, gives these bacteria a better opportunity to act on the food residues, and increases their effect. Some foods, especially vegetables of the leguminous class, appear to be provocative of excessive intestinal fermentations. Flatulence, and even toxic poisoning may be the result of great bacterial activity in the digestive tract. It is hardly possible to check this by administering septics, but purging is of value in removing the fermentative material. At one time it was held that the bile has a specific antiseptic effect, but later researches throw doubt on this conclusion. Probably the bad results of a restricted flow of bile are indirect, the less perfect digestion giving the bacteria a greater opportunity. Free hydrochloric acid restrains bacterial fermentation and has this effect in the stomach, but this influence can hardly extend to the intestines, for the free acid is neutralized before it reaches that point. Particular foods, especially milk and kephir, have been shown to have a preventive action on putrefaction.

113. Digestion of food as a whole. — From what has preceded we learn that several liquids and certain organisms participate in producing the complex changes that food undergoes during digestion. Some of these liquids have certain common functions, as for instance, proteins are dissolved both in the stomach and by the pancreatic juice. Moreover, the various digesting fluids appear to act coöperatively. This is made plain by following the course of the food changes. After the food has remained in the stomach for a short period of time, it is gradually discharged into the small intestine, the rate of discharge varying with the kind of food, that is, with the promptness and rapidity of digestion, which differs with different foods. The progress made up to this point in food transference, so far as we have definite knowledge, is chiefly the cleavage of the proteins into various stages of hydrolysis, the resulting bodies being proteoses and peptones. All proteins appear to be acted on in the stomach, but to different degrees and probably at different rates. It seems probable that the simple proteins are as fully dissolved as any, while some of the conjugated and derived proteins, such as the nucleo-proteins and those that are coagulated by heat, are at least more slowly, and in some cases less perfectly broken up. Starch, already somewhat dissolved by the saliva, is not further acted upon by the stomach enzyms, neither are the solid and liquid fats affected to any discoverable extent. Simple sugars are not acted upon by the gastric juice, but it seems probable that the di-sugars may be split into simple ones by the hydrochloric acid. It appears then, that in the intestines protein digestion must be completed, the larger part of the starch transformed to sugar and the digestion of the fats wholly accomplished or mainly so. As a matter of fact, the partial solution in the stomach of the proteins and the swelling of the undissolved part to a gelatinous mass may be considered as a preparation of the food for intestinal digestion, for through these changes the proteins present a larger surface to the attack of trypsin and other intestinal enzyms and digestion proceeds more promptly than would be the case with the freshly ingested food. Moreover, the compounds in the chyme, especially the acid, react on the liver and pancreas, and cause an abundant flow of digestive fluids from these glands.

As soon as the chyme mixes with the bile and pancreatic juice, the mass is changed from an acid to an alkaline condition. This seems to be essential to the effective operation of the pancreatic ferments. While the pancreatic juice will carry on digestion by itself, this is not satisfactory in the absence of bile, for when the latter is not permitted to enter the small intestine, the digestion of fats is very imperfect. It seems essential that these two liquids act together. The bile aids in rendering the digesting mass alkaline, contributes to the formation and solution of the fatty acids and soaps, and in these ways and others not altogether explainable promotes the activity of the pancreas enzyms. The juices that flow from the small glands in the intestinal walls appear to essentially supplement the work of the bile and pancreatic juice. In the first place, they probably contain a substance that makes active the mother substance of trypsin, in the second place, they aid in splitting the peptones into simpler bodies, and lastly, they convert the sugars into the final form (dextrose) in which they are absorbed into the blood circulation. If we consider the digestion of the food compounds by classes, the following is a summary of the ways in which they are acted upon : pepsin, trypsin, and terepsin secreted by the stomach, pancreas, and intestinal glands act on the proteins; ptyalin in the saliva, amylopsin from the pancreas, and lactase, maltase, and sucrase in intestinal secretions act on the carbohydrates, and the fats are acted on mainly by the lipase of the pancreatic juice.

The bacteria are not surely known to have necessary specific functions, unless it be their solvent action on the cellulose. The various enzym activities finally prepare the food for absorption into the blood circulation, not merely by solution, but by such rearrangement of the ingested food compounds as to fit them for constructive purposes in the animal body or for supplying the energy that is required for internal and external work.

E. ABSORPTION OF THE FOOD

From the time the food enters the stomach, during nearly its entire course along the alimentary canal, there is a constant production of soluble compounds, which progressively disappear into other channels, so that when the anus is reached only a small portion of the original dry matter is found in the residue. In some way, not wholly explainable in all its details, the digested food has been absorbed and received into vessels through which it is distributed to the various parts of the body.

114. Function of lacteals and blood vessels in absorption. — A merely casual observation shows us that the inner surface of the walls of the digestive organs are covered by numerous projections. The anatomist, by a careful study of these, has learned that imbedded in their tissue, especially in the intestines, are the minute branches

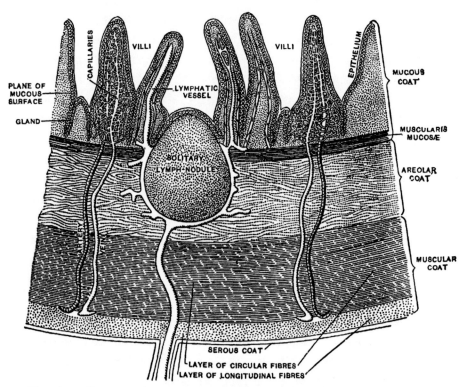

Fig. 5.— Cross section mucous membrane of small intestine, showing capillaries and lacteals. (GERRISH.)

of two systems of vessels. One set is the lacteals, belonging to the so-called lymphatic system, and the other set is the capillaries of the blood system. The lymphatic vessels or tubes all lead to a main tube or reservoir, the thoracic duct, which extends along the spinal column and finally enters one of the main blood-vessels. Any material, therefore, taken up by the lacteals ultimately reaches the blood. The capillaries all converge to a larger blood vessel, known as the portal vein, which enters the liver, carrying with it whatever material the capillaries have absorbed.

The manner in which the soluble food is absorbed has been explained in part on common physical grounds. When two solutions of different densities, containing diffusible compounds, are separated by a permeable membrane, diffusion through this membrane from the denser to the lighter liquid will always occur. Such a condition as this prevails in the intestines, we may believe. The intestinal solution, the denser one, is separated from a less concentrated liquid, the blood, which is constantly flowing on the other side of a thin dividing membrane. Under these conditions there occurs the passage into the blood of certain parts of the digested food. It is held that in this

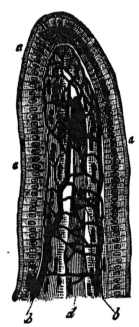

Fig. 6. — Intestinal villus, showing: *a*, epithelium; *b*, capillaries; *c*, lacteal vessel.

way water, soluble mineral salts, and sugar pass directly into the blood-vessels. The peptones are also taken up by the capillaries, and the fats enter the blood through the lacteals.

115. Changes in the walls of the intestinal tract. — In the absorption of peptones and fats, at least, we en-

counter forces other than the osmotic transference of substances in solution, the operation of which is still more or
less unexplained.

As we have learned, the ingested proteins are changed
in the stomach and intestines to peptones, and in part, perhaps mainly, to simpler compounds resulting from the cleavage of peptones. The fats are split partly, or entirely, into
fatty acids and glycerin, with the subsequent formation
of soaps by the union of the free acids with the alkaline
bases of the bile. There is good evidence that in the passage of these new compounds through the walls of the
intestine changes occur of a synthetical character, with a
partial or total reconstruction of the proteins and fats into
forms similar to those in the ingested food. The rebuilding of fats and their transference into the lacteals is regarded as being accomplished through the activity of
cells lying in the mucous lining of the intestine. It
seems, then, that the vital forces residing in the living
cells play a part in transferring the nutrients into
the blood circulation, and that this absorption can no
longer be explained wholly on the basis of osmotic pressure.

116. Place of maximum absorption. — Absorption of
digested food undoubtedly takes place in the stomach,
but the main transference of the products of digestion into
the blood is from the intestines, particularly the small
intestine. Much of the water that passes into the large
intestine is absorbed there, together with the products
of digestion not already absorbed and those products that
result from bacterial action. It is a question of importance whether there is an absorption of proteins when
the lower intestine is flooded with an enema containing

proteins such as the white of an egg. The evidence is that under these circumstances protein absorption occurs and furnishes a very fortunate means of nourishing a patient when the ordinary method of digestion is not possible.

F. FECES

. The soluble and insoluble portions of the intestinal contents become separated gradually, and the undissolved part arrives finally at the last stage of its journey along the alimentary canal, and is expelled as the solid excrement, or feces. This is made up of the undigested food and other matter, such as residues from the bile and other digestive juices, mucus, and more or less of the epithelial cells which have become detached from the walls of

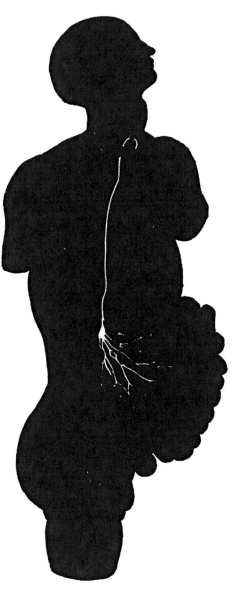

Fig. 7. — Lacteals during digestion. (COLLINS.)

I

the stomach and intestines. Dead and living bacteria
appear to constitute a considerable portion of the fecal
matter. These organisms are not taken in with the food
to any great extent, but are the result of their continuous
growth in the lower intestines. Small quantities of fermentation products are present, which give to the feces
its offensive odor. The incidental or waste products may
properly be considered as belonging to the wear and tear
of digestion.

The ordinary conception of the fecal residue is that it
is only the part of the food that has resisted the action of
the digestive fluids, but in fact it is much more than that.
Not only does it include the various waste products previously referred to, but also compounds that have been
absorbed into the blood circulation and returned to the
alimentary canal for excretion. It has been shown that
when a phosphorus compound was injected subcutane-
ously into a sheep, the phosphorus was excreted in the
feces in another combination. It is also proven that
mineral compounds absorbed from the intestinal tract may
afterwards appear in the feces.

G. The Relation of the Different Food Compounds to the Digestive Processes

Numerous digestion experiments with a large variety
of foods have abundantly established the fact that these
materials differ greatly in their solubility in the digestive
juices. This is an important matter, and one which should
be well understood, for we must consider both the weight
of the food eaten and its availability in determining its

nutritive value. Variations in digestibility are caused primarily by variations in composition, therefore, we must deal fundamentally with the susceptibility of the various single constituents of foods to the dissolving action of the several digestive ferments.

In this connection, we need to pay little attention to the mineral compounds. They do not undergo fermentative changes in the way that the carbon compounds do, but pass into simple solution either in the water accompanying the food, or in the juices with which they come in contact.

117. Digestibility of the proteins. — As has been noted, protein is a mixture of nitrogenous compounds. The gluten of wheat contains at least five of these bodies, and other seeds as many. What is the relative susceptibility of these single proteins to ferment action either as to rapidity or completeness of change does not appear to be known. Some proteins are practically all digested by artificial methods, and probably are in natural digestion. It is a fact, however, that protein is much more completely dissolved from some foods than from others. That of milk and meat is practically all digestible, that of some grains very largely so, while with vegetables quite a large proportion escapes solution. Whether this is due to a differing degree of solubility on the part of the character- istic protein compounds of the various foods is not quite determined. The fact that highly fibrous materials show the lowest proportion of digestible protein suggests as an explanation that the nitrogen compounds of plant tissue are so protected by the fiber present that they escape the full action of the digestive juices. It is certain, however, that the protein in plant tissue is less fully digested than that from milk, meat, and eggs.

118. Digestibility of the Carbohydrates. — In the case of the carbohydrates, our knowledge of the relative susceptibility of the individual compounds to enzym action is more definite.   First of all, the necessary modification of the sugars, which are already soluble, is slight, and they are wholly digested.   In the second place, we have learned in two ways that the starches are wholly transformed to diffusible compounds, first by submitting them in an artificial way to the action of various diastatic ferments, and, second, by discovering a complete absence of starch or its products in normal human feces.   We can say, therefore, that under normal conditions the unprotected starches, like the sugars, are completely digestible.

Digestibility must be considered, however, from the standpoints both of rapidity and of completeness.   As to the former factor, starches from unlike sources exhibit some remarkable differences.   Investigations by Stone, who submitted a number of these bodies to the action of several diastatic ferments, show that " this variation reaches such a degree that under precisely the same conditions certain of the starches require eighty times as long as others for complete solution."   The potato starches appear to be acted upon much more rapidly than those from the cereal grains.

Other carbohydrates, cellulose and hemicelluloses, such as pentosans, galactan and mannan and related bodies, show great variations in digestibility according to their source, these variations ranging in observations by Swartz from 0 to 100 per cent.   The extent to which these substances disappear from the alimentary canal appears to be dependent on their solubility and their susceptibility to attack by bacteria.

119. Digestibility of the fats. — The extent of the digestion and absorption of the fats or oils is also not definitely known. If we were to accept the figures given for ether-extract in tables of digestion coefficients as applying to the real fats, we would believe that their digestibility varies from less than one-third to the total amount. It is unfortunately true that these coefficients mean but very little. The ether-extract from some foods is only partially fat or oil, as we have seen, and the inaccuracy of a digestion trial is still further aggravated by the presence in the feces of bile residues and other bodies which are soluble in ether, so that the difference between the ether-extract in the ingested food and that in the feces does not give accurate information as to what has happened to the actual fats. It seems very probable that pure vegetable fats and oils and all mixed animal fats are quite completely absorbed.

The foregoing statements make it plain that when the general composition of a food is known, it is possible to predict with a good degree of certainty whether its rate of digestibility is high or low. The larger the proportion of starch, sugar, milk, meat and eggs and the smaller the percentage of gums and fiber, the more complete will be the solution.

H. FACTORS WHICH MAY INFLUENCE DIGESTION

Digestion has an important relation to the nutritive efficiency of food, and to the physical welfare of the individual. On the one hand, only that portion of the food that is digested and absorbed can serve the purposes of growth and the maintenance of the vital functions, and on the other hand, bad digestion causes discomfort and disease.

120. Meaning of " digestibility." — In discussing the factors that may influence the digestion of food, it is essential to understand clearly what is involved in the term digestion as it is used in science and in common speech. The term is made to include three elements, completeness of solution and absorption of the food nutrients, rate of digestion, and comfort of digestion. In science, the figures that are given for the digestibility of various foods refer to the completeness or extent to which the food is dissolved and transferred to the circulation. But different foods from which come the same proportion of undigested dry matter may differ materially in the rate at which they undergo digestive changes, and in this sense their digestibility is unlike. Again, when for any cause digestion causes discomfort, the sufferer declares that the particular food eaten is not digestible. As a matter of fact, the ultimate completeness of solution in the digestive fluids may not be influenced either by the rate or the discomfort attending the process. Among the numerous factors that may modify digestion, the following are among the most important : —

121. Kind of food. — The kind of food, other things being equal, determines the completeness and also, we may believe, the rate of digestion. Investigation has shown, as already noted, that vegetable foods are less fully digested than those of animal origin, a fact due probably, to the inclosure of the protein and other nutrients in the fibrous tissue of much vegetable substance. It is entirely rational to claim, too, that this association of the nutrients with a cellulose framework retards digestion by protecting the protein and other compounds from attack. If no allowance is made for the metabolic products in the feces, the digestibility of the various classes of foods is calculated to be as follows : —

TABLE XIX

	PROTEINS	CARBO-HYDRATES	FATS
	Per Cent	Per Cent	Per Cent
Animal foods	98	100	97
Cereals	85	98	90
Vegetables and fruits . .	80	95	90

The individual nutrients differ in their susceptibility to attack by the digestive fluids. We have seen that potato starch is hydrolyzed more rapidly than that from the cereal grains. In the case of the fats the higher their melting point the more slowly they are likely to be decomposed and emulsified. It is probable that tallow requires a longer time for complete digestion than does butter or the salad oils, and may be less completely absorbed. This point may well be raised touching the digestibility of imitation butter that is made, in part at least, from the body fats of bovines and swine.

This influence of the melting point is quite clearly indicated by the following figures : — [1]

[1] " Metabolism and Practical Medicine," Von Noorden, Vol. I, p. 56.

TABLE XX

Kind of Fat	Melting Point	Per Cent Loss in the Feces
	C°	
Stearin	60	91 to 86
Stearin and almond oil . . .	55	10.6
Spermaceti	53	31.0
Mutton fat	50–51	9.2
Mutton fatty acids	56	13 to 20
Mutton fat	49	7.4
Lard	43	2.6
Pork fat	34	2.8
Goose fat	25	2.5
Olive oil	fluid	2.3

122. Influence of food on secretions. — The more recent investigations reveal the fact that the kind of food has an influence not only on the abundance, but on the kind of digestive secretions, which is important, because an abundant supply of digestive juices is necessary to good digestion. The conclusion is, or better perhaps the theory, that certain chemical excitants are conveyed to the secreting glands through the blood circulation, and excite the flow of the several digestive fluids, and that the formation of these excitants is caused by the reaction of food compounds on the inner membranes of the stomach and intestines, this reaction being more pronounced with some food materials than with others. Broths, meat extracts, milk, dextrin, maltose, and dextrose exert a pronounced influence in this way in the stomach, which makes rational the taking of soups or bouillon as the first dinner course, or the eating of toasted bread and zwieback by persons with weak digestion. On the other hand, fats tend to inhibit gastric secretion, so that an excessive proportion of fat in the meat might weaken digestion in the stomach.

Food may exert an indirect influence on the pancreatic secretion. The acid in the chyme stimulates the flow of the pancreatic juice. Any diet, therefore, that has the effect of diminishing or of neutralizing the stomach acid which otherwise would reach the small intestine is unfavorable to . pancreatic digestion. Mendel [1] states that " the activity of the enzyms of the pancreatic juice seems to be correlated in a marvelous way with the corresponding elements of the diet. A regimen rich in fat calls forth a secretion containing a relative abundance of the lipolytic (fat-splitting) enzyme ; with a meat diet, the proteolytic enzymes preponderate, and so forth. Furthermore, this regulative action can apparently be modified by the conditions of the diet. One is almost inclined to speak of a physiologic education of the digestive glands, and to conceive of them as being trained for fat, or proteid, or carbohydrate digestion powers by the presence of the corresponding compounds in the alimentary canal. Indeed, this conception has already been raised above the realm of mere fancy." Such facts as these are significant, and we may reasonably hope that some time in the future bad digestion and the habit of constipation may be relieved through the diet, rather than through medicines.

[1] "Some Aspects of the Newer Physiology of the Gastrointestinal Canal," p. 6.

123. Mechanical condition of ingested food. — It is generally held that thorough mastication of food promotes good digestion. This is rational; although involving chemical changes, digestion is broadly considered a means of rendering the nutrients soluble, that is, transferable through the walls of the alimentary canal. The doctrine has been taught, in one notable instance at least, that excessive mastication greatly increases the efficiency of the food. If this is true, it must be because of increased thoroughness of digestion. Observation does not show this result. It is concluded from experimental evidence " that any dietetic practice, therefore, such as excessive mastication, which may be claimed to result in greater economy in the utilization of food so far as it relates to thoroughness of digestion, must improve upon a condition in which there is already almost complete utilization." While in a normal subject, careful mastication may not increase the proportion of nutrients that will ultimately be digested and absorbed, fineness of division of the food particles makes for promptness, and therefore comfort, of digestion, because the larger the food surface which the digestive fluids may attack, the more rapidly will solution be effected, which is highly desirable. Of course bolting the food in coarse pieces may result not only in incomplete, but uncomfortable, digestion. In comparing the digestibility of breads from different kinds of flour, that from coarse flour, that is, whole wheat flour, is found to be less completely digested than bread from fine flour, but this is due, not so much to the degree of fineness as to the presence in the coarse flour of more cellulose (crude fiber) which serves to protect the other constituents of the flour from the action of the various juices.

124. Relish for food. — This involves two elements, the vigor of appetite and the attractiveness of the food in appearance and taste. When a person is hungry, in other words, has a " good appetite " and the food meets his approval in its kind and in the way it is prepared, the psychic condition is favorable to abundant secretions in the digestive tract. When, on the other hand, the appetite is " poor " or the food is distasteful, the necessary activity of the secretory glands receives no such stimulus. Forced nutrition does not conform to the best conditions for efficient nutrition. Unskillful or slovenly cooking, or an unwise selection of food may neutralize a vigorous appetite, or even breed dyspepsia.

125. The amount eaten. — The evidence concerning the effect of the amount eaten at one meal upon the completeness of digestion is somewhat conflicting, but indicates that a full meal is somewhat less perfectly digested than when food is taken sparingly. Snyder[1] found this to be so, though his results were not uniform. Sherman[2] found a slight difference in protein digestion in favor of the restricted diet. It is fair to assume that with heavy eating the completion of digestion would require longer than when but little food is to be acted upon. Nevertheless, there is no evidence to show that with normal digestion there is any large amount of waste when food is taken in generous, but reasonable, amounts.

126. Effect of work. — It is quite generally agreed on the basis of considerable experimental evidence that even severe labor does not depress digestion. In other words, a man at rest does not digest his food differently than when at work.

[1] Bul. 101, O.E.S., p. 64.　　　　[2] Bul. 121, O.E.S., p. 47.

127. Influence of accessory articles of food. — These include condiments, flavors, and stimulants which are used, not for their food value, which is small, but as a means of rendering food more attractive to the taste. It cannot be said that these, including alcoholic drinks, when used in reasonable quantity, depress digestibility. In fact, when properly used, they may, and probably do, exert a favorable influence upon digestion by promoting an increased flow of gastric juice through the psychic effect of a pleasing taste and through their reaction on the stomach membranes. Physicians use condimental substances to excite the secretions in cases of weak digestion. The essential conditions of good digestion do not justify the prevalent excessive and growing demand for such condiments as the peppers, garlic, mustard and vinegar, the long, intemperate use of which produces conditions on the part of the user that are unnatural and ruinous to the stomach.

128. Influence of cooking food. — In considering this factor, it is necessary to understand the effect of heat on different classes of food. As we have learned, certain proteins, especially the albumins, are coagulated and hardened by heat, even at a temperature considerably below the boiling point. Cooking also hardens, that is, makes more fibrous, many animal tissues. On the other hand, the effect of boiling and baking upon vegetable tissue is to disintegrate it, liberate starch grains from their cell inclosures, and make them available to the action of the digestive fluids, more or less dextrinize starch, and in some cases cause hydrolytic changes, as when in the cooking of apples and other fruits the pectins are changed to pectoses.

These facts lead to the conclusion, which is also sustained to some extent by experimental evidence, that the cooking of meats retards digestion, while with fruits and vegetables the same cause accelerates digestion. The advocates of raw vegetable foods should appeal only to persons with strong digestive powers. That such foods promote digestion as compared with those that are cooked, in the light of existing knowledge is an absurd proposition.

129. Influence of individual peculiarities. — It is a fact of common experience that certain persons do not comfortably digest certain foods, whatever may be the ultimate proportion that is digested. Definite and proven explanations of this fact are not available. It is not improbable that a mental attitude toward a given food sometimes has its influence, although this can hardly explain why certain individuals are made uncomfortable from eating strawberries or pork, or some other food. This may be due to an enzym deficiency in some part of the digestive tract, or to a peculiar reaction upon the individual of particular compounds present in the offending food; but these suggestions are speculative.

130. The extent to which different classes of foods are digested. — A large amount of experimenting shows that the following are approximately the proportions of the nutrients that are digested in the different classes of foods. These figures refer to apparent digestibility and not to actual. If the metabolic products in the feces were accounted for, the proportions would be higher, especially for protein. The satisfactory separation of the real undigested portion of the food from the accompanying waste products is not yet accomplished.

TABLE XXI

KIND OF FOOD	PROTEIN	CARBO-HYDRATES	FATS
	Per Cent	Per Cent	Per Cent
Meats and fish	97		95
Eggs	97		95
Dairy products	97	98	95
Animal foods (mixed diet) . . .	97	98	95
Cereals	85	98	95
Legumes (dried)	78	97	90
Sugars		98	
Starches		98	
Vegetables	83	95	90
Fruits	85	90	90
Vegetable foods (mixed diet) . .	84	97	90
Total food (mixed diet)	92	97	95

CHAPTER VI

THE DISTRIBUTION AND TRANSFORMA-TIONS OF THE DIGESTED FOOD

THE digested food, after absorption, all passes into the blood, either directly or indirectly, and mixes with it. The materials which are to serve the purposes of nutrition are now taken up by a stream of liquid that is in constant motion throughout the minutest divisions of every part of the animal. Flowing in regular channels, the blood reaches not only the bones and muscular tissues, but it passes through several special organs and glands, where the nutrients it is carrying and certain of its own constituents meet with profound changes. It is here that we discover the manner in which food is applied to use, and what are some of the transformations which the proteins, carbohydrates, and fats undergo in performing their functions.

In order to follow intelligently this most interesting phase of nutrition, we must know something of the blood and of the organs — the lungs, liver, and kidneys — through which it passes.

A. THE BLOOD

The blood, when in a fresh state, is apparently colored and opaque, but if a minute portion is examined with a microscope, it is seen to be a comparatively clear liquid in which float numerous reddish disk-like bodies known as corpuscles, also blood plates and blood granules. These bodies give to the blood its bright red color. The liquid in which they are suspended, a clear amber yellow liquid, is called the plasma.

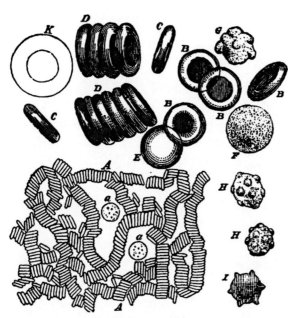

FIG. 8. — Red and white corpuscles of blood (magnified). *A*, red corpuscles; *a, a*, white corpuscles; *B, C, D*, red corpuscles, much magnified; *F, G*, white corpuscles, much magnified.

131. Corpuscles. — The corpuscles are not mere masses of unformed matter, but they are minute bodies having a definite form and structure. They make up from 35 to 40 per cent of the blood, and contain over 30 per cent of dry matter. This dry matter consists mostly of hæmoglobin, a compound that is peculiar to the blood, and equips it for one of its most important offices.

132. Hæmoglobin. — Hæmoglobin, as before stated, is made up of a protein (globin), and a coloring matter (hæmatin), in the latter of which is combined a definite proportion of iron. The peculiar property of this compound, which renders it so useful a constituent of the blood, is its power of taking up oxygen and holding it in a loose combination until it is needed for use throughout the body. When thus charged, it is known as oxyhæmoglobin. Because of this function of their most prominent constituent, blood corpuscles become the carriers of oxygen to all parts of the body. They are also concerned in gathering up one of the waste products of the nutritive changes, viz., carbon dioxid, which is conveyed by them in loose chemical combination to the point where it may be thrown off from the body. Hæmatin may also unite with other compounds, as, for instance, carbon monoxid, which displaces and excludes oxygen and is disastrous in its effects.

133. Leucocytes. — The blood also contains amœba-like bodies know as white corpuscles, that are variable in shape and constantly changing in form. These are sometimes called leucocytes, and are regarded as having an important function. They may increase with extraordinary rapidity, especially around centers of infection and inflammation, and it is regarded as proven that they endeavor to destroy foreign bodies in the blood and also render harmless the injurious products coming from the activity of micro-organisms. They evidently have other functions not well understood, for it is noticed that they accumulate in large numbers during intestinal digestion. Very likely they act as a means of transportation, and they probably play some part in metabolism in accomplishing certain exchanges of nutrient substances.

134. The plasma. — The plasma is about nine-tenths water, so that it easily holds in solution whatever soluble nutrients are discharged into it from the alimentary canal.

K

Among its constituents are found members of all the classes of compounds that are important in this connection, — ash, protein, carbohydrates, and fats. The proportion of ash is about 1 per cent, three-fourths of it being common salt, and the remainder consisting of phosphoric acid, lime, and other important mineral compounds. The solid matter of the plasma is rich in proteins, including the fibrinogen, which is the mother substance of fibrin, and several albumins and globulins. These proteids make up about 80 per cent of the total dry substance of the plasma. Sugar and fats are also present, their proportions varying somewhat with the extent to which they are being absorbed from the digestion of food. In fact, the blood carries not only its characteristic and permanent constituents, but also the nutrients absorbed from the alimentary canal. It is evident that the blood is charged with those materials which we recognize as necessary to the construction and maintenance of the animal body. The plasma also constantly contains very small proportions of the end products of metabolism, such as urea and uric acid and waste bile products which are being transported to the points of excretion. It also holds in solution, or as carbonates, some of the carbon dioxid gathered up in the circulation of the blood through the tissues.

B. The Heart

In quantity, the blood is from 3 to 4 per cent of the total weight of the human body. It is contained in the heart and in two sets of vessels, one set called the arteries, leading from the heart by various ramifications to all

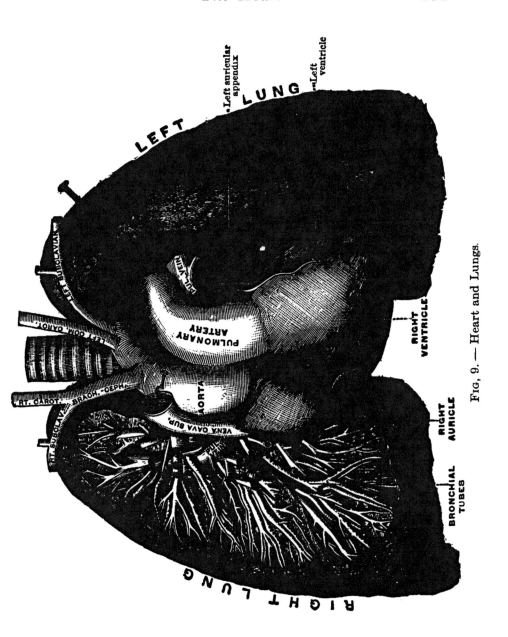

FIG. 9. — Heart and Lungs.

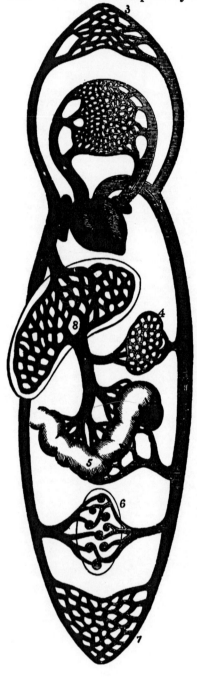

parts of the body, and the other set called the veins, leading from all parts of the body back to the heart.

135. Circulation.—Through these vessels the blood is moving in a constant stream, which we call the circulation. It does not move of itself, but is forced along by a very powerful pump, the heart. This is a highly muscular organ divided into four chambers, which are separated by valves and partitions, the two upper chambers being called the right and left auricles, and the two lower, the right and left ventricles. The right auricle is above the right ventricle, and is separated from it by a valve, and the same is true of the left auricle and ventricle. Out of the left ventricle, the blood is pumped into the arteries, and after reaching the arterial

FIG. 10. — Diagram of circulation. *1*, heart; *2*, lungs; *3*, head and upper extremities; *4*, spleen; *5*, intestine; *6*, kidney; *7*, lower extremities; *8*, liver. (COLLINS.)

capillaries throughout the entire body, it passes from these into the smallest divisions of the veins and comes back to the heart along the venous system, entering the right auricle. It is then carried to the lungs by way of the right ventricle and is returned to the left auricle to be sent to the left ventricle, and from there to again start on its journey through the body. As we shall see, the arterial blood carries to the body food nutrients and oxygen, and the venous blood brings back the wastes. The principal facts pertaining to the blood and its circulation have been reviewed in this simple manner as an aid to the discussing of other considerations somewhat pertinent to our subject.

136. Entrance of nutrients. — The nutrients, as prepared for use by digestion, enter the blood on its return flow to the heart, coming into the venous cavity by way of the hepatic (liver) vein and the thoracic duct as previously described. When, therefore, the right side of the heart is reached, a new accession of food material is on its way to sustain the various functions of nutrition.

We are more interested in the object of blood circulation than we are in its mechanism. Somehow the digested food disappears into these constantly moving blood currents, and the only evidence of its effect which comes to us from ordinary observation is the warmth, motion, and perhaps growth, of the animal that is nourished.

C. The Lungs

The first point where important changes occur is the lungs. Here the blood loses the purplish hue which it always has after being used in the body tissues, and takes on a bright scarlet, — a phenomenon that is more easily understood when we understand the lung structure.

137. Object of breathing. — Breathing is a matter of common experience. We all know how air is drawn into

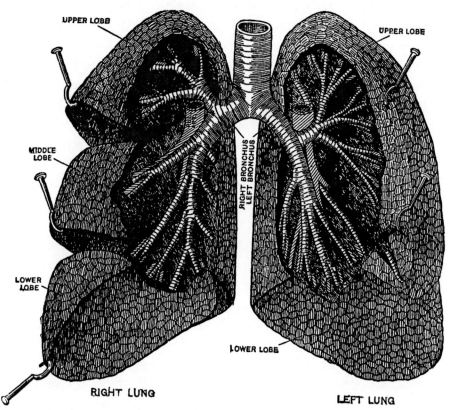

FIG. 11. — Air tubes of lungs. (GERRISH.)

the lungs at regular intervals, and equivalent volumes of modified air being as regularly forced out. The mechanism of respiration (breathing) we will not discuss at length. It will aid us, however, if we know that the passage which the air follows to and from the lungs, the trachea (windpipe), divides into two branches, one to each lung, and these divide and subdivide until they branch into numerous fine tubes. Each of these tubes ends in an elongated dilation which is made up of air cells opening into a common cavity. These cells are so numerous in the lung tissues that only a very thin wall separates adjoining ones, and in this wall are carried the capillaries or fine divisions of the blood-vessels leading from the heart. This arrangement permits the (venous) blood, as it flows along, to take up oxygen from the respired air and transfer certain wastes into the lung cavities, and thus be made ready to go back to the body carrying a joint load of digested food and of oxygen that is held in combination with the hæmatin. Of course the air that passes out of the lungs is less rich in oxygen than when it was taken in, and there have been added to it certain materials which we will notice later.

It is easily understood from these facts that respiration stands in a fundamental relation to nutrition. The lungs are to the body what the draft is to the furnace. Food can no more be used without the supply of oxygen through the lungs than can coal be burned without an access of air to the fuel box.

D. THE USE OF FOOD

The revivified (arterial) blood now passes to all parts of the body and is brought into the most intimate relation with the minutest portion of every tissue. Several things happen in the course of time, all of which, whether the combination or cleavage of food compounds, or the oxidations that result in complete combustion, are brought about by the protoplasmic activity of the cells of which the body tissues are an aggregation.

138. Builds tissue. — In the first place, the new supply of nutritive substances is used by the living cells in a way we do not wholly understand, to rebuild worn-out tissue and to form new growth. With the young animal, much material is appropriated in the latter way. In the case of mammals, there is furnished to the mammary gland the nutrients out of which the milk is formed through the special activities of that gland.

139. Function of oxygen. — Moreover, it is in the tissues that the oxygen which was taken up in the lungs is used to slowly oxidize a portion of the food. This combustion is believed not to take place by contact of the oxygen and nutrients in the blood-vessels, but it occurs through cell activity by progressive steps throughout the minute divisions of the muscles and other tissues of the body. The tissue cells undoubtedly obtain their energy from oxidation of the nutriment furnished to them. Notwithstanding this oxidation may be very gradual and occupy much time, its ultimate products are, for the most part, similar to those which result from the rapid combustion of fuel. In the fireplace, starch, sugar, cellulose, fats, and similar bodies would be burned to carbonic acid and water, and this is what takes place in the animal to the extent that these nutrients are not used constructively.

140. Protein not wholly oxidized. — When the protein is not stored as such, but is broken up, the result in the animal is somewhat different from that in the furnace, because in the former the oxidation is not complete. In the animal, the proteins are partially oxidized to carbonic acid and water, but a portion of their substance passes from the body principally in the form of urea and uric acid, which are the prominent constituents of urine. These compounds carry with them a certain proportion of carbon and hydrogen which, in ordinary fuel combustion, would more fully unite with oxygen. The heat production from protein is therefore less in the animal than in the furnace.

Oxidations in the human body are continuous, but not uniform. They vary with the mass, age, and habits of the individual, with the exercise the individual is taking, and with the amount of food that must be disposed of. The quantity of oxygen needed is therefore variable, and when the demand for it with a given individual is largely increased, the heart pumps faster, more blood passes through the lungs, the breathing is more rapid, and the supply of oxygen is in this way augmented.

E. ELIMINATION OF WASTES

The various waste products from this combustion of the digested nutrients and from the breaking up of the proteins within the animal body evidently must be disposed of in some manner. If not eliminated from the body, they would cause results of a most serious character, as, for instance, when an accumulation of urea in the blood produces uræmic poisoning. The blood, therefore, not only carries to the tissues the necessary nutrients and oxygen, but it has laid upon it the burden of taking into its currents the waste products of combustion and growth, and carrying them to the points where they are thrown off.

141. Urea. -- One of the branches of the arterial system of blood-vessels runs to the kidneys, and, by repeatedly rebranching, traverses all their substance. The main function of the kidneys is to secrete the urine, a liquid in which all the waste nitrogen from the digested protein finds its way out of the body in the form of urea and other nitrogen compounds. The blood that enters them carries with it the urea and uric acid which have resulted from a breaking down of protein, and, in a most wonderful manner, these compounds are filtered out so that they are not present in the outgoing blood.

142. Mineral compounds. — The mineral ingredients of the food in excess of storage in the body are excreted both through the kidneys and in the feces. Compounds of potassium and sodium appear almost wholly in the urine. Phosphorus, calcium, and magnesium are divided between the urine and feces, the two former being more largely excreted by way of the intestines, while practically all the iron goes out by way of the feces.

143. Carbon dioxid. — The carbon dioxid must in some way also be eliminated from the body. This is not accomplished to any extent until the venous blood containing it reaches the lungs, where it is exchanged for a new supply of oxygen and passes off in the expired air. In the case of man, the air " breathed out " is nearly a hundred times richer in carbonic acid than the air " breathed in."

144. Water. — Water may be regarded from one point of view as a waste, for it is produced in the oxidation of the food, and this passes off from the lungs as vapor, through the skin as sensible or insensible perspiration, and in considerable quantities through the kidneys. Benedict and Carpenter have shown, on the basis of a large number of determinations, an average loss of 960 grams of water from the lungs and skin by a person at rest, during twenty-four hours ; a little less than two-thirds of this loss coming from the surface of the body. This " insensible perspiration " is 60 per cent as much as the water excretion through the kidneys. A man at hard work may lose several times as much water from the lungs and skin as through the kidneys.

To summarize, it may be said that the blood is constantly undergoing gain and loss. The gain comes from the food (including water and oxygen), and the loss consists of urea, carbonic acid, and water given off through various channels.

F. THE LIVER

One part of the arterial system of blood-vessels runs to the stomach and intestines, and is distributed over their walls in fine divisions. These connect with the capillaries of the portal vein, which leads to the liver. During this passage of the blood from one system to the other, part of the digested food is taken up. Now it is very evident that the quantity of material thus absorbed must vary greatly at different times according to the nature and amount of food supply and the activity of the digestive processes. If, therefore, the blood from the alimentary canal was allowed to pass directly into the general circulation, the supply to the tissues of the nutrients, especially the carbohydrates, would be very uneven.

145. Function of liver. — Just here comes in a liver function. In that organ there is found a starch-like body known as glycogen (see p. 73), which appears in increased quantity following the abundant absorption of sugar from the intestines. It is believed, because of this and other facts, that the liver acts as a regulator of the

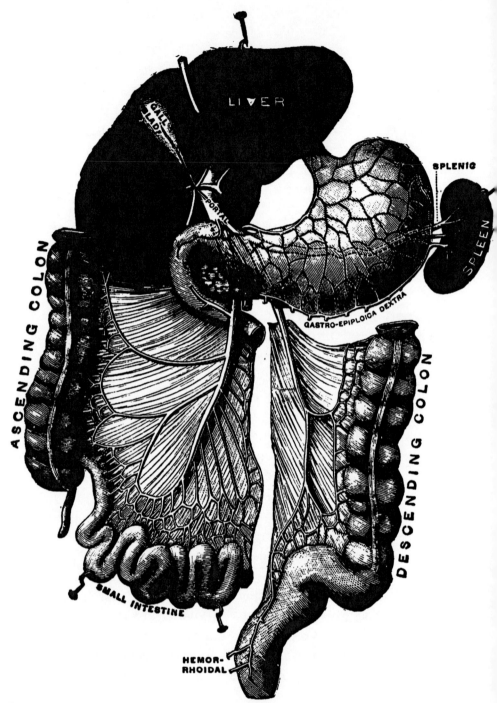

FIG. 12. — Portal system of veins. Showing how absorbed nutrients are collected from intestinal tract and carried to liver by portal vein.

carbohydrate supply to the general tissues of the body, storing a temporary excess of the sugar in the form of glycogen, which is gradually given up to the general circulation as it is needed after first being transformed back to sugar. Glycogen is also stored in the muscles, in an amount equal to or greater than that in the liver.

CHAPTER VII

THE FUNCTIONS OF FOOD COMPOUNDS

A. Scientific Methods of Inquiry

The discussion of human nutrition on a scientific basis requires an understanding of what are the physiological needs of the human organism under various conditions and how these may be met most efficiently and economically. Before stating present views of the functions of the several nutrients, it will be well to gain some conception of how we have arrived at the knowledge upon which our conclusions are based, for such a consideration of methods will doubtless strengthen confidence in the conclusions.

146. A determination of the elements essential to the construction of the human body. — Definite information as to the constructive elements of the tissues of the human body has been obtained by chemical analysis. It is a fair assumption that whatever is uniformly found present in a normally nourished organ or tissue is essential either to its construction or welfare. To be sure, the human body may retain certain substances in quantities that are not only unnecessary, but injurious, as, for instance, arsenic; but when a salt of potassium is found in the muscular tissue in practically constant proportions under all conditions of nourishment, it is fair to assume that normal muscles could not exist without it. Indeed, we know that the absence of certain elements would make impossible the presence in the human body of those compounds that are essential to its very existence.

147. Methods of ascertaining the functions of the various nutrients and the needs of the human body under varying conditions. — Our understanding of the functions of the food compounds and of the most efficient, and physiologically most economical, administration of dietaries under varying conditions is still incomplete. The exact knowledge we do possess is the result of many years of laborious investigation. We still lack much essential information concerning the special physiological relations and reactions of the individual compounds found in human food, but the general metabolism, or food exchange and use, in the animal organism is now sufficiently well understood to admit of many safe and important conclusions.

Children and adults who are living under varying conditions of age, environment, and activity consume individually a given amount of food daily. Certain questions arise. Is the food sufficient in quantity? Is it of the right kind from the physiological point of view ; that is, are the nutrients of the right kind and in the right proportion? A general practical answer to these two questions might be found in an observation as to the health and physical status of the individual, which are the facts of ultimate importance. The laws of nutrition cannot be established by such general observations, however. Even changes in body weight are not a safe basis for concluding whether a given diet is meeting the nutritive demands of a given individual. A loss of fat may be replaced by a gain of water. It has been shown also [1] " that a change from a diet poor in carbohydrates to one rich in carbohydrates is accompanied by a considerable retention of water in the tissues of the body." In these ways we learn nothing of processes or how the physiological needs of the individual must be met, and we could not reason from one case of apparently successful nourishment to know how to meet the needs of another individual under entirely different conditions.

148. Necessary measurements. — It is clear that first of all it is necessary to measure both the income of the body, that is, the food plus water and oxygen, and also the outgo, that is, the excretions which, as we have learned, are practically all included in what passes out through the lungs, the skin, the kidneys, and in the feces. We must do this not only that we may determine whether with a given diet the individual is losing or gaining body substance, but we must also in this way ascertain in what the body gain or loss consists, whether of protein or of fat. In being able to measure the balance in this way, it is possible to determine what is the minimum amount of food that will maintain an individual under given conditions of activity without loss of body substance, and also whether a given ratio of nutrients is efficient. Indeed, it is by this method that we have learned how and to what extent the body substance is utilized to supplement food deficiencies, whether of kind or quantity. It is also possible to determine the extent to which nutrients of one class may be

[1] " Metabolism and Energy Transformations of Healthy Man during Rest," Benedict and Thorne, p. 110.

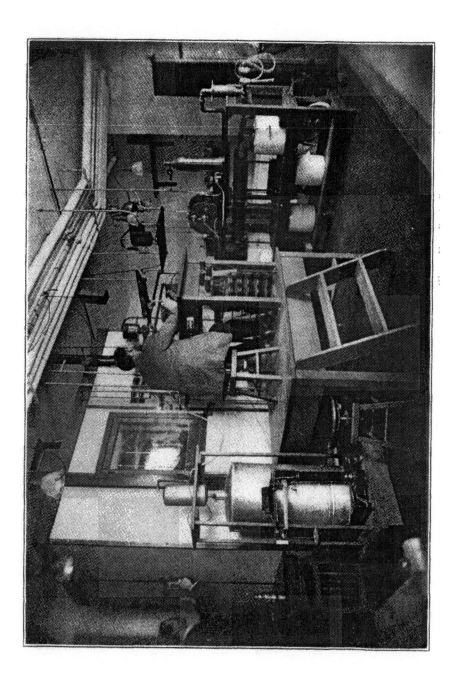

substituted for, or cȯnserve, those of another class, or what is the effect of omitting from the diet all of one class of compounds.

149. How measurements are made. Respiration calorimeter. — Let us consider more in detail how it is possible to arrive at a balance between the income and outgo of the body. It is a mere matter of weighing and chemical analysis to ascertain what enters the body in the food and drink, — the quantities of carbon, nitrogen, phosphorus, sulfur, and all the other elements. Recently it has become possible to measure the oxygen consumed in breathing. The food, drink, and oxygen constitute the income. Of the outgo, viz., the feces, urine, carbon dioxid from the lungs, and water from the lungs and skin, the feces and urine can be weighed and analyzed, as is done with the food. For measuring the carbon dioxid and water excreted, a special apparatus has been devised, which also now measures the oxygen consumed and heat given off. This apparatus is known as a *respiration calorimeter*. By means of the respiration apparatus it is possible to measure, not only the gaseous excreta delivered to the air or the respiration chamber, but also to discover what particular nutrients are being oxidized at any given time. This is done by determining what is known as the *respiratory quotient*, which is obtained by dividing the volume of carbon dioxid evolved by the volume of oxygen used. If a carbohydrate alone is oxidized, the two volumes are equal and the quotient is 1.00. If fat alone is being burned, the carbon dioxid is less in volume than the oxygen, and the quotient is approximately .70. When a mixture of fat and carbohydrates is being

L

utilized, the quotient will range somewhere between 1.00 and .70 and the relative proportion of these two classes of nutrients that are undergoing oxidation can be determined by calculation.

150. Food balances. — The fundamental facts upon which a food balance is based are the following: The general balance of gain or loss of tissue is obtained by comparing the income and outgo of carbon. All organic compounds, whether in the plant or animal, contain carbon, and cannot be formed without it. If, therefore, the carbon taken into the body is more than that given off through the various channels, it is proof that the body substance has increased. If the balance is the other way, there has been a loss of body tissue.

It is possible to know the kind of tissue that is lost or gained. All the nitrogen excreted from the body passes out in the urine and feces, that in the urine coming from the digested protein. No protein tissues can be formed without the use of nitrogen, and no other tissues require its retention. If, therefore, the body retains nitrogen, it is evidence that muscular tissue or some other form of nitrogenous substance has been deposited. If at the same time the body has retained more carbon than would be required for the increase of protein tissue, then it is necessary to conclude there has been also a deposition of fat or other non-nitrogenous material. By such means it is possible, for instance, to discover the effect of a given dietary upon protein storage, or to learn if a change in activity, such as passing from rest to hard work, causes a greater utilization of protein, or whether the increased need for food to sustain increased labor may be met by eating more carbohydrates. The ratio in which one nutrient may replace another is also an important consideration that the respiration calorimeter has made it possible to study.

151. Energy balance and use. — Very delicate modern apparatus now accurately measures the potential energy of various food compounds; that is, the energy that they give up in the form of heat or motion when burned. The respiration calorimeter measures the heat given off from the human body, heat being the end product of all vital activity. This may be done with the subject both at rest and at work. If, then, by the *metabolic* balance it is shown how much food has been oxidized and how much has been retained, conclusions may be drawn as to the food energy utilized for the vital processes of the subject, and, by taking such measurements with the subject at rest and doing different amounts of work, it is possible to learn how much food is needed to accomplish a given amount of work. By such means the law of the correlation and conservation of energy has been shown to hold with human machines as well as with those of wood and iron.

B. The Functions of the Nutrients

The digestion, absorption, and distribution of food are not its use, — they are the preliminaries necessary to use. Not until the nutrients have been converted to available forms and have passed into the blood do they in the slightest degree furnish energy or building material to the animal organism. We have followed to a certain extent the chemical changes which the digested food suffers, but no detailed statements have been made as to the part taken by each class of nutrients in constructing the human body and in maintaining its complex activities.

152. Food used in two general ways. — The animal organism uses food in two general ways: viz., for constructive purposes, which involve the building or repair of tissue and the formation of milk; and as fuel for supplying different forms of energy mainly through oxidation of the food nutrients. The tissues which are to be formed are of several kinds; principally the mineral portion of the bone; the nitrogenous tissue of the muscles, tendons, skin, hair, and various organs and membranes; and the deposits of fat which are quite generally distributed throughout the body substance.

153. Forms of energy. — Energy in the forms in which it is used by the animal organism may appear as muscular activity, such as walking, working, breathing, the beating of the heart, the movements of the stomach and intestines, as heat, and as chemical energy necessary for carrying on digestion and other metabolic changes. The human body is certainly the seat of greatly varied and complex constructive and destructive activities, which are sustained by the matter and potential energy of the food. How this is done we do not fully understand, but we know many facts which are of great scientific and practical importance and which must be consciously or unconsciously recognized if we would not come into conflict with immutable laws.

154. Functions of water. — Water fills an important place in the nutrition of all forms of life. In both plants and animals it acts as a solvent of the building materials which it carries from one part of the organism to another. It also serves as a carrier of wastes, particularly those excreted through the kidneys, and the free use of water is recommended as promoting thorough cleansing of the tissues. It is proper to speak of water as building material for the animal body, for it is an abundant constituent of animal tissue and takes part in chemical changes such as hydrolysis. It fills an essential office in regulating the heat processes of the body through varying rates of evaporation (see p. 168).

155. Functions of the mineral compounds. — We have learned that mineral compounds are abundant in the human body. The tissues, the blood, digestive fluids, and especially the body framework, contain a variety of these bodies, which are as essential as any other substances to the building and maintenance of the animal organism. Bone formation without phosphoric acid and lime is not possible, and to deprive the gastric juice of the chlorine which it contains would be to destroy its usefulness. Sodium salts are an essential part of the bile, iron must be supplied to the hæmatin of the blood, and potassium phosphate is always present in muscular tissue. Children would fail to develop if given no mineral food, and adults, if entirely deprived of even one substance, sodium chloride, would become weak, inactive, and finally die. Not only must the growing child have the ash compounds for constructive purposes, but the mature man must be supplied with them in order to sustain the nutritive functions. It is especially true of mammalian females, which store combinations of phosphoric acid, lime, and potash so abundantly in the milk that they must have an adequate supply of these substances.   Nothing is clearer than that these materials must of necessity be furnished in the food.   They cannot originate in the animal organism, neither can carbon compounds take their place.

Mineral compounds evidently have important offices outside of supplying constructive material.   Their physiological influence or reactions must also be taken into account.   While the whole subject is not well understood, abundant evidence exists that the chemical environment of animal tissues has an important influence in several directions.   It has been shown that the eggs of certain marine fishes multiply (segment) normally only in water containing a mixture of certain salts of a certain concentration.   In the same way muscular contractions are greatly influenced by the salts that are in contact with the tissues.   Osmotic pressure or the rate of transfer of liquids in the animal body is also influenced by the inorganic salts present.   Indefinite as our knowledge is, it is quite evident that the soluble salts of calcium, magnesium, potassium, and sodium play an important rôle in the vital activities of the animal organism, other than for constructive purposes.

156. Phosphorus and brain power. — It was at one time popularly taught that phosphorus has a special relation to brain activity and because fish was supposed to contain much phosphorus it was commonly spoken of as " brain food."   As a matter of fact, it has never been shown that this element has an especial relation to brain activity, and, moreover, fish is no richer in phosphorus than many other foods, such as meats, milk, cheese, and certain grains (see p. 387).   To be sure, the nerve tissue is relatively rich in phosphorus, but other elements are just as essential to the structure of the brain.

157. Foods supplying mineral compounds. — Nature seems to have adapted our needs to the compounds furnished by the natural food products, such as the cereal grains, milk, meat, and other unmodified materials, as they supply a complete variety of the needed inorganic substances. Milk, which is the exclusive food of infants, is especially adapted to rapid bone formation. It is only when modified (artificial) foods are largely eaten, foods from which the mineral salts have been extracted by manufacturing processes, that we need fear a deficiency of the necessary mineral compounds. (See pp. 210–211.)

Much is written about the proper proportion of protein and carbohydrate in the food, but it is to be feared that the equally critical matter of the supply of the so-called mineral ingredients does not receive attention commensurate with its importance.

158. Functions of protein. — While there are at present many unsolved problems relative to the nutritive offices of protein, there is no reasonable doubt that the food proteins are the only source of similar substances in the animal body. This is equivalent to a statement that from the food proteins are formed the muscles, the connective tissues, the skin, hair, and the major part of the tissues of the secretive and excretive organs ; in short, that they are the source of a large proportion of all the working parts of the human body. So far, scientific research has not succeeded in demonstrating that a protein is ever synthesized (built up from simple compounds) outside of the plant. It appears that bodies of this class must come to animal life fully elaborated, for when protein is absent from the food, the body protein is utilized to maintain the vital functions, even if nitrogen compounds of a lower order are present.   This is a truth of great significance in its relation to the nutrition of man.   The nitrogenous tissues are those that largely determine the vigor and quality of any individual, and as these are formed rapidly in the early stages of growth, a normal and unrestricted development demands an adequate supply of protein food.

The proteins are a source to the body of two important ash constituents, viz., phosphorus and sulfur.   There are reasons for believing that these two elements enter into the building of the protein tissues only when they are supplied in the food in their protein combinations.   It does not seem to be definitely proven that their inorganic salts may be used by the animal organism for synthesizing phosphorus and sulfur-bearing proteins.

159. Relative efficiency of different proteins. — The relative efficiency of protein according to its source is one of importance.   Have vegetable proteins as large constructive value as those of animal origin?   Is a larger proportion of the proteins of milk and meat available for the building of animal tissue than when derived from the cereal grains?   We have seen that the " building stones " of animal proteins differ materially in proportion from those of vegetable proteins.   Abderhalden [1] calls attention in the following table to the much larger proportion of glutamic acid in the proteins of plant origin as related to their value for constructive purposes : —

[1] "Phys. Chemistry," 1908, p. 653. See Note, p. 199,

TABLE XXII

GLUTAMIC ACID IN 100 GRAMS PROTEIN

	GRAMS
Gliadin (wheat)	37.17
Gliadin (rye)	33.81
Hordein (barley)	36.35
Zein (maize)	16.87
Glutenin	23.42
Legumin	16.6
Vignin (peas)	16.89
Conglutin (lupine)	20.96
Casein	10.7
Egg albumin	8.0
Albumin (fish muscle)	8.9
Albumin (ox muscle)	11.9
Serum-albumin	7.7
Serum-globulin	8.5

These figures indicate that flesh foods are relatively more economical for tissue formation than vegetable foods. The proteins of flesh foods are themselves like the proteins that must be built into the animal body, and it seems plausible that their building stones can be used with less waste than can proteins of quite unlike constitution.

Von Noorden,[1] an authority of note, estimates that sucklings are able to convert 90 per cent of food protein into body protein, but suggests that the proteins of milk are particularly well adapted to reconstitution.

The same author also suggests on theoretical grounds that, in general,[2] " no more than 80 grams of body protein

[1] " Metabolism and Practical Medicine," Von Noorden, Vol. I, p. 71.
[2] Loc. cit., p. 70.

could be formed from 100 grams of protein in the food."
This whole question must for the present be considered on
a theoretical basis, but, at the same time, we are justified
in believing that [1] " a given quantity of protein in the food
cannot yield an equal amount of body protein, and also
that animal proteins are more efficient in this respect
than vegetable proteins."

160. Protein used in a variety of ways. — The functions
of the proteins are not restricted, however, to the use
already described. According to existing views, they are
utilized in more ways than any other class of nutrients.
It was held at one time by prominent scientists that outside the vegetable fats the proteins are the sole source
of animal fats, and this view was, not so very long ago,
to some extent accepted. Indisputable proof to the contrary is now in our possession, and some investigators even
go so far as to deny the possibility of the formation of fat
from protein. On this point, opinion is divided. Certainly
we must be convinced that nitrogen compounds of the
food are, with some species, not the most important
source of animal fat, for various investigators, such as
Lawes and Gilbert, Soxhlet, and others, have shown
upon the basis of searching experiments that sometimes
over four-fifths of the fat stored by pigs must have had its
origin outside the food protein and fat. Besides all this,
the common experience of feeders of animals that foods
highly non-nitrogenous are often the most efficient for
fattening purposes is good evidence that fat formation is
not greatly dependent upon the protein supply. Nevertheless, the possibility of producing animal fat from

[1] Loc. cit., p. 69.

protein is not disproved, and there are several considerations which make it seem probable that under certain conditions, this does occur.

Protein can unquestionably serve as fuel, or, in other words, as a source of energy. (See p. 162.) The amount so used depends much upon the subject and character of the ration. In the case of mature carnivorous animals and adult persons who neither gain nor lose in flesh, the protein eaten serves as a source of energy rather than of constructive material. When a portion of the protein is required for milk formation or for building tissue in the growing body, a varying quantity escapes oxidation.

The formation in the animal of carbohydrates from protein appears to be proven. We have seen that the sugar formed during digestion may be stored as glycogen, and that this glycogen in the liver and muscles is a reserve store of fuel to maintain the activities of the animal body, and it is important to know whether the contribution of energy from the digested protein is through the same avenue. There are now good grounds for believing that this may be the case.

In the plant, the amino acids which are the building stones of the proteins are synthesized from the carbohydrates and lower nitrogen compounds, and there seems to be no reason why a reverse process may not take place. Much investigation has been directed at this problem that did not furnish a conclusive answer, although in some experiments the sugar formed when a pure protein diet was fed, can be accounted for only by deciding that it was due to protein cleavage. Nevertheless, the question will bear further study.

161. Functions of carbohydrates. — Carbohydrates are usually characterized as the fuel portion of the food, or that part which is burned to produce the various forms of energy. This conception of the function of these bodies is correct in the sense that in many dietaries they constitute the larger part of the fuel, although not the whole of it, and in some dietaries less than half. For instance, the diet of a certain ball team contained on the average daily 181 grams of protein, 557 grams of carbohydrates, and 292 grams of fat. If the young men neither lost nor gained in flesh, the protein of their diet supplied about one-eighth of the fuel energy that they expended, the remainder coming about equally from the carbohydrates and fats.

In contrast to this, Japanese students in the cadet school at Tokyo were found to eat 83 grams of protein, 631 grams of carbohydrates, and 14 grams of fat. In this case, over 80 per cent of the fuel energy came from the carbohydrates. As we shall see later (pp. 161–162) all the nutrients may serve as fuel in the body, but in the dietaries of many classes of people the carbohydrates are the chief source of the energy that comes from food oxidation.

162. Carbohydrates a source of animal fats. — Contrary to views that held for a time, it is now well established that the animal fats may have their source in the carbohydrates; in other words, starch and sugar and related bodies may serve the main purpose in producing body fat. In many experiments, notably those with swine, the protein and fat of the food have fallen far short of accounting for the fat in the body increase, sometimes much the greater part of the latter having no possible source other than the carbohydrates. A practical expression of this general conclusion concerning the fat-forming function of carbohydrates is seen in the well-recognized value of corn meal as a fattening food, a feeding stuff nearly seven-tenths of which consists of starch. Recent experiments with milch cows leave no doubt that milk fat may also be derived from carbohydrates.

163. Functions of the fats and oils. — So far as is at present known, the possible uses of the food fats and oils and of the carbohydrates ,are similar. In other words, both may serve as fuel, and both may be a source of animal fat. The differences are that the supply of carbohydrates is much the larger, and the fuel value of a unit weight of fat much the greater. Moreover, it seems possible for a vegetable fat to become deposited in the animal without essential change, whereas fat formation from carbohydrates involves complex chemical transformations.

C. FOOD AS A SOURCE OF ENERGY

The fact that all the organic compounds of the food may serve as a source of energy, and as the larger portion of the food is utilized for energy purposes, it seems wise to give this phase of nutrition a somewhat special consideration. The living animal, either as a whole or in some of its parts, is constantly in motion. This means that the animal mechanism is ceaselessly performing work. Even if the body is apparently quiet, the heart beats, pumping blood to all parts of the body, the lungs are expanded and contracted, and the stomach and intestines keep up the movements which are essential to digestion. Besides, a living body is the seat of continuous, invisible, and complex chemical and physical changes, such as the breaking up of compounds in digestion and their rebuilding in assimilation, that, if not work in the common meaning of the term, are its equivalent. Walking, pulling, lifting, pumping blood, breathing, masticating, digesting and assimilating food, represent, then, a great variety of operations of living machines.

Now work requires the expenditure of energy. The projection of a rifle ball through space at the rate of two thousand feet per second is .work. The ball does not move of itself, but is propelled by the application of the energy stored in a powerful explosive. Back of every one of our great mechanical operations, such as pumping, grinding, and moving railroad trains, will always be found some sort of energy, and what is true of machinery made of wood and iron is equally true of that made of bone and muscle. The fact that the mechanism is alive does not abrogate a single physical law, so that the fundamental principles of energy as applied to machines are directly applicable to the activities of animal life.

It is safe to go farther, and say that the animal organism does not originate energy. Among the fundamental conceptions upon which all our knowledge of chemical and physical laws rests is this, that energy and matter are indestructible, and, moreover, that the sum total of these in the universe is unchangeable. If, then, man expends the muscular energy necessary to propel a bicycle over one hundred miles of road, the equivalent of this must have been supplied to his body from some outside source. He could not create it. We know that this is so, and we also know it must be conveyed to him in his food.

164. Manifestations of energy. — In considering this subject it is natural to first ask, what is energy? This is a difficult question to answer in a popular way, and the physicists' definition would hardly serve our purpose. All we can do, perhaps, is to illustrate it by pointing out some of its manifestations. Let us resort to an old illustration. Every farmer's boy has doubtless seen a blacksmith hammer an iron rod until it was red-hot. The motion of the hammer-head descending with great velocity was suddenly arrested when it came in contact with the rod. This descent of the hammer-head illustrated one form of active energy, viz., motion of a mass of matter. When the hammer met the iron rod on the anvil, the mass motion ceased. Was the energy therefore lost? Not unless our fundamental conception is wrong, and we find that in this case it is not. The physicist teaches us that the energy represented by the moving mass of matter, that is, the hammer-head, was communicated to the molecules of the iron rod, and as the vibrations of the molecule increased in rapidity, the rod grew hotter and hotter. Here we have another illustration of energy, viz., the motion of the molecule or heat into which the energy of mass motion has been transformed. The iron rod might have been heated in another way, — by plunging it into burning charcoal, and here the heat energy would come from the combustion of the carbon. Somehow, when it is deposited in the plant, there becomes stored in this carbon, in a way about which we can only theorize, what perhaps we may call the chemical energy of the atom, which, when combustion occurs, is changed into heat or molecular motion.

Perhaps another illustration may still further serve our purpose. A small dynamo is being run by a pair of horses working in a tread power such as is used for threshing grain. The horses are constantly climbing up a moving treadway and thereby communicating muscle energy to motion of machinery. This motion is, by the dynamo, converted into electricity, which, by passing through the carbon film of an incandescent lamp and there meeting resistance, is in part, at least, transformed into heat. We have then, in a chain, muscular vibration, motion of the mass (pulleys, wheels, etc.), electricity and heat, all active energies and all transferable the one into the other. This is a fairly good picture of what goes on with the horse or man, externally and internally, in sustaining life and performing labor. From these phenomena we learn that not only are there several forms of energy, but that one form is transferable into another.

165. Energy stored in plant substance. — Back of it all, and this is what interests us, is the animal's food. As a result of years of patient investigation, it has become known that through the combustion of the carbon compounds of vegetable and animal origin, which serve as nutrients, chemical energy may be transformed into those other forms that are manifested in the activities of living beings. When we ask from whence comes the energy given up by the plant compounds, we arrive at our last stage of inquiry. Here we enter the domain of plant life, and it is a notable triumph of the human intellect that we are able to declare with certainty that the ceaseless and multiple activities of life on this planet are sustained by an energy which comes to the plant in the sun's rays through almost limitless space.

166. Energy unit. — It is obvious that if the internal and external work performed by man is sustained by the food, it is desirable to measure the energy available in different foods, provided, of course, that they differ in this respect, as we know they do. In order to measure anything, we must have a standard or unit of measurement. In this case, it cannot be a unit of space or of mass; that is, we cannot declare that wheat flour contains so many cubic feet or pounds of available energy. Energy has neither dimensions nor weight. If we measure it at all, it must be by units of temperature or of work performed. Units of this kind are applied to the measurement of food energy. The one most commonly in use is the calorie, this being the energy which, in terms of heat, is sufficient to raise the temperature of one pound of water 4° F. Expressed in terms of work, the calorie is very nearly 1.53 foot tons, or, in other words, it is equivalent to the work involved in lifting one ton 1.53 feet.

167. Energy units in food compounds. — The total energy or heat units developed in the combustion of human foods is determined in an apparatus called a calorimeter. The latest form of this device is one in which food material is burned under pressure in the presence of pure oxygen, and the heat ·evolved is all used in warming a known weight of water. Data are thus obtained from which it is possible to calculate the calories in the particular material burned. The energy value of single compounds,

M

such as albumin, starch, and sugar, may also be found in the same way, as has been done in a large number of instances. These data show that the heat resulting from the combustion of the compounds of the same class is not the same in all cases. The value in calories of one gram (about one-twenty-eighth of an ounce) of the several nutrients is shown in the following table : —

TABLE XXIII

ENERGY VALUES OF FOOD COMPOUNDS

Proteins

	Cal.		Cal.
Wheat gluten	5.99	Egg albumin	5.73
Gliadin	5.92	Muscle (pure)	5.72
Glutenin	5.88	Blood fibrin	5.64
Plant fibrin	5.94	Peptone	5.30
Serum-albumin . . .	5.92	Wool	5.51
Milk casein	5.86	Gelatin	5.27
Yolk of egg	5.84	Asparagin (amide) . .	3.45

Carbohydrates	Cal.	*Fats*	Cal.
Starch	4.18	Of swine	9.38
Cellulose . . ´ . . .	4.18	Of oxen	9.38
Glucose	3.74	Of sheep	9.41
Cane sugar	3.95	Maize oil	9.28
Milk sugar	3.95	Olive oil	9.47
Maltose	3.95	Ether extract of oats .	8.93
Zylose	3.74	Ether extract of barley .	9.07

For illustration, the energy value of a pound of edible material from a few foodstuffs is given as follows : —

	Cal.		Cal.
Sirloin steak	1210	Wheat flour	1645
Corned beef	1655	Oat meal	1845
Fresh codfish	310	Sugar	1820
Eggs	720	Molasses	1360
Milk	325	Potatoes	375
Butter	3615	Squash (canned) . .	250
Oysters	260	Apples	320

These figures mean that when a pound of each of these foods is wholly burned, the heat produced is as stated. It has been demonstrated, too, by severe and elaborate investigations that the law of the correlation and conservation of energy holds in the animal organism as it does with machinery, or, in other words, the energy given off as animal heat has been measured and found to be exactly equivalent to the food energy minus that in the various excreta.

168: Available energy. — We must distinguish, however, between the heat produced when any food substance is wholly oxidized in a calorimeter, and the heat or energy which is available when the same material is applied to physiological uses. It never happens that the combustible portion of a ration is entirely burned in the animal.

In the first place, food is practically never all digested, and, as only the digested portion furnishes energy, the available fuel value of a ration must be based primarily, not upon the total quantity of dry matter it represents, but upon the amount which is dissolved and passes into the blood. If all foods were digested in the same proportion and with the same ease, their total fuel values might show their relative energy worth, but as digestion coefficients for the various food materials vary greatly, it is evident that the fuel waste in the feces is not uniform.

In the second place, the digested proteins are never fully burned. A portion of these compounds always passes off in the urine unoxidized, the fuel value of which is lost to the animal. For this reason, the available energy of the digested protein is about one-fourth less than the total.

In the third place, there is an escape from the alimentary canal of unconsumed gases, due to the fermentations which take place during the latter states of digestion. These gases, mostly methane (marsh gas), have their source mostly in the carbohydrates. With farm animals the loss of energy in gases has been found to vary from 10 to 20 per cent of the digested dry substance of the food. With the human species, the loss is much less and is perhaps almost negligible.

We are to understand, then, that the *available* energy of food is represented by the fuel value of the dry matter which is digested from it, minus the dry matter of the urine and that lost in gases.

If, however, we wish to know the actual energy gain from a particular diet, we must go farther than a determination of its available energy.

169. Net energy. — Within a comparatively short time we have begun to speak of the *net* energy of foods, and as this is a practical consideration which is likely to be the subject of much future discussion, it is well to notice it in an explanatory way. As we have learned, food is not applied to use until it reaches the blood. Between the time when it is taken into the mouth and when it passes into the circulation, it must have work expended on it in the way of mastication, solution, and moving it along the digestive tract, and it appears highly probable that the amount of this work per pound of food must vary greatly in different cases. In fact, we know this is so from the result of some masterly investigations conducted by Zuntz in Germany. By means of various devices and methods, a description of which would be out of place here, he measured the oxygen consumption necessary to sustain the mechanical energy of mastication and digestion with a horse, and he calculates from his determinations that the following heat units represented the energy used in chewing certain feeding stuffs:—

	CAL.		CAL.
1 lb. hay	76	1 lb. corn	$6\frac{1}{3}$
1 lb. oats	21	Green fodder equal to 1 lb.	
		hay	47

The differences revealed by these figures are interesting and important. Chewing green food cost in labor only about 62 per cent of the effort required to masticate its equivalent of dry hay, the proportions of labor for hay, oats, and corn being in the ratio of 100, 27, and $8\frac{1}{3}$.

This author goes farther and calculates that the work of mastication and digestion combined is 48 per cent of the energy value of the digested material from hay and 19.7 per cent of that from oats. To be sure, these results were obtained with a horse and do not apply to man, but they serve to illustrate the fact that the mastication and digestion of food is work and requires an expenditure of energy. The fact is also evident that the expenditure of energy varies with the mechanical condition of the foods, though not to the same extent perhaps.   All these deductions are based upon the excess of oxygen used when the work of chewing and digestion is going on over that used in the absence of such effort.

If we wish to ascertain the comparative energy worth of two unlike foods, it would obviously be incorrect to multiply the total quantities of protein, carbohydrates, and fats in each, by the unit heat values, in order to ascertain the relative energy gain to the animal body.

To recapitulate, we may define *available* energy as total energy minus that which is lost in the excreta and in gases which escape, and *net* energy as available energy minus the cost of digestion and of preparing the food for use.   Net energy is the balance of profit to the body.

170. Factors used in computing food values. — It is shown on pp. 161–162 that the different food compounds, even of the same class, have somewhat different heat values.   These are total values, also, and make no allowance for losses in the urine solids and in digestion.   Rübner, basing his figures on experiments with dogs, adopted certain factors for the calorific values of the several classes of nutrients.   Sherman,[1] in a very recent publication, suggests somewhat smaller factors as more nearly representing the net value of the constituents of foods.   Both sets of factors are given below.

	RÜBNER	SHERMAN
Protein	4.1	4.0
Carbohydrates	4.1	4.0
Fats	9.3	9.0

[1] " Chemistry of Food Nutrition," p. 125.

171. Energy relations of the several nutrients. — As has been pointed out, the animal body is the field of numerous mechanical activities which are sustained by the energy derived from the food. What is the relation of the several nutrients to these manifestations of vital energy is an interesting and, in some ways, an intensely practical matter. For instance, has protein a peculiar function in the maintenance of muscular activity which no other nutrients have? The belief prevailed at one time that muscular contraction caused a wasting of the muscle substance which must be replaced by the protein compounds of the food; in other words, protein alone was believed to sustain the work of the animal body, both internal and external. It would follow from this that the more work is done, the more protein is needed. This view is no longer held. The more exact methods of modern research have revealed the fact that an increase of muscular effort, even up to a severe point, increases but little, if any, the nitrogen compounds of the urine, these being the measure of the protein that is destroyed. There has come to light a corresponding fact that the consumption of fuel in the body other than proteins increases proportionately with the increase of work. This means that mechanical work is largely sustained through the combustion of carbohydrates and fats, and that while, for reasons we do not yet wholly understand, a fairly generous amount of protein seems to promote the well-being of the laborer, the non-nitrogenous nutrients mostly supply the extra energy demanded for the labor.

172. Heat relations. — The question is very naturally asked, as no energy is lost, into what is the energy of muscular contraction converted, as, for instance, that required for walking, the beating of the heart and the work of the intestines? It is concluded by physiologists that muscular energy used by the living organism is partly transformed into external motion and partly into heat, and this certainly is consistent with facts as observed. Violent exercise by the animal greatly increases the production of heat. We know this is so, because, under these conditions, an increased amount of blood is thrown to the surface of the body, thereby greatly increasing the loss of heat by radiation; perspiration sets in, and with it the consequent evaporation of much more moisture, thus disposing of much heat. Accurate determinations[1] reveal an increase of insensible perspiration (from lungs and skin) from an average of 960 grams of water per day for men at rest, to an average of 4272 grams for men at work. This shows what an important factor is the evaporation of water from the body in heat regulation. The dog, and sometimes other animals, pants and thereby causes a large loss of heat from the expanded surface of the moist tongue. All this occurs without reducing the body temperature below the normal. In fact, nature adopts these various devices, such as increased circulation of the blood and perspiration, in order to regulate the body temperature and prevent its rising above the proper point. The explanation of this greater heat during labor is that the mechanical energy manifested by the muscles is converted to heat, which, under circumstances of severe exercise, is more than enough to keep the body at its usual temperature and

[1] " Metabolism and Energy Transformations of Healthy Man during Rest," Benedict and Carpenter, p. 114.

maintain the usual radiation. When it is severely cold, on the other hand, vigorous exercise is sometimes necessary in order to keep sufficiently warm.

The view is now held that all body heat is a secondary product, that combustion first supports muscular activity with heat as the waste product; in fact, that, under the majority of conditions, no food is burned primarily to keep the animal warm. There is much evidence to support this position.

173. The critical temperature. — The possible combustion of food for the purpose of warming the animal body should not be denied, however. Recent investigations indicate that under given conditions there is an air temperature called the *critical temperature*, at which metabolism (oxidation) reaches a minimum. If the air temperature falls below this point, thus causing a greater radiation of heat from the body surface, increased oxidation occurs. If the temperature rises above this point, there is no diminution of oxidation, but rather a slight increase; hence the conclusion that there is a minimum oxidation necessary to the maintenance of the vital functions which must go on, however much the demands for the radiation of heat may be lessened by a rise of the air temperature. Down to a certain temperature point, the oxidation necessary for maintaining the work of the body gives off enough heat as a waste product to keep the body temperature up to 98.6° C. Above the critical temperature an excess of heat must be disposed of. What this critical temperature is for man does not appear to have been determined. Whichever way the air temperature moves from the critical point, there is heat regulation, this being *chemical* for the lower temperature, and *physical* for the higher.

D. The Nutritive Interrelation of the Food Compounds and the Need of combining These in the Diet

As we have seen, the conclusion reached by many extended and severe investigations is that the compounds of foods have certain functions in common. For instance, the proteins, carbohydrates, and fats are all oxidized wholly or in part to supply the necessary energy for muscular activity. The proteins then serve both constructive and fuel purposes. Carbohydrates and fats are alike in being sources of energy through oxidation, and in being utilized for the deposition of animal fat. In view of these facts, the question arises whether the physical welfare of the human subject requires the mixture of nutrients that commonly exist in the average human diet and that is enforced in the dietary standards that are recommended by students of human nutrition. It is certain that some species of animals may exist wholly on a flesh diet which is practically devoid of carbohydrates. Even man himself, in the wild state or when confined to game as a source of food, is able to subsist for a considerable period of time on animal food alone.

174. Carbohydrates physiologically economical. — Why do food standards call for a large proportion of non-nitrogenous material, particularly carbohydrates? The necessity of protein in the diet is abundantly demonstrated. Many investigations have shown that when the food contains no protein, the waste of nitrogen continues, no matter how abundant is the supply of carbohydrates and fats. In other words, a continuous protein cleavage is demanded by the animal organism, and no other nutrients can serve as a substitute for protein in meeting this demand. If the food contains no protein, body tissue will be depleted. It cannot be said that either carbohydrates or fats are an essential part of the diet in the sense protein is, because it is possible as energy producers to substitute one for the other and protein for both.

In spite of these facts, it is safe to assert that the welfare of the human organism is best promoted by a food carrying a mixture of the three classes of nutrients. The larger part of man's food is used for the production of energy, and it is physiologically economical that this energy be supplied by the non-nitrogenous nutrients, particularly carbohydrates. If the proteins are broken down to supply energy, there is always a definite proportion of urea and uric acid residue that must be eliminated through the kidneys. An exclusive protein diet would burden these organs beyond their accustomed habit, and flooding the system with these nitrogenous wastes, in the opinion of medical experts, increases the tendency to gout and other forms of rheumatism. On the other hand, the carbohydrates, when not stored as fat, are completely oxidized to the simplest compounds, carbon dioxid and water, which are eliminated through the lungs and skin, possibly part of the water so formed acting as a solvent of the urinary compounds. Investigation seems to prove conclusively that the animal body has a physiological preference for carbohydrates over the fats or other nutrients as a source of energy. After the free ingestion of sugar the respiratory quotient in certain experiments has become 1.00 when just previously it was much less than 1.00. This demonstrates that while fat was being oxidized before the sugar was taken, the oxidation immediately changed wholly to the sugar. This indicates the physiological adaptability of starches and sugars for maintaining muscular activity.

175. Protein sparers. — The carbohydrates and fats are sometimes classed as "protein sparers." This means that, with an adequate supply of these bodies in the food, protein destruction may be reduced to the lowest possible limit. To illustrate, if a man doing moderate work were maintaining an energy balance when eating of digestible nutrients 218 grams of protein, 400 grams of carbohydrates, and 56 grams of fat, and 100 grams of digestible carbohydrates were added to the daily food, approximately 100 grams of digestible protein could undoubtedly be withdrawn from the daily food without causing any drain upon body protein to meet the demands of the organism. As stated, however, such a substitution cannot be carried beyond certain limits without depressing the protein supply below the body needs for maintenance. Fats are not as efficient protein sparers as are carbohydrates. To be more explicit, fats and carbohydrates do not replace protein in proportion to their energy equivalents, carbohydrates being the more efficient. In brief, then, experience and science both indicate that carbohydrates are the most healthful, and physiologically the most economical, source of a large proportion of the food energy used by the human subject. There is every justification for the relative abundance of starch foods in man's diet.

CHAPTER VIII

LAWS OF NUTRITION

THE preceding pages have been devoted to a discussion of the origin of human foods : what they are in substance, how their nutrients are made available, and how used. So far no attempt has been made to summarize into a systematic statement what may be called the fundamental principles or laws of nutrition, some of which we have not yet directly formulated, but which are inferences from the facts presented. It is desirable to do this, however, before passing to the consideration of the practical side of human nutrition.

176. Food source of all energy and building material. — All energy and building material applied to the maintenance and growth of the human body come from the food, water and oxygen being included in this term. The human organism originates neither matter nor force.

177. Only digested food available. — Only that portion of the food which is digested, *i.e.*, that which is dissolved by the digestive fluids and rendered soluble and diffusible so that it passes into the blood, is available for any use whatever. This fact is especially important in view of the greatly varying digestibility of different foods.

178. Avenues of excretion. — The undigested food and the wastes from the digested food pass from the body in some direction.   The undigested part appears in the solid excrement or feces.   The urea and other nitrogenous compounds which are the unoxidized portion of the digested protein, pass out wholly in the urine.   All digested nitrogen not stored is found here.   The carbon dioxid is eliminated through the skin and lungs, chiefly the latter, and water is disposed of through the kidneys, skin, and lungs.

179. Uses of digested food. — The digested food is used in two general directions : (*a*) for the production of energy, and (*b*) for constructive purposes.   (*a*) The food energy is made available through combustion, *i.e.*, the oxidation of the carbon compounds of the food to simpler substances, carbon dioxid and water, thus liberating the energy stored in the plant during its growth.   Protein is never fully oxidized, but carbohydrates and fats may be.   All the organic nutrients may be oxidized to produce energy, the available heat values of protein, carbohydrates, and fats being approximately as 1, 1, 2.25.   This liberated energy finds expression in the animal organism in various ways, as heat, mechanical energy or motion, and chemical transformations.   The total energy of food is never all available for use because of a loss in the excreta and gases. Moreover, the net energy gain seems not to be proportional to the available energy, but is dependent upon the work of digestion, which varies somewhat with different foods.

(*b*) The food compounds are used for constructive purposes, either without changing their general character, as, for instance, the building of muscular tissue from the plant proteins, or they may be reorganized into bodies of a very different character, as in the formation of animal fats from starch and sugar. The proteins are used to construct muscular tissue; in fact, all the nitrogenous parts of the human body, and they are perhaps a source of fat. Carbohydrates can only be used constructively for the formation of fat, and the same is true of food fats or oils. Mineral matter is needed for the formation of bone, is distributed through the soft tissues, and has important functions in digestion.

180. Food balance. — The matter of the digested food, including water and oxygen, is exactly equal to that stored in the body or in milk, or both, plus that in waste products, — feces, water, carbonic acid, and urine solids. Such a balance may not be maintained for any particular day, but will ultimately be found to exist.

181. Food requirements definite. — Under given conditions of species, sex, age, climate, and use, a definite amount of digested organic matter is necessary to maintain a particular person without gain or loss of body substance. This means simply that tissue wastes must be replaced, and the fuel supply must be kept up.

If an individual receives no food, or less than the amount needed for maintenance purposes, tissue waste and the production of energy do not cease, but go on wholly or in part at the expense of the body substance, and, as it is commonly expressed, the person " grows thin."

182. Production. — Food supplied above a needed maintenance quantity may be utilized for the production of new substances or work. In the proper sense of the term, no production ever occurs without an excess of food above the maintenance requirement. Milk formation may sometimes go on at the expense of the body substance, but with proper feeding, milk, flesh or muscular work are produced at the expense of food supplied in excess of that needed for maintenance.

183. Specific requirements. — Regard must be had to the supply of particular nutrients as well as of total food. Even with a person doing no work a certain amount of protein will be broken up constantly into urea and similar compounds, an amount which will be withdrawn from the body tissues to the extent that it is not supplied by the food. In addition to this, nursing mothers, for instance, must have protein for the formation of the nitrogen compounds of milk, or a growing child, for the growth of bone and flesh in a quantity proportional to the production, and food must supply it. There is, therefore, a minimum supply of protein, which, in a particular case, is necessary for maintenance and for constructive purposes, less than which ultimately diminishes production to the extent of the deficiency, or else requires the use of body tissue.

184. Nutrients interchangeable in part. — The different classes of nutrients are to some extent interchangeable in their functions. That is to say, all the organic nutrients may be burned to supply energy. Protein may be so used, even to withdrawing it from the purposes to which it is necessary, unless the carbohydrates or fats are sufficient to protect it from being consumed as fuel. A proper supply of the non-nitrogenous nutrients is required, therefore, to insure the application of the necessary minimum of food protein to its peculiar uses. Carbohydrates seem to have a special physiological adaptation to energy production.

PART II

PRACTICAL DIETETICS

CHAPTER IX

GENERAL CONSIDERATIONS

THE ultimate aim of scientific knowledge relating to human nutrition should be to promote the healthful and economical use of food. Unless this knowledge has a practical application, it serves merely as an object of intellectual interest. A person may determine what he shall eat from two points of view, viz., he may select his food on the basis of rational considerations of health and economy, or he may sensuously follow the dictates of appetite. It is to be feared that the latter point of view largely prevails. Man does not seem to regulate his diet wisely by an intuitive sense of what is best for his physical welfare, but in a large number of cases is the unfortunate victim of unbridled indulgence in that which most delights his taste, but eventually ruins his health. If reason dominates, then many questions come to the front, some of which are the following : —

1. The amounts and proportions of the various foods that best meet the physiological requirements of different classes of persons in their varying conditions of age, activity, and environment.

2. The selection of food materials that will supply a diet physiologically adequate and efficient for a given purpose.

3. The economical purchase of a food supply.

4. Methods of preparing foods to secure dietetic efficiency
and the minimum waste.

5. The preservation of food.

6. Food sanitation.

*Our physiological food requirements and the influence of
various conditions of age, activity, and environment upon
these requirements, as shown by eating habits.*

It is hoped that in the preceding pages it has been made
clear that through the matter and energy supplied in food
the human body is constructed and its activities maintained.
It should also be plain that as the different food compounds
have unlike functions, all of these must be found in a diet
that will build and sustain a normal human body. We
cannot avoid the conclusion either, that as food supplies
the raw material for the growth of body tissue as well as
the fuel used to maintain the work performed by the human
machine both internally and externally, food consumption must necessarily vary greatly with different individuals.

A. How Standard Dietaries have been Established

Food requirements — in other words, dietaries — have
been the subject of a large amount of study. Several
methods of inquiry have been used, perhaps the most common one being to determine what amounts of nutrients are
actually being consumed by individuals or groups of individuals living under various conditions of age, environment,
and activity.   In this way there has been studied the food
consumption of children, the two sexes, professional men

and women, persons engaging in labor of unlike severity and persons living under varying environments or engaged in special occupations.

185. Method of study. — The general procedure in these studies has been to weigh, and, as far as possible, analyze, the food materials purchased for the individual or group of individuals, and weigh and analyze all the unconsumed materials. The difference between the purchased food and that unconsumed represents what is actually eaten. In many cases, as for, instance, with meats bought in large bulk, the purchased materials have been assumed to have an average composition. In this manner a widespread study has been made of the dietaries of different classes of people in the United States where habit, inclination, the limitation of means, and a local food supply have had their full and unrestrained influence. Similar studies have been carried on in an extensive way by European investigators.

186. Standard dietaries. — Based upon the results of these observations, with possibly certain modifications indicated by general principles, the following so-called *standard dietaries* have been suggested which are given in terms of protein, carbohydrates, and fats, together with the aggregate energy of the nutrients in each dietary. The dietaries in Tables XXIV and XXV are a statement of food consumption, and not of the amounts of the nutrients digested.

In the table [1] immediately following may be found the standards suggested some years ago by European investigators : —

[1] "Chemistry and Economy of Food," Bul. 21, O.E.S., p. 210.

TABLE XXIV

EUROPEAN STANDARDS FOR DAILY DIETARIES FOR PEOPLE OF DIFFERENT CLASSES

	NUTRIENTS				POTEN-TIAL ENERGY
	Protein	Fats	Carbo-hydrates	Total	
	Grams	Grams	Grams	Grams	Calories
Children:					
1 to 2 years, average	28	37	75	140	765
2 to 6 years, average	55	40	200	295	1420
6 to 15 years, average . . .	75	43	325	443	2040
Aged woman	80	50	260	390	1860
Aged man	100	68	350	518	2475
Woman at moderate work . . .	92	44	400	536	2425
Man at moderate work (Voit) .	118	56	500	674	3055
Man at hard work (Voit) . . .	145	100	450	695	3370
Man at moderate work (Mole-schott)	130	40	550	720	3160
Man at moderate work (Wolff) .	125	35	540	700	3030
Subsistence diet (Playfair) . .	57	14	341	412	1760
Diet in quietude (Playfair) . .	71	28	341	440	1950
Adult in full health (Playfair) .	119	51	531	701	3140
Active laborers (Playfair) . . .	156	71	568	795	3630
Hard-worked laborers (Playfair) .	185	71	568	824	3750

Dr. W. O. Atwater,[1] after an extensive study of dietary conditions in the United States, suggested the following for the conditions prevailing here, which may be regarded as a compromise with the European standards: —

[1] Loc. cit., p. 213.

TABLE XXV

STANDARDS FOR DAILY DIETARIES (AMERICAN)

	PRO-TEIN	FUEL VALUE	NUTRI-TIVE RATIO
	Grams	Calories	1 :
Woman with light, muscular exercise . .	90	2400	5.5
Woman with moderate muscular work .	100	2700	5.6
Man without muscular work			
Man with light muscular work	112	3000	5.5
Man with moderate muscular work . . .	125	3500	5.8
Man with hard muscular work	150	4500	6.3

It is to be observed that Dr. Atwater's standards are rather more generous than the European. This is to be expected in standards based upon eating habits, for the relatively larger supply of food materials in the United States and the higher wage of our laboring classes conduces to more generous and more expensive eating habits.

It is to be noted that these tables differ in the terms in which the standards are stated. The earlier standards are given in terms of total nutrients in the food eaten. Later only total protein and the energy of the total food are stated, while Dr. Langworthy gives the standards in terms of digestible protein and utilizable energy.

An excellent and quite complete summary of the results of dietary studies throughout the world has been presented by Dr. Langworthy.[1]

[1] Year Book, U. S. Dept. Agr., 1907, p. 366.

TABLE XXVI

RESULTS OF DIETARY STUDIES IN THE UNITED STATES AND
OTHER COUNTRIES

PERSONS	TOTAL PROTEIN EATEN	ENERGY OF TOTAL DIET	DIGESTED PROTEIN	ENERGY UTILIZED
United States:	Grams	Calories	Grams	Calories
Men at hard muscular work: Artisans, laborers, etc., average of 24 studies	177	6485	162	6000
Athletes, average of 19 studies	198	4980	182	4510
Men at moderate muscular work: Farmers, artisans, laborers, etc., average of 162 studies	100	3685	92	3425
Men not employed at muscular occupations: Business men, students, etc., average of 51 studies	106	3560	98	3285
Men with little or no muscular work: Inmates of institutions, average of 49 studies	86	2820	80	2600
Very poor working people, average of 15 studies	69	2275	64	2100
Canada: Factory hands, average of 13 studies	108	3735	99	3480
West Indies:				
Farmers, light work, Leeward Islands	82	——	75	3085
Ireland: Workingmen	98	——	90	3107
England: Workingmen	89	——	82	2685
Scotland:				
Workingmen	108	——	99	3228
Students	143	——	132	3979
Finland:				
Workingmen	114	——	105	3011
Workingmen (hard work)	167	——	150	4378
Students	157	——	144	3984
Sweden:				
Workingmen	134	——	123	3281
Workingmen (hard work)	189	——	174	4557
Students	127	——	117	3032

TABLE XXVI — *Continued*

RESULTS OF DIETARY STUDIES IN THE UNITED STATES AND
OTHER COUNTRIES — *Continued*

PERSONS	TOTAL PRO-TEIN EATEN	ENERGY OF TOTAL DIET	DI-GESTED PRO-TEIN	EN-ERGY UTIL-IZED
	Grams	Calories	Grams	Calories
Russia:				
Factory hands	119	—	109	3194
Miners (hard work)	155	—	143 ·	4000
Northern Italy: Laborers	125	—	115	3655
Southern Italy: Laborers	148	—	136	4400
Italy: Farmers and mechanics	125	—	115	3400
Germany:				
Workingmen (hard work)	134	—	123	3061
Farmers	137	—	126	4530
Professional men	111	—	102	2511
France:				
Men (light work)	110	—	101	2750
Farmers (south of France)	149	—	137	4570
Belgium:				
Workingmen	92	—	84	3000
Farmers	136	—	125	4370
Poland: Well-to-do families	121	—	111	3015
Japan:				
Laborers	118	—	103	4415
Laborers (hard work)	158	—	137	5050
Professional and business men	87	—	75	2190
Students	98	—	88	2800
Java: Men (light work)	73	—	67	2500
China, Lao-Kay: Laborers	91	—	83	3400
Anam: Laborers	134	—	123	3866
Egypt: Native laborers	112	—	103	2825
Congo: Native laborers	108	—	90	2812

187. Influence of conditions. — A study of the fore-going tables reveals facts of importance, principally two : (1) that age and occupation have a very marked influence upon actual food consumption, and (2) that food consumption in different countries under unlike physical and economic conditions differs greatly even with persons of the same class and kind of occupation. The first fact is in accordance with the bio-chemical facts we have been considering. If the food must supply the energy used in internal and external work, then the more units of work are performed, the more food is required. The child is growing rapidly and requires building material which the adult does not. The second fact of the unlike consumption of food in different lands, for instance, students or men at hard work, is related in part to certain economic conditions such as food supply and wages, but at the same time it opens a question of large import which will be quite fully considered later.

B. Actual Food Consumption as a Basis for Standard Dietaries

In view of the evident variations in the amount of food consumed by different persons, even those of the same class, the question is very properly raised whether the measurement of what persons of various classes actually eat gives a proper basis for establishing food standards. It is popularly asserted that most persons eat too much, and that less food would conduce to better health and adequately sustain the fullest activities. This claim is also made by scientists of established reputation, and carefully considered evidence is presented to support it. It must be confessed that the aim of scientific investigation should be to find out what are the real physiological requirements of persons in the several conditions and occupations of life, and it is not safe to assume that the eating habits of those individuals selected for observation are necessarily correct. We know it to be true that many persons have acquired luxurious table habits even to gluttony, and we are sure that much disease and suffering are due to excessive or ill-advised eating. It is not so evident, however, that the great mass of persons in mediocre circumstances and of sober, well-ordered lives could eat much less to the physical advantage of themselves and the race. In discussing this question, facts both of general observation and those derived from scientific inquiry should be considered.

188. The test of experience. — In the first place, it must be conceded that in many cases where unrestrained food selection and consumption have prevailed, generation after generation of men and women have grown to a normal, well-developed, and healthy type. We have no reason for supposing that among those people who have shown a persistence of type and vigor there has not been a free satisfaction of appetite, or, conversely, that there has been either a voluntary or an involuntary limitation of food to a minimum. Moreover, an excess of food over and above real physiological needs must certainly be a physiological burden, and if excessive eating is generally indulged in, we could hardly expect such instances of apparently perfect health and great vigor in persons who freely indulge in a generous diet. It should be admitted that these arguments are of a popular character and are not scientific proof. Let us turn for a moment to arguments of similar nature on the other side.

189. Variable individual demands. — The advocates of a restricted diet point to the greatly variable food consumption by different individuals of apparently healthy and normal life as good evidence that some must certainly eat more than they need. It has been conceded that there is much overeating, which is the cause of many physical ills. On the other hand unlike eating is not evidence of overeating on the part of some individuals. The activities of the human organism internal and external are very complex and are greatly unlike with different persons without the fact being apparent. One person sits quietly, walks with the least effort, and uses the minimum effort in performing a given amount of work, while another is of a restless, nervous temperament, is constantly moving, and uses unnecessary exertion in accomplishing a physical task. When we remember that all physical activity of whatever kind is sustained by an exact equivalent of food energy, it is easy to understand why the real food needs of different individuals may vary greatly because of unrecognized differences in muscular activity.

190. Fate of excess food. — Again, if a person consumes carbohydrates and fat in excess of the maintenance needs of the body, what is their fate? The scientific evidence is that there is no increase in energy exchange; that is, in the final transference of the potential energy of the food into heat, which is the measure of such exchange, but that the surplus is stored in the body. It is hardly conceivable, anyway, that the energy of excess food would be exactly disposed of in the work of getting rid of the excess.

If this were the case, then the necessary energy expenditure would be directly proportional to the amount of food digested, unless storage in the body occurs, — an absurd proportion.

191. Experimental evidence. — Those who argue for a restriction of the diet below the ordinary eating practices point to certain experimental observations as furnishing proof of the correctness of their position. Reference is not here made to the claims of food " faddists " who, without any adequate knowledge of scientific fundamentals and without accurate observations, proclaim the blessings of a minimum diet. Their unsustained assertions may be passed by without discussion, for so far as they have been investigated they have proved unreliable.

When, however, such a distinguished scientist as Dr. Chittenden of Yale University advocates greater moderation in eating and presents a mass of carefully observed data to sustain his views, the matter becomes worthy of careful consideration. The work of Chittenden[1] was undertaken primarily to investigate the minimal necessary supply of protein, but the data permit observations on the energy supply. It seems that he succeeded in maintaining a uniform body weight on what he estimated to be a food energy of approximately 1600 calories daily. Under the change in diet his weight fell from 144 pounds to about 126.5 pounds, after what it remained practically constant. Observations were made by Dr. Chittenden on four other subjects who maintained a fairly uniform body weight on food estimated to furnish daily from 2000 to 2500 calories. These figures seem low when it is recalled that calorimeter

[1] " Physiological Economy in Nutrition," pp. 19–51.

measurements of energy exchange by several subjects of varying weight (43 to 82 kg.), in absolute muscular rest and in a hunger condition, showed a daily heat production of 1214 to 1656 calories, while the exchange of somewhat heavier persons when asleep has been found to vary between 1418 and 1853 calories.[1] (See Table XXVII.)

Chittenden's five subjects, though active, were engaged in mental rather than physical labor, and were of light weight, from 126 to 143 pounds (57.3 to 65 kg.) It has been shown that mental labor does not require an amount of food energy that is appreciable through calorimetric measurements. Further experiments were conducted by Chittenden[2] with seven college athletes which continued during five months. In these experiments the protein food taken was deliberately made much below the quantity usually consumed at the training table, and the total quantity of food eaten was also diminished. Seven-day balance trials having for their object a determination of the intake and outgo of nitrogen show that seven of these, weighing from 123 to 171 pounds apiece, are estimated to have presumably received food varying in energy from 2174 to 3091 calories. These figures are much below the standards obtained from a study of the actual dietaries of equally active persons in ordinary life.

192. Possible errors. — Two facts should be recognized in discussing Dr. Chittenden's conclusions ; first, his athletes confessedly ate less during the periods when the nitrogen balance was accurately determined, and second, the energy values were estimated. It is unsafe to conclude,

---

[1] " Metabolism and Practical Medicine," Von Noorden, Vol. I, pp. 260–261.   [2] " Physiological Economy in Nutrition." pp. 327–454.

TABLE XXVII

HEAT PRODUCTION (ENERGY USE) DURING 24 HOURS[1]

Subjects in Fasting Condition

NAME	WEIGHT SUBJECT, KG.	HEAT IN 24 HOURS, CALORIES	CALORIES PER HOUR AND KG.	CONSTITUTION
Rud.	43.2	1333	1.29	Very small and thin.
Dr. Sch.	48.0	1214	1.05	Small, thin, good muscles.
Rutt.	53.0	1527	1.20	Poor in fat.
B.	58.0	1510	1.08	Normal.
Dr. K.	64.0	1656	1.07	
Dr. M. L.	67.5	1608	0.99	Poor in fat, very muscular
Dr. Jaq.	82.0	1556	0.79	Rich in fat, not corpulent; good muscles.

HEAT PRODUCTION IN SLEEP DURING 24 HOURS[1]

NAME	WEIGHT SUBJECT, KG.	HEAT IN 24 HOURS, CALORIES	CALORIES PER HOUR AND KG.	CONSTITUTION
Dr. Anderson . . .	90.4	1773	.82	Small amount of fat, very strong.
J. C. W.	76.0	1853 / 1798	1.02 / 0.99	Medium, highly trained.
Stud. Md.	72.7	1657	0.95	
Engineer	71.2	1787	1.05	Poor in fat, very good muscles.
Cand, M.D. . . .	64.9	1475	.95	Slight, good muscles, highly trained.
Dr. Bjerre	63.0	1418	0.94	Slight, normal.
Dr. Bergman . . .	57.1	1560	1.14	Slight, strong.

[1] " Metabolism and Practical Medicine," Von Noorden, Vol. 1, pp. 260-1.

therefore, that the energy values of the average diet of the athletes when under observation was as low as is given. This view is strengthened by the fact that although Dr. Chittenden estimated at 1700 calories the food-energy consumption of Mr. Fletcher, who maintained an apparent body equilibrium while he was given the " drastic exercises " of the Yale University crew, when this subject was tested in the respiration calorimeter in a state of inactivity, his heat output was 1896 calories, 536 calories more than his food contained.[1] Dr. Benedict in commenting on this says with good reason that Mr. Fletcher's use of energy when taking the Yale exercises could not have been less than 3000 calories, part of which was at the expense of his body. The maintenance of a nitrogen equilibrium and of uniform body weight, as in Mr. Fletcher's case, is not evidence that the body has not lost substance, for muscular exercise in excess of the food supply is sustained by the body fat as long as it lasts, and weight may be maintained even during a loss of body fat, for this loss may be replaced by water. Moreover, the estimation of available food energy on the basis of the average composition and digestibility is a precarious method. Exact measurements are necessary for exact conclusions.

193. Minimum nutrition. — But after all, is minimum nutrition desirable? (The question of the desirable protein intake will be considered later.) Certainly much disease is caused by overeating. Many persons should practice greater moderation in satisfying their appetite. Those who take on excessive fat would do well to eat less, exercise freely, and thus draw upon the food for the maintenance

[1] *Am. Jour. Phys.*, Vol. 16, p. 433.

of muscular activity, thereby preventing the storage of fat. It is especially true of those who live sedentary lives and store body substance beyond what may be regarded as a normal weight, that they would do well to be more abstemious. Doubtless by so doing in many cases bodily comfort would be promoted, the tendency to disease would be less, and mental efficiency would be increased. The case is different with that large number of persons who practically keep in nutritive equilibrium.

194. Energy requirement determined by energy output. — In discussing this we must constantly keep in mind the fundamental fact that " the energy output is practically the energy requirement," under given conditions, of course, and the expenditure caused by the muscular activity of a particular individual cannot be reduced without affecting the work done or causing loss of body substance. Stated another way, it is necessary to conclude that when the body is maintained in equilibrium, neither gaining or losing, there is an exact balance between the intake of available food energy and the expenditure of energy on the part of the organism. If an individual maintaining this balance is to continue a given energy expenditure and not lose flesh, he must continue to receive its food equivalent; or if he is to eat less food and not lose flesh, he must diminish the energy expenditure. The question is, then, can those of us who are active eat less, that is, can we effect a diminution in the necessary energy exchange of our bodies, and if we can, how is it to be done?

195. Reduction of energy requirement. — Of course, if the diet of any person is so light as to cause a loss of weight, then energy needs are diminished, because, other

o

things being equal, the greater the body mass the greater the food needs. Moreover, when less food is eaten, the work of digestion is lowered. This is a minor factor, however. The most effective way of materially diminishing the work of the body is to restrict its muscular exertion; but with a person who continues a given occupation, it is scarcely possible for him to so modify his activities that his food needs are lowered to any appreciable extent. If a person undertook to restrict his daily and habitual movements, even though they might be purposeless, it would be at a sacrifice of comfort and with no certainty of its accruing to his physical advantage simply because it would be possible to eat less.

It is certain that a lower maintenance diet means, in general, a lower range of activity in some direction or other, unless we conclude that the human organism may be induced to take on new metabolic habits, with a larger net result of work accomplished in proportion to the food eaten. If we have confidence in the law of the conservation and correlation of energy, we must conclude that this cannot happen. It has been suggested that there is what may be called a race habit in the use of food. Doubtless this is so, but it would be absurd to expect that one race will accomplish more units of work with a given expenditure of energy than another. It may be true, however, that the racial habits of life or nervous temperament may so differ as to give one race preëminence in the proportion of food energy that is converted into productive work.

196. Relation of food and body type. — One question has not been answered. We do not know what the effect on the physical type of man would be if generation after generation was to adopt food minima as a practice. If we reason by analogy, the results would not be desirable. Farm animals are not reared to their best estate or made most productive by studying to reduce their rations. We recognize the value of full-fed animals. It is fair to raise the question whether the full-fed man, with his reserve of energy is not the type upon which the virility, even the intellectual strength, of a nation must depend.

C. THE NECESSARY PROTEIN SUPPLY

Apart from the question of the total food requirements of the human body, there is much discussion over the necessary protein supply. Investigation has shown there is a necessary daily minimum protein use. Even with persons in starvation, a certain protein destruction goes on, which, after a time, draws on the tissues. When insufficient protein is taken in the food, the necessary balance will be supplied from the body. On the other hand, where there is no growth of tissue or temporary storage of protein, any excess of protein above this minimum requirement is also broken down. In other words, the body maintains a nitrogen balance, the excretion of nitrogen compounds in the urine fluctuating with the intake of protein.

197. Fixed and circulatory protein. — Bio-chemists have come to regard the protein of the animal organism as existing in two general conditions, viz., what may be called the " fixed," " stable," or " tissue " protein, and the " circulatory " or " labile " protein. It is the latter that does not resist disintegration, and it probably consists in part of that surplus protein which is immediately derived from the food and which has not become deposited in the tissue form. This is the type of protein that fluctuates according to the food supply, and it is by the disintegration of this that the body keeps in protein balance when sufficiently long periods of time are considered. A sudden increase of food protein may cause a temporary storage, for there appears to be a " lag " in the adjustment of the supply to the expenditure, but the adjustment comes more or less gradually.

198. Protein standards. — The food standards which are based upon observations of practice call for not less than 100 grams of protein daily for professional men, and 175 grams for men at severe labor. Voit gave 118 grams as the standard for a strong man doing moderate work. Notwithstanding these estimates, men in various occupations have been found to maintain a protein balance, that is, no loss of protein occurred from the body, when the intake was much less than the standards set. Dr. Chittenden, a teacher, was able after some training to keep in protein equilibrium on 40 grams of protein per day. Five of the college athletes he experimented with even made a slight gain of protein (nitrogen) on from 55 to 72 grams of protein daily. Several instances are on record where men of moderate size made a daily use of only from 33 to 50 grams. Unquestionably a protein equilibrium may be maintained, temporarily at least, on much less of an intake than is called for by the dietary standards.

199. Demands on protein supply. — Is the protein in the dietary standards in excess of what in a few investigations has been found to be a minimum requirement, necessary or even desirable? Would it be to our advantage to eat less meat, fish, cheese, milk, or eggs? We shall see that when an individual passes from a state of comparative inactivity to severe labor, protein exchange is not materially increased, provided carbohydrates and fats are supplied in sufficient quantity. In other words, the source of muscular energy is not in the destruction of protein compounds, but may come almost entirely from the oxidation of the non-nitrogenous parts of the food. A large protein supply, then, does not appear to be necessary to the laborer, as a means of repairing waste of muscle tissue, although it must be confessed that in ordinary dietetic practice he consumes protein foods somewhat in proportion to the severity of his labor.

200. Protein and health. — The arguments in favor of a restricted consumption of protein are based chiefly on the benefits to health. It is urged that as all protein wastes, of whatever kind, must be eliminated through the kidneys, a generous protein consumption places a heavy burden upon these organs at which they are said to rebel, and there occurs an accumulation of nitrogen wastes in the organism that is dangerous to health. Rheumatism and gout have been regarded as related to uric acid accumulation, and nitrogenous bodies are believed to often cause "auto-intoxication," bringing on biliousness and low forms of fever. Unquestionably much physical suffering and disability arises in these and other ways from the excessive consumption of protein foods, especially meats. The question turns on what is excessive. Are the dietary standards excessive? Dr. Chittenden claims for himself and the other subjects with whom he experimented that a material reduction of the protein intake resulted in a betterment of condition both physical and mental. There is also much popular testimony to the same effect, although the most of this relatès to the total food consumption rather than to the mere diminution of the protein intake.

201. Arguments against minimum protein supply. — But students of human nutrition do not all agree that so radical a diminution of protein in the food is desirable. In the first place, there is some reason for believing that protein serves the mature animal organism in other ways than merely repairing tissue waste, and that the physiological needs are less efficiently served when the protein supply is held down to the minimum that just makes good the unavoidable protein destruction. General facts of observation and experience are cited. It is held to be significant that the communities holding leading positions in the world consume a liberal quantity of protein, or, conversely, that communities with an inferior physical and mental status use a low proportion of protein in the diet. We certainly cannot ignore the facts of long continued experience. It is asserted with great force, that we do not know what would be the effect of a low protein diet if continued through many generations. We do know that people of great physical strength have developed and lived in whose diet animal foods occupied a prominent place. If we argue from analogies in feeding farm animals, — and physically man is an animal, — generous protein feeding is desirable for the growth and maintenance of vigorous organisms and a satisfactory rate of production. It is regarded as significant by one critic of Dr. Chittenden that all the athletes used in his tests returned to practically their former diet, which they would hardly have been allowed to do if the low protein diet had been found to be so greatly superior. The question is a complex one, and is by no means settled. Certainly no facts appear which show with any conclusiveness that the dietary standard of 118 grams of protein per day for a moderately active person of average size may not be followed with safety and advantage to health and vigor.

NOTE.[1] — It is probable that the source of protein has much to do with the efficiency of a given quantity, especially when the purposes of growth must be served. Since paragraph 159, p. 152, Chap. VII, was written Osborne and Mendel have published the results of extensive studies on the efficiency of individual proteins. The experimental animals used were albino rats, the technique and control being such as to inspire confidence in the data secured. The authors call attention to the fact that gelatin has long been known as a protein inadequate of itself for sustaining life. Other individual proteins can now be studied. Observations were made with rations containing the following proteins : casein, lactalbumin, glycinin, excelsin, legumin, edestin, glutenin, gliadin, zein, hordein, and perhaps others. It was concluded that in the earlier experiments the failure to produce growth or even to permanently maintain life, where the artificial food mixture contained only a single protein, was due to the inadequacy of the mixture of non-protein compounds and inorganic salts accompanying the protein. Later experiments where the single proteins were fed with protein-free milk (casein and lactalbumin removed) showed that adequate growth was secured with casein, lactalbumin, egg albumin, edestin, glutenin, and glycinin. Growth was not secured but life was maintained when the following proteins were fed with protein-free milk : gliadin of wheat, and hordein of barley, while zein from corn proved to be insufficient for the maintenance requirement. It is hardly to be expected that these results would have any significance as related to ordinary dietaries that are made up of a mixture of animal and vegetable foods. It seems possible, however, that the development of the human body may be modified when the diet is largely of one material such as rice or corn. As a side issue, the authors point to the fact that the synthesis of conjugated proteins (nucleo proteins, hæmoglobin) from simple proteins and inorganic salts must have taken place.

[1] Science, 1911, pp. 722–732.

CHAPTER X

THE SELECTION OF FOOD, OR THE REGULATION OF DIET

IT is useless to expect that the eating habits of the general mass of persons can ever be brought to a dead level established by scientific principles. Individual tastes and physiological dissimilarities will always play an important part in the use of food, and this fact should have a free recognition. On the other hand, we should frankly admit the irrational, luxurious, and health-destroying dietetic habits in which the American people so largely indulge. Besides, the economics and sanitation of the food supply are matters of great importance. There is every reason why our use of food, upon which our physical welfare so fully depends, should be given the same rational consideration that we give to business, education, or any other important relation.

202. Limitations of food standards. — But this does not mean that diet should be regulated by rule or mathematical formulæ; in fact, this is not necessary. In special cases, such as " food cures," the training table and the food supply of institutions, a careful consideration of the composition and combination of foods is wise and even essential to the best or most economical results, but it is fanciful to suppose that the daily eating habits of the great mass of people will be voluntarily brought under scientific regulation. At the same time it is reasonable to hope that through education and the diffusion of certain fundamental principles and facts, a more rational general point of view may be established than now seems to prevail.

The application in a practical way to the dietary of a family of the scientific facts and principles of human nutrition, when the members of the family differ in age, activity, tastes, and food adaptations, is not a simple matter. How shall the housewife meet the situation in a way that is not burdensome? Much will depend upon her equipment of knowledge. If she is well informed as to the general needs of the human body in its various ages and conditions, and understands what nutrients are supplied by the different classes of foods, knowledge that should be imparted to every young woman, she will find no great difficulty in selecting a combination of foods that is nutritively efficient and at the same time is simple and economical. She can at least avoid the gross errors so often observed in the eating habits of many families. There are some general facts that should be kept in mind as a guide to practice.

203. Classes of food. — In order to render clear statements that will be made concerning the regulation of diet, we should at this point gain definite information concerning the food-stuffs from which a diet may be selected.

Food materials are classified in a general way, and without a very definite division between the classes, into watery foods, protein foods, carbohydrate foods, and fatty foods. This does not mean that some food materials contain water and others do not, or that one class consists wholly of protein or carbohydrates or fat. To be sure, the sugars and the starches are wholly carbohydrate, and butter and salad oil practically all fats; but the great bulk of food materials are mixtures of all classes of nutrients, and we use the classifying terms to indicate that a relatively large proportion of water or protein or carbohydrates or fats is present in the dry matter of the class designated by one of these-terms. The real facts are best illustrated by the following table of selected foods arranged by classes. For a fuller knowledge, the full table at end of volume may be consulted.

TABLE XXVIII

CLASSES OF FOOD

Protein Foods

	WATER	ASH	PROTEIN	CARBO-HYDRATES	FATS
	Per Cent	Per Cent	Per Cent	Per Cent	Per Cent
Sirloin steak (free from visible fat) . . .	74.0	1.2	22.1	——	3.1
Round steak (lean) .	70.0	1.1	21.3	——	7.9
Veal, leg, medium fat	70.0	1.2	20.2	——	9.0
Ham (smoked, lean) .	53.5	5.5	19.8	——	20.8
Liver	71.4	1.4	21.3	——	4.5
Chicken (broiler) . .	74.8	1.1	21.5	——	2.5
Codfish (fresh) . .	82.6	1.2	16.5	——	.4
Codfish (fresh) . .	53.5	24.7	24.9	——	0.8
Mackerel (fresh) . .	73.4	1.2	18.7	——	7.1
Lobster	79.2	2.2	16.4	0.4	1.8
Eggs (without shell) .	73.7	1.0	13.4	——	10.5
Cheese (full cream) .	34.2	3.8	25.9	——	33.7
Milk (cow's, average)	87.0	0.7	3.3	5.0	4.0

Carbohydrate Foods

	WATER	ASH	PROTEIN	CARBO-HYDRATES	FATS
	Per Cent	Per Cent	Per Cent	Per Cent	Per Cent
Breakfast foods . .					
White bread . . .	35.3	1.1	9.2	53.1	1.3
Crackers	6.8	1.8	10.7	71,9	8.8
Gingerbread . . .	18.8	2.9	5.8	63.5	9.0
Tapioca pudding . .	64.6	0.8	3.3	28.2	3.2
Potatoes (cooked) .	75.5	1.0	2.5	20.9	0.1
Squash	88.3	0.8	1.4	9.0	0.5
Molasses	25.1	3.2	2.4	69.3	——
Honey	18.2	0.2	0.4	81.2	——
(Sugar cane) . . .	——	——	——	100.0	——
Tapioca	11.4	0.1	0.4	88.0	0.1
Apples	84.6	0.3	0.4	14.2	0.5

Fat Foods

	WATER	ASH	PROTEIN	CARBO-HYDRATES	FATS
Salt pork	7.9	3.9	1.9	——	86.2
Bacon (smoked) . .	18.8	4.4	9.9	——	67.4
Cream	——	——	——	——	
Butter	11.0	3.0	1.0	——	85.0
Salad oil	——	——	——	——	100.0

Watery Foods

	WATER	ASH	PROTEIN	CARBO-HYDRATES	FATS
Asparagus	94.0	0.7	1.8	· 3.3	0.2
Beets	87.5	1.1	1.6	9.7	0.1
Peas	74.6	1.0	7.0	16.9	0.5
Apples	84.6	0.3	0.4	14.2	0.5
Strawberries . . .	90.4	0.7	1.0	7.4	0.6
Beef soup	92.9	1.2	4.4	——	0.4
Consomme	96.0	1.1	2.5	0.4	——
Oysters (edible portion)	86.9	2.0	6.2	3.7	1.2
Milk	87.0	0.7	3.3	5.0	4.0

Dry Foods

	WATER	ASH	PROTEIN	CARBO-HYDRATES	FATS
	Per Cent	Per Cent	Per Cent	Per Cent	Per Cent
Breakfast foods . .					
Crackers (average) .	6.8	1.8	10.7	71.9	8.8
White bread . . .	35.3	1.1	9.2	53.1	1.3
Cookies (molasses) .	6.2	2.2	7.2	75.7	8.7
Zwieback	5.8	1.0	9.8	73.5	9.9
Doughnuts	18.3	0.9	6.7	53.1	21.0
Bacon	20.2	5.1	10.5	——	64.8
Salt pork (fat) . . .	7.9	3.9	1.9	——	86.2
Cheese	34.2	3.8	25.9	——	33.7
Butter	11.0	3.0	1.0	——	85.0

The foregoing are simply illustrations of the types of foods. · There are numerous combinations of the raw food materials which contain the nutrients in a great variety of proportions, such as soups, breads, salads, puddings, pies, and cakes. It is evident, however, that a regulation of diet must be accomplished through selection of the uncooked materials.

204. Facts for guidance. — The housewife who keeps the following facts in mind may combine foods in an approximate way that will fully meet the needs of the human organism of whatever age or condition.

1. Fresh vegetables, fruits, milk, fresh meats, fish, and shellfish contain large percentages of water.

2. Bread, flours and meals, crackers, breakfast foods, pastry (mostly), nuts, dried fruits, cakes, syrups, cured meats, cheese, butter, contain relatively large percentages of dry matter.

3. Animal foods, such as lean meats of all kinds, fish, excepting certain very fat species, shellfish, eggs, cheese, and milk furnish dry matter containing relatively high percentages of protein.

4. Legumes and certain nuts supply relatively more protein than other vegetable foods.

5. The cereal grains, vegetables, and fruits, while containing material percentages of protein, are made up largely of carbohydrates or allied bodies having a similar nutritive function.

6. The unmodified foods, such as grains, vegetables, fruits, meat, eggs, and milk, may be depended upon to supply in kind all the necessary elements to sustain the growth, functions, and wastes of the human body. On the other hand, the foods which it is proper to designate as " artificial " are not only not essential to an adequate diet, but they are those which, when used freely, may render a diet very one-sided or deficient.

7. Certain foods that are manufactured may be entirely devoid of one or more of the classes of nutrients, or have a very one-sided composition. For instance, such materials as corn starch, sago, tapioca, the syrups and sugars, butter, lard, and salad oils contain no ash or protein, excepting that ash elements may be present in the syrups.

8. Foods may be so selected as to give an abundant supply of the mineral ingredients. For instance, the dry substance of certain vegetables like asparagus, lettuce, and spinach, and animal foods such as eggs and beef extract, are relatively rich in iron compounds, just as the dry substance of leguminous seeds, carrots, and some other vege-

tables, milk and cheese is comparatively rich in calcium compounds.

9. Lean meats, milk and its products, flours and meals from the cereal grains, and especially cereal preparations that have been dextrinized through heat or malting, are more easily and more fully digested than the fibrous vegetable foods.

205. Regulation of diet as to quantity of dry matter eaten. — The ordinary measure of food consumption is the bulk of material taken into the stomach. This may be a most inaccurate measurement of the actual nutriment consumed. In estimating a given ration, account must be taken of the amount of dry matter it contains. While water is an essential ingredient of our food, and is abundant in the human body, it is not a

TABLE XXIX

Two Meals of Equal Weight, but greatly Unlike in their Content of Dry Matter

Order No. 1	Wt.	Dry Matter	Order No. 2	Wt.	Dry Matter
	Oz.	Oz.		Oz.	Oz.
Clam chowder . .	8	0.904	Ham	3	1.395
White bread . . .	2	1.294	Potato (boiled) .	4	0.976
Butter	½	0.425	White bread . . .	2	1.294
Strawberries . . .	4	0.584	Butter	1	0.850
Sugar [1]	½	0.500	Apple sauce . . .	4	1.556
Cream [1]	2	0.600	Crackers . . .	1	0.930
Total	17	4.307	Cheese .	1	0.658
			Cream [2] . .	½	0.150
			Sugar	½	0.500
			Total	17	8.309

[1] On strawberries.   [2] In coffee.

tissue-builder in the true sense, neither does it supply energy, so that the determination of food values is based on what is left in an article of diet after the water is eliminated.

It is possible to greatly vary the real supply of nutriment, and at the same time maintain a good degree of uniformity in the bulk or weight of food eaten. This is readily observed in an *à la carte* restaurant where orders like the two on p. 206 are not infrequently noted. These would have the same weight, No. 1 being the more bulky, but they would be greatly unlike in their content of dry matter.

If the above foods were of average composition, Order No. 2 would supply more than twice the dry matter in Order No. 1, although probably less in bulk. This illustrates how easy it is to vary the diet in its essentials, and, at the same time, consume a satisfying bulk of food. Those who feel the necessity of reducing their diet may do so by selecting foods carrying a high proportion of water. In this way, the meal may be made more satisfying than a much smaller bulk of dry food, and at the same time, hold the intake of nutriment to the desired minimum. The free use of soups and fresh vegetables as against meats, cheese, bread, cake, sweets, and similar materials is wise for those persons who have a tendency to overindulgence in eating. On the other hand, men at severe labor, such as wood choppers and " river drivers," are not permanently satisfied with a food supply containing watery food in any large proportion, but demand the old-fashioned diet of pork and beans and flour bread. Invalids receiving liquid preparations such as beef juice,

clam juice, or broths are not as generously nourished
as the bulk of food would indicate to the uninformed.
While such preparations are admirably adapted to the
weak condition of a convalescent and to frequent feeding, the fact that they often contain only from three
to four per cent of dry matter shows a very low food
value.

**206. Regulation of diet with reference to the combina-
tion of nutrients.** — The number of combinations of food
materials that may be devised is almost endless, even of
those that are rational from every point of view.   It is
not the purpose in this connection to give numerous examples of possible approved dietaries, but simply to illustrate
how the principles herein set forth may be applied.   The
following menus for two days are suggested by a practical
dietitian as examples of meals well combined, healthful,
and economical.[1]

No. 1

Breakfast   *Lunch*

Oatmeal   Milk   Sugar   Pea soup   Crackers
        Codfish balls   Macaroni and cheese
   Toast   Butter   Graham bread and butter
        Coffee   Tea   Cookies

Dinner
Mutton stew — dumplings
Riced potatoes, bread and butter
Poor man's rice pudding
Coffee

[1] For a list of raw materials required see pp. 232–233.

No. 2

Breakfast		*Dinner*

Pancakes   Syrup   Corned beef

Tea   Potatoes   Lima beans

Bread   Butter

Bread pudding

Supper

Baked omelet

Creamed potatoes

Toast

Cheese   Milk

In day No. 1 the mutton, codfish, milk and cheese are the distinctively protein foods, and in day No. 2 the proteins are supplied mainly from the corned beef, skimmed milk, eggs and cheese. The carbohydrates are supplied in abundance from the flour, bread, vegetables, and sugar, while the fats are introduced mostly in the meats, cheese, and butter. Such combinations would not be deficient in the ash elements.

The economy of these food combinations, both nutritively and as to money cost, will be discussed later (see pp. 231–234).

207. How an ill-considered diet may fail to meet physiological requirements. — It is not necessary to recount here the number of elements that are necessary to the building and maintenance of the human body, or to review the nutritive functions of the many compounds that are found in human foods, in order to point out possible errors in the selection of food and the ways in which various dangers may be avoided.

P

Experience shows and science corroborates the fact, that the majority of persons, young and mature, are supplied with nutriment sufficient in quantity and kind to meet the needs of their bodies reasonably well. So many kinds of materials are ordinarily supplied to the table that in many families, at least, no physiological need is left unsatisfied. If man's diet included only the various products of the soil and of animal life in an unmodified condition except the cooking, there would doubtless be little danger that any one, however ignorant, would suffer from incomplete nutrition. But human foods are now so largely made up of what may be called "artificial" products, that is, materials so modified by some manufacturing process as to almost wholly lack nutrients of one or more classes, it is easy for a child, or even an adult, to so select his diet on the basis of pleasurable taste as to be badly nourished.

208. Artificial foods. — It is not difficult to illustrate how this may happen by a glance at what occurs in manufacturing certain food materials that are much used in cookery. Wheat flour enters largely into the diet of every family. In producing it the outer coating of the wheat kernel is removed, thus throwing into the milling offals that portion of the kernel that is most heavily charged with the mineral ingredients, particularly phosphorus, potassium, calcium, and magnesium. The proportion of digestible protein in white flour is not less than in whole wheat flour, as is so often claimed. The starches and gums, such as corn-starch, sago, and tapioca, are separated from the other compounds that accompany them in the plants in which they are produced, and as almost pure carbohydrates are extensively used in foods. The sugars in the solid form and in molasses and syrups, of which such immense quantities are consumed in various articles of diet and in candies, are extracted from sugar cane and the sugar beet, and to some extent from the sap of the sugar maple, the accompanying compounds being rejected. Milk fat is divorced from the other compounds of the milk, and in the form of butter is eaten as an almost pure fat. Lard is " rendered " from portions of the pig's carcass, and the salad oils are extracted from olives, cotton-seed, and other sources. These nearly pure forms of the starches, gums, sugars, and fats form a large part of such foods as puddings, sauces, cakes, and various pastries. In fact, many of these articles of diet may properly be considered as concentrations of non-nitrogenous food com-pounds, with the partial elimination of the mineral ingre-dients and the proteins. As such combinations are delight-ful to the taste and tempt the appetite, they are often allowed to form a generous portion of a meal. They are especially attractive to children; and where these are allowed an almost unrestrained choice of food, as is the case in many homes, such articles of diet are a menace to the normal development and vigor of the young, because they are nutritively unbalanced and may easily fail to supply in sufficient abundance the needed elements of growth, and may also fail to furnish to the secretory glands and tissues the compounds and chemical environment best adapted to active metabolism.

209. Two lunches for a boy compared. — Both children and adults are most fully nourished when their diet con-sists mainly of meat, fish, milk, cereals, vegetables, and fruits rather than pastries, cakes, and fancy dishes so

largely sugars, starches, and fats. The foregoing statements may be illustrated by a concrete example. If an
average boy were offered his choice between a lunch of
bread and honey, or even molasses, or one of bread and
milk, he would, without doubt, choose the former. Let
us see whether or not his choice would be wise. It is
estimated that he would eat as follows : —

TABLE XXIX a

BREAD AND HONEY

		DRY MAT- TER	ASH .	PRO- TEIN	CARBO- HY- DRATES	FATS
	Oz.	Oz.	Oz.	Oz.	Oz.	Oz.
White bread	4	2.536	.04	.364	2.084	.048
Honey	3	2.454	.006	.012	2.436	
	7	4.990	.046	.376	4.520	.048

BREAD AND MILK

		DRY MAT- TER	ASH	PRO- TEIN	CARBO- HY- DRATES	FATS
	Oz.	Oz.	Oz.	Oz.	Oz.	Oz.
White bread	4	2.536	.04	.364	2.084	.048
Milk	16	2.080	.112	.528	0.800	.640
	20	4.616	.152	.892	2.884	.688

The nutriment in the two combinations is greatly
different. More than 90 per cent of the dry matter in the
bread and honey consists of carbohydrates and fats, while
in the bread and milk the proportion is about 77 per cent.

The combination of bread and milk has three times the mineral matter, over twice the protein, and as much food energy as is found in the bread and honey. There is no question but the former would more completely supply the complex demands of a growing boy or girl. Those children who are allowed to partake freely of sweets, including candy between meals, may not be expected to develop with maximum vigor. Such foods not only are incomplete in themselves, but they spoil the appetite for the plainer, more nutritious articles of diet. Certainly farm animals could not be developed to their best estate on a system of feeding so irrational, and there is no reason to suppose it is possible with growing children.

CHAPTER XI

THE RELATION OF DIET TO THE VARYING CONDITIONS OF LIFE

THE fact is almost self-evident that, as food supports bodily activity and growth, the necessary amount of nutrition must vary greatly with different classes of persons. It is, therefore, no less important than interesting to understand the relation of age, size, sex, disposition, occupation, and other conditions to nutritive demands. Fortunately, through the use of the respiration calorimeter, considerable reliable data have been secured concerning the influence of these factors.

210. Childhood. — At no period of life is gaseous exchange (food oxidation) so vigorous or so large in proportion to weight as during childhood. Children are peculiarly active, being constantly in motion during their waking hours. It has been found that a child two and one-half years old, weighing 25 pounds uses, when at rest, half as much oxygen as an adult weighing 150 pounds, and nearly three times as much for each unit of weight. This means that the demand for food energy would be in these proportions, which for young children of varying ages is from 2 to 3 times as much per unit of weight as it is for adults.

The following table shows very clearly how age affects metabolic activity: —

TABLE XXX

Oxygen Use per Minute (Energy Requirement) for Persons of Different Ages[1]

Age Yrs.	Weight Kg.	Oxygen consumed, C.C.	Oxygen use per Kg. weight	Relative Value Oxygen Consumption by Boys	
				Per Kg. of weight	Per sq. meter of surface
2½	11.5	112.2	9.76	285	160
6	18.4	139.9	7.61	223	145
9	21.8	148.0	6.79	199	137
14	36.1	188.1	5.21	152	125
17	44.3	212.7	4.80	140	123
22–43 (adults)	66.7	227.9	3.41	100	100

It appears that, whether we consider weight or body surface, the child appropriates more oxygen, that is, gives off more heat per unit of weight or of surface, than either the adult or the aged. Besides, the rapidly developing child stores in his tissues protein and inorganic salts which must come from the food. For these reasons the liberal, and sometimes seemingly excessive, amounts of food eaten by children, especially between the ages of ten and sixteen, are not irrational, and those who dictate school dietaries should keep these facts in mind.

211. Old age. — With advancing years, generally after the age of 70 or 75 is passed, there is a marked decrease in vitality and bodily activity. The demand for food is correspondingly diminished. Von Noorden [2] states, on the basis of exact observations, that the gaseous exchange is

[1] " Metabolism and Practical Medicine," Von Noorden, Vol. I, p. 268.
[2] *Loc. cit.*, p. 267.

found to be about 20 per cent less with old persons than with those in middle life. This refers evidently to the resting condition. There is no definite point at which " old age " begins, and the stage of life at which metabolic activity starts on the down grade varies with different persons.

212. Weight. — The amount of food required to sustain persons in a resting condition increases with their weight, though not proportionately, that is, a heavy man doing no work uses more total food than a light one, but he uses less per pound of weight. The energy demand for 24 hours has varied in experimental observations from 9 calories per pound of body weight with large individuals, to 14 calories with small; but it only requires 30 per cent or 40 per cent increase of energy expenditure when the weight doubles. The energy use is more nearly proportional to body surface.

TABLE XXXI
Effect of Weight on Energy Use

Persons in Absolute Rest			Persons Asleep		
Weight Kg.	Calories in 24 Hr.	Energy used per Kg. of weight in 24 Hr.	Weight Kg.	Calories in 24 Hr.	Energy used per Kg. of weight in 24 Hr.
82.0	1556	19.0	90.4	1773	19.6
73.0	1584	21.7	83.5	1670	20.0
67.5	1621	24.0	76.0	1853	24.4
50.8	1315	25.9	62.5	1431	23.0
48.0	1214	25.6	57.2	1560	27.2
43.2	1333	30.9	55.0	1590	29.0

The above table [1] illustrates clearly the facts that have been stated. One exception should be made to these general statements, viz., that increased weight, due to the laying on of fat, does not cause an increase of total energy used by the resting individual. If the obese person is active or does external work, then he uses more energy because more is required to move the body around.

213. Sex. — There is a belief that men require more food than women; and if this refers only to total food consumption, it is true, because men weigh more generally, are more active physically, and perform more external work. It is not true, however, when we consider only the demands for the maintenance of what may be called physiological activity. Investigation shows that when the oxygen use of men and women of similar weight in a resting condition is compared, the gaseous exchange is practically the same.

TABLE XXXII

ENERGY EXCHANGE (OXYGEN USE) OF MEN AND WOMEN IN RESTING STATE [2]

WOMEN		MEN	
Weight Kg.	Oxygen used per Kg. per minute C.C.	Weight Kg.	Oxygen used per Kg. per minute C.C.
38.5	4.85 ⎫ 4.36	——	——
48.7	4.03 ⎭	43.2	4.53
54.0	3.91	53.4	3.93
61.7	3.79	58.0	3.81
68.0	3.40	66.7	3.42

[1] " Metabolism and Practical Medicine," Von Noorden, Vol. I, pp. 260–261. [2] *Loc. cit.*, p. 270.

Of course, when laboring the additional oxygen consumption is proportional with both sexes to the work performed, and because man is in a general way of higher muscular development than woman, he uses a much larger total energy. It has been claimed that trained muscles, even when not in use, have greater metabolic activity than the untrained. The similarity of oxygen use, per unit of weight, by the two sexes does not sustain this conclusion.

214. Disposition. — The temperament of an individual has much to do with his food requirements. Persons of a sanguine type, being more active, use more energy than the phlegmatic. Bodily movement, whether deliberate, or due to nervous activity, constitutes work, and must be sustained by an equivalent of energy derived either from food or body substance.

215. Work. — All activity of the human body, whether in the maintenance of its functions or in the performance of labor, is work. The forcing of the blood through the arteries and veins, the digestion of food and its assimilation, we speak of as *internal* work, while walking, running, lifting, the use of tools, the moving about of various objects, and other forms of visible physical activity are designated as *external* work. The two forms of work may also be classified as *physiological* and *mechanical*. Nothing in nutrition is more important than the relation of food to work. This is true, not only because a larger proportion of the nutriment we take is expended in sustaining our external activities, but because we should understand the conditions bringing about an unnecessary expenditure of food energy. Indeed, outside of the storage of body substance, which amounts to but little except in the case of the young, all food energy goes to sustain work, either physiological or mechanical. In this connection, it is proposed to discuss only the relations of food to *mechanical work*.

216. Increased use of oxygen from work. — No one can have failed to notice that physical exertion, especially if it is quite severe, is attended with more rapid breathing, a quicker pulse, and in warm weather a flushed face and abundant perspiration. An interesting table which has been compiled from data given by Benedict and Carpenter[1] shows the relation of pulse-beat to heat production and carbon-dioxid elimination : —

TABLE XXXIII

INCREASED CARBON DIOXID	INCREASED HEAT PRODUCTION	INCREASED PULSE BEAT
Per Cent	Per Cent	Per Cent
38.9	52.0	35.7
8.9	10.2	16.1
29.0	31.2	19.6
49.2	53.0	22.9
37.9	34.5	12.9
13.0	13.1	21.1
30.0	38.0	25.0

There is an entirely rational explanation for these phenomena. Increased work requires an increased expenditure of energy, that is, an increased use of oxygen for

[1] " Metabolism and Energy Transformations of Healthy Man during Rest," p. 250.

developing the potential energy of the absorbed food.   As heat is the final or waste product of muscular energy, an increase of mechanical work performed by the muscles causes an increase of heat, which must be radiated from the body.   The relation of muscular exercise to the use of oxygen and heat production is made clear by the following table [1] (Sitting = 100) : —

TABLE XXXIV

Effect of Muscular Exercise on Energy Use

	Carbon Dioxid Eliminated	Oxygen Absorbed	Heat Produced
	Per Cent	Per Cent	Per Cent
Man at rest, sleeping	70	79	73
Man at rest, awake, sitting . .	100	100	100
Man at rest, standing	112	116	117
Man at severe muscular exercise .	746	786	673

Above eight times more oxygen is used, and seven times more heat evolved during heavy work than during rest.

217. Increased respiration and blood flow. — For these reasons, there occurs more frequent respiration and a more rapid passage of the blood through the lungs where it comes in contact with the respired air.   Still further, the blood is more fully thrown to the surface of the body where it may cool more rapidly, and perspiration also occurs in order that its evaporation may aid in ridding the body of the excess of heat (see p. 168).   All this means more food, somewhat in proportion to the work done, the

[1] *Loc. cit.*, p. 252.

energy of which is expended not only to carry on external work, but also in part to support the work attending the increase of breathing and blood flow. More external work causes more physiological or internal work.

Additional data may be cited to support the above statements. In the case of two men, it was found that in climbing up a steep incline the inspired air increased not less than five times in volume over the use when resting. When a person is walking rapidly or cycling, the number of respirations per minute is at least doubled, and the depth of respiration is increased several times, so that the volume of each breath becomes greater than under rest conditions. Even the work of dressing and undressing, with the attendant influence of a period of nakedness, caused in twenty-one observations an average increase in oxygen use of 34 per cent and an increase in heat radiation of 18 per cent.[1]

218. Fuel efficiency with man. — Measurements of the oxygen consumption under various conditions show that one foot-pound increase of mechanical labor costs in extra food energy approximately the equivalent of three foot-pounds of food energy, that is, the factor of efficiency of human food as fuel is about 33 per cent.[2] This shows that the living human machine is relatively a most efficient one. Practically the same factor holds for work animals.

219. How fuel efficiency is modified. — Several conditions materially modify this factor of efficiency. When a

[1] " Metabolism and Energy Transformations of Healthy Man during Rest," Benedict and Carpenter, p. 247.

[2] Benedict and Carpenter calculate the factor of efficiency to be 20.9 per cent, that is, that proportion of excess food energy above maintenance is realized in labor performed.

person takes up mechanical operations with which he is not familiar, or enters upon work that exercises a new set of muscles, a unit of work accomplished costs more in food energy than is the case with operatives whose muscles are trained to do a particular thing. Trained workmen will do a given amount of labor on less food than the untrained. Very strenuous exercise, like athletic contests, is wasteful of food energy. The general rule is that the energy cost of a unit of work increases with the rate of work above what would be the natural movement. The figures of the table on the following page show this.

Unnaturally slow movements also are expensive of energy. After a continuance of the same labor for hours, there is an increase in the energy expenditure per unit of work performed, and fatigue, whether it comes after a shorter or longer time, has a similar effect.

Economy in the use of the energy that the food supplies to the body, which is equivalent to economy in the use of the body itself, is most fully secured when the movements in labor are at the natural rate, neither hurried nor restrained, and when periods of intense effort do not occur, and when labor is not too long continued and is not carried to the point of extreme fatigue. In considering the general nature of the diet for sustaining work, it should be remembered that the non-nitrogenous constituents of the food, the carbohydrates and fats, furnish the main supply of energy (see pp. 156, 171).

220. Obesity. — Obesity, or the excessive accumulation of body fat, is an occasion of great discomfort to many persons. The intense desire of the excessively corpulent to be freed from this condition has opened the way for the

TABLE XXXV

ENERGY AND FOOD REQUIREMENTS OF A MAN (70 KILOGRAMS WEIGHT WITH CLOTHING) FOR DIFFERENT KINDS OF MUSCULAR WORK [1]

MUSCULAR WORK PER HOUR	ENERGY EXPENDITURE PER UNIT OF WORK	INCREASE OF METABOLISM DURING ONE HOUR'S WORK	
		Cal.	Gms. Fat used up
3.6 kilometers over level road .	40.3 per km.	144	16
6.0 kilometers over level road .	47.2 per km.	283	30
8.4 kilometers over level road .	78.6 per km.	660	70
6.0 kilometers over level road, with 25 kilogram load . . .	64.1 per km.	385	41
4.8 kilometers over level road with 25 kilogram load . . .	59.3 per km.	285	30
Climbing 300 meters (30 per cent gradient; easy climb) . . .	49.0 per 100 m.	147	16
Climbing 300 meters, stiff climb (over 30 per cent)	58.0 per 100 m.	174	18
Ascent of stair — 300 meters in a distance of 3000 meters— 10 per cent rise	89.0 per 100 m.	267	28
9 kilometers cycle ride on level road	20.3 per km.	183	19
15 kilometers cycle ride on level road	20.8 per km.	313	33
22 kilometers cycle ride on level road	25.9 per km.	571	60
9 kilometers cycle ride with 3 per cent ascent	38.3 per km.	345	36
15 kilometers cycle ride on level road, with a head-wind of 10 meters per second . . .	40.1 per km.	601	64

[1] "Metabolism and Practical Medicine," Von Noorden, Vol. I, p. 229.

sale of " fat cures " that mostly deplete the store of cash rather than of adipose tissue.

It seems reasonably certain that in a large percentage of cases the cause and cure of obesity are entirely within the control of the afflicted individual. With many obese persons, perhaps a majority, the laying on of excessive fat is the result of a disparity between the food consumed and the energy expenditure. In other words, certain individuals, especially men in the professions not requiring physical activity and those doing office work at a desk, eat more than is needed to sustain the energy expenditure. It is noticeable that when an individual becomes less active without diminishing his food he grows fatter, and the same occurs with an increase of food without a corresponding increase in the physical activity.

The remedy for obesity with individuals whose metabolism is normal is either less food or more exercise. A reduction in the food taken may require a rigorous control of appetite, especially at first, but after a time the eating habit will probably become readjusted. A material increase in physical exercise will accomplish the same result as a decrease of the food taken.

It does not now seem possible to explain all cases of corpulency on the basis of overeating or deficient physical exercise. These instances where very corpulent persons maintain their weight without loss on an amount of food less than the customary requirement for such individuals, laying on of fat by animals on which castration or ovariotomy has been performed, and the influence of life conditions with women, seem to indicate a modified metabolism.

Studies of such cases of obesity have so far failed to establish the fact of abnormal life processes, for the use of oxygen (energy exchange), protein metabolism, and digestion appear to have been normal. An explanation of all cases of obesity does not seem to have been reached.

CHAPTER XII

FOOD ECONOMICS

A. Regulation of Diet with Reference to Economy of Expenditure

THE cost of a meal for an individual or a family is made up of two main factors: the money cost of the raw food materials, and the time and other expense required for preparing and serving the food. In both these directions considerations of economy seem to have very little weight with the average American family as compared with either sensuous desire or habits that are determined by custom and social demands. Well-to-do Americans extravagantly satisfy epicurean tastes, and their menus, when rationally judged, are seen to be more luxurious and wasteful than almost any other department of family expenditure. Even families of the middle class that, because of moderate means, feel the necessity of practicing rigid economy in dress, house furnishing, 'education, reading matter, and social life are often extravagant in the purchase of table supplies, though ignorantly so, perhaps. The fact is, we are so accustomed to certain eating habits that we do not realize how unnecessarily expensive they are.

221. The cost of raw food materials. — The proper basis for estimating the relative cost of nutriment in the various raw materials is the amount of energy that may be bought in the edible food solids of different materials for a unit sum of money. Many articles of food as purchased are made up in part of substance that is not edible, as, for instance, the bones and legs of a dressed fowl, the skin and bones of a fish, or the paring and core of an apple. All raw food materials, with very few exceptions, contain water varying in proportion from 5 per cent or less to over 90 per cent. Both the refuse and water must be subtracted from the total weight in order to learn the weight of edible solids. The following table shows that a pound of bluefish as purchased was made up of .486 pound of refuse, .403 pound of water in the edible portion, and .111 pound of edible solids, this amount of solids having a food energy equal to 210 calories. At 18 cents a pound for the fish as purchased, one dollar would buy only .61 pound of edible food solids. In comparison with this, wheat flour has no refuse, and in one pound only .128 pound of water, leaving .872 pound of edible solids, containing energy equal to 1640 calories. At 3.4 cents per pound for the flour, one dollar would purchase 25.6 pounds of edible solids as against .61 pound in the bluefish. This means that at the prices given one dollar will purchase about forty-two times as much edible food solids in wheat flour as in bluefish. But a comparison on the basis of the weights of edible solids purchased for a unit sum of money is inaccurate and misleading, because the energy value of the edible solids in different foods is greatly unlike. The water-free edible nutrients of bacon, for instance, would furnish over 90 per cent more energy from a unit weight than would the nutrients of wheat flour. For this reason our comparison must be made on the basis of the energy purchased in the edible food for one dollar. For blue-fish this would be 1166 calories and for wheat flour 48,230 calories.

The table which follows has been made up from the analyses and energy values given in the revised edition of Bulletin 28, O.E.S., U. S. Department of Agriculture, and the prices are those at which foodstuffs were sold in the city of Geneva, N. Y., during July, 1910. Food prices vary from year to year and in different localities, but the figures given indicate in a general way the cost of nutriment from the several classes of foods.

TABLE XXXVI

COST OF NUTRIENTS IN VARIOUS HUMAN FOODSTUFFS

NAME	POUND PRICE	REFUSE IN ONE POUND	WATER IN ONE POUND OF EDIBLE PORTION	EDIBLE SOLIDS IN ONE POUND	EDIBLE SOLIDS FOR $1.00	FOOD ENERGY FOR $1.00
	Cents	Pounds	Pounds	Pounds	Pounds	Calories
Corn meal	3.0	——	0.125	0.875	29.17	55,166
Wheat flour	3.4	——	0.128	0.872	25.65	48,230
Rolled oats(in bulk)	5.0	——	0.077	0.923	18.46	37,000
Hominy	5.0	——	0.118	0.882	17.64	33,000
Sugar	6.0	——	——	1.00	16.66	31,000
Molasses (can)	5.0	——	0.251	0.749	14.96	25,800
Lard	18.0	——	——	1.00	5.55	23,444
White bread	5.33	——	0.353	0.647	12.13	22,790
Cookies	10.0	——	0.081	0.919	9.19	19,100
Crackers	11.0	——	0.068	0.932	8.48	17,320
Pork (fat)	18.0	0.081	0.159	0.760	4.25	16,390
Corning beef (cheap)	8.0	0.055	0.561	0.384	4.80	14,815
Coffee cake	14.0	——	0.213	0.787	5.62	11,609
Butter	32.0	——	0.110	0.890	2.78	11,265
Mutton chops	14.0	0.148	0.404	0.448	3.20	11,250
Cheese, full cream	18.0	——	0.342	0.658	3.65	10,833
Bacon	25.0	0.087	0.184	0.729	2.54	10,732
Milk	3.67	——	0.870	0.130	3.54	8,855
Ham, fresh	18.0	0.103	0.451	0.446	2.48	8,444
Grapes	4.0	0.250	0.58	0.170	4.25	8,375

Cost of Nutrients in Various Human Foodstuffs — Continued

Name	Pound Price	Refuse in One Pound	Water in One Pound of Edible Portion	Edible Solids in One Pound	Edible Solids for $1.00	Food Energy for $1.00
	Cents	Pounds	Pounds	Pounds	Pounds	Calories
Ham, smoked	22.0	0.122	0.358	0.520	2.36	7,600
Pork, roast	18.0	0.193	0.408	0.399	2.22	7,444
Plums	5.0	0.05	0.745	0.205	4.10	7,400
Corning beef, good	18.0	0.055	0.561	0.384	2.13	6,583
Rib roast, beef	20.0	0.201	0.453	0.346	1.73	5,550
Apples	4.0	0.250	0.633	0.117	2.92	5,500
Lamb chops	25.0	0.148	0.453	0.399	1.60	5,260
Steak, round	20.0	0.072	0.607	0.321	1.60	4,475
Steak, porterhouse	25.0	0.127	0.524	0.349	1.40	4,440
Eggs	17.0	0.112	0.655	0.233	1.37	3,735
Corn, green, canned	12.5	—	0.761	0.239	1.91	3,640
Fish, salt	15.0	0.016	0.548	0.436	2.90	3,635
Turkey	30.0	0.227	0.424	0.349	1.16	3,585
Tongue, beef	16.0	0.265	0.518	0.217	1.36	3,406
Chicken, canned	50.0	—	0.469	0.531	1.06	3,310
Ham, deviled	60.0	—	0.441	0.559	0.93	2,983
Tomatoes, canned	4.0	—	0.940	0.060	1.50	2,625
Halibut	18.0	0.177	0.619	0.204	1.13	2,611
Fowls	30.0	0.259	0.471	0.270	0.90	2,583
Liver	25.0	—	0.714	0.286	1.14	2,460
Trout (lake)	18.0	0.485	0.366	0.149	0.83	2,139
Raspberries	15.0	—	0.840	0.160	1.07	2,066
Oranges	8.33	0.270	0.634	0.096	1.15	2,041
Mackerel	18.0	0.447	0.404	0.149	0.83	2,027
White fish	18.0	0.535	0.325	0.140	0.78	1,805
Peas, green, canned	15.0	—	0.853	0.147	0.98	1,700
Oysters	15.0	—	0.883	0.117	.580	1,533
Strawberries	12.5	0.05	0.859	0.091	0.73	1,400
Bluefish	18.0	0.486	0.403	0.111	0.61	1,166
Chicken, broilers	50.0	0.446	0.437	0.147	0.29	590
Beans, string, canned	16.5	—	0.937	0.063	0.38	575
Lobster, whole	35.0	0.617	0.307	0.076	0.22	400

222. Cheap and costly foods. — This table reveals several interesting and important facts. It is emphatically true that at present prices the products of plant growth, such as flours, meals, rolled oats, hominy, and sugar are by far the cheapest source of nutrition. Among animal foods pork and dairy products supply the cheapest nutriment, excepting possibly mutton. While the public might concede the relative cheapness of pork products, the general impression appears to be that milk, butter, and cheese are comparatively expensive, which is not true at the present time. The most costly foods of plant origin as a source of energy are certain fresh and canned vegetables and some fruits, including string beans, peas, tomatoes, strawberries, and raspberries. It should be recognized, of course, that fruits and vegetables are healthful foods, and are an essential part of well-regulated dietaries, but it is well for those who must economize to know that they are comparatively costly fuel. As their use safeguards health, they have a value not accounted for on the fuel basis. The costly animal foods are fish and shellfish. The common meats like beefsteak of various kinds, lamb chops, and beef and lamb roasts occupy a middle ground among animal foods as to expensiveness, not differing greatly from eggs and poultry. The table shows clearly that the cheapest diet is the one into which cereal grain foods enter most largely, also that the cost of living is increased when fish, shellfish, and chicken broilers take the place of dairy products and the ordinary meats. In the matter of economy the vegetarian who makes a free use of cereal products has a great advantage over the meat eater, but whether he has other advantages will be discussed elsewhere. Fruits, however healthful they may be, excepting possibly grapes and plums, furnish comparatively high cost nutrition. Of course prices are not fixed, and as they change the relative expensiveness of foods changes.

One or two points are worthy of special notice. From the standpoint of food value, white bread is more than twice as costly as the wheat flour that is used to make it. A barrel of flour, 196 pounds, will make on the average about 315 five-cent loaves of bread. The bread costs the consumer $15.75, whereas the flour can be bought at the time of writing for $6.50. For some years the sale of skimmed milk has been prohibited in the city of New York. When sold at two cents per quart, it supplies nutrients twice as cheaply as whole milk at six cents per quart.

Notable examples of luxurious living are the payment of $.50 to $.75 per pound for butter of an especially high flavor when good creamery butter may be bought for $.30 or $.35, the purchase at high prices of the first fruits and vegetables that come into the spring market, or the purchase of anything at an unusual price simply because it excels in flavor or appearance. Such expenditures mean the payment of a heavy tribute to appetite. Exquisite flavor may serve to excite a desire for food, may even overstimulate appetite, but only to that extent is it a nutritive asset.

223. Cheap and costly meals. — There has previously been given (see p. 209) examples of food combinations that were presented as types of an efficient and economical diet. The meals suggested are simple according to present standards of living but are much more elaborate than the diet upon which countless numbers of men and women have been well nourished. The table which follows gives the quantities of raw materials which these menus would require to feed a family of six persons for one day, and there is also shown the actual nutriment supplied with its cost : —

TABLE XXXVII

No. 1

A DAY'S SUPPLY OF FOOD FOR A FAMILY OF SIX PERSONS

(See menu, p. 208)

MATERIALS	PROTEIN	FAT	CARBO-HYDRATES	COST
Oz.	Oz.	Oz.	Oz.	
4 Rolled oats	0.64	0.29	2.70	$0.025
8 Flour (Graham)	1.06	0.176	5.71	0.017
8 Flour (white)	0.89	0.08	6.00	0.017
40 Lean mutton	5.72	5.24	——	0.250
34 Milk	1.12	1.36	1.70	0.080
12 Butter	0.16	10.20	——	0.240
48 Potatoes	0.864	0.048	7.06	0.060
4 Rice	0.32	0.012	3.16	0.025
4 Macaroni	0.536	0.036	2.96	0.040
4 Cheese	1.036	1.348	0.01	0.050
8 Sugar	——	——	0.50	0.030
8 Crackers	0.880	0.680	5.69	0.055
40 Bread	3.68	0.520	21.23	0.120
4½ Codfish	1.10	0.012	——	0.040
16 Peas	3.94	0.160	9.92	0.075
Tea	——	——	——	0.005
Coffee	——	——	——	0.010
	20.86	20.16	66.14	$1.14
Grams per person	98.5	98.2	312.5	——
Calories per person	——	——	——	2570
Cost per person for one day	——	——	——	$0.19

No. 2

A Day's Supply of Food for a Family of Six Persons

(See menu, p. 209)

MATERIALS	PROTEIN	FATS	CARBO-HYDRATES	COST
Oz.	Oz.	Oz.	Oz.	
40 Corned beef	6.19	9.52	——	$0.30
32 Flour	3.58	0.32	24.00	0.068
32 Potato	0.57	——	4.74	0.04
8 Lima beans	1.45	0.12	5.27	0.05
64 Skimmed milk	2.18	0.49	3.26	0.08
12 Eggs	1.43	1.12	——	0.16
32 Bread	2.94	0.42	17.00	0.08
8 Butter	——	6.80	——	0.15
5⅔ Cheese	1.38	1.79	——	0.06
8 Sugar	——	——	8.00	0.005
	19.72	25.58	62.27	$0.993
Grams per person	98.18	97.2	294.2	——
Calories per person . . .	——	——	——	2492
Cost per person for one day	——	——	——	$0.165

The above are examples of materials sufficient for eighteen meals for one person that are simple in character, easy to prepare, nutritious and inexpensive. Such a diet would support an average-sized person at moderate labor and is greatly abundant for professional men or those doing office work. Many similar food combinations could be arranged, equally nutritious and economical.

It is possible to criticize the food supply in these two menus on the ground that it lacks both fruit and succulent vegetables. While the healthfulness of fresh fruit and vegetables must be conceded, and when the family means justify it, they should be included in the dietetic scheme, it is also indisputable that they do not furnish economical nutrition. Limited means predicate their limited use, especially when they must be bought in a city market.

In contrast to the foregoing examples of simple and inexpensive diet are the two following dinner menus, one of which is much more elaborate than the other : —

Dinner No. 1	*Dinner No. 2*
Oysters on half-shell	Clear soup
Clear soup	Baked bluefish
Broiled chicken	Mashed potatoes
Mashed potatoes Turnip	Cucumber and tomato salad
Celery Cranberry jelly	Saltines
Lettuce salad	Sliced fruit Cookies
Saltines	Coffee
Chocolate ice cream	
Cake Coffee	
Cheese Crackers	
Salted nuts	

It is estimated by an experienced dietitian that approximately the following supply of raw materials would be needed for the two dinners, the cost of which is given in Table XXXVIII. Reference to Table XXXVI shows that these dinners are made up of raw materials that in most instances are costly in proportion to the nutriment they supply. In addition to this the number of courses, especially in No. 1, requires a great variety of raw materials, and the labor of preparation and serving is correspondingly large. Such meals are consistent only with the possession of generous means, unless the expenditures of the family are to be unwisely distributed among its real needs.

TABLE XXXVIII

Two Dinners Compared

Dinner No. 1 *for Six Persons*		*Dinner No. 2* *for Six Persons*	
MATERIALS	COST	MATERIALS	COST
18 Oysters	$0.30	1 lb. Beef shank . .	$0.15
1 lb. Beef shank . . .	0.15	Seasoning	0.05
Seasoning	0.05	2 Eggs	0.04
3 Eggs	0.06	4 lb. Bluefish . . .	0.72
12 Crackers, saltines .	0.03	2½ lb. Potatoes . . .	0.05
4½ lb. Chicken . . .	1.35	2 Cucumbers . . .	0.10
2 lb. Potatoes . . .	0.04	3 Tomatoes	0.06
2 lb. Turnip	0.04	1 head Lettuce . . .	0.05
1 bunch Celery . . .	0.10	½ lb. Malagas . . .	0.10
1 pint Cranberries . .	0.05	3 Oranges	0.10
1 head Lettuce . . .	0.10	¼ lb. Coffee	0.08
1 qt. Thin Cream . .	0.30	½ lb. Butter	0.16
⅛ lb. Chocolate . . .	0.05	½ lb. Bread	0.03
2 lb. Sugar	0.12	¾ lb. Sugar	0.045
2 lb. Salt (Freezing) .	0.04	½ lb. Flour	0.017
¼ lb. Coffee	0.08	¼ lb. Cream	0.05
¼ lb. Cheese	0.05	12 Saltines	0.03
½ lb. Nuts	0.10		$1.832
½ lb. Flour	0.017	Cost per person . .	0.305
Baking powder . . .	0.01		
3 oz. Salad oil . . .	0.09		
2 oz. Vinegar	0.02		
¾ lb. Butter	0.24		
¼ lb. Bread	0.015		
	$3.402		
Cost per person . .	0.58		

It seems that, for dinner No. 1, it would take twenty-six kinds of raw material, and for dinner No. 2, eighteen kinds. The cost per person for the raw materials of dinner No. 1 would be $0.58 and for dinner No. 2 $0.305. The one meal is nearly twice as expensive as the other, not reckoning

the extra labor of preparing. The contrast with two days'
simple diet previously given, where cost of the raw materials
per person for one day was $0.17 and $0.19, is still more
marked, with no disadvantage in the simple fare as to
nutritive efficiency and a probable advantage as to health.

224. Rational food selection. — Several objections may
be raised to gauging the values of human food by the number of calories bought for one dollar. In the first place,
it may be said that the edible solids of one food are greatly
unlike those of another food and may be more important
in the animal economy, as, for instance, beefsteak has more
protein than wheat flour, and will go farther in sustaining
tissue growth or repairing tissue waste. This is granted,
but it is still held that cheese or milk is a cheaper source of
protein than fresh fish, oysters, lobster, or broiler chickens,
and that the necessary protein supply may be selected with
reference to economy. It may be urged with truth, too,
that with adults food is very largely used to furnish energy,
and may consist chiefly of non-nitrogenous materials, and
that energy from wheat flour is as efficient, if not more so,
and costs greatly less, when it comes from this source rather
than from lake trout or green string beans. Other objections to these mathematical measurements of food values
are that we should not be confined to a few articles of diet
simply because they are cheap, that we should consider
the enjoyment of eating as well as the economy, that
individual tastes differ, that some persons cannot digest
certain foods with comfort, and that health demands a
variety in the diet, including vegetables and fruit which
are comparatively costly. These are facts that should be
admitted, but they are not necessarily obstacles to the

practice of economy in selecting food. There is a sufficient variety of the desirable and less costly materials to satisfy fully the demands of a normal appetite, individual idiosyncrasies, or the requirements of good health. Moreover, it is not rational for families of moderate means to indulge in table luxuries on a par with rich dress fabrics, Turkish rugs, or expensive furniture. Good judgment calls for restraint of table indulgence as much as of the desire for social display.

It is admitted that a variety of food is essential to the best dietetic results, and that the table cannot be wholly supplied with the cheaper materials. It is necessary to use some foods that are comparatively costly. This does not annul the fact, however, that the palatableness and nutritive effectiveness of two dietaries may be entirely out of proportion to their cost, due wholly to a wiser selection of raw materials in one case than in the other. At the same time, the writer disclaims any sympathy with those extremists who point out the low relative cost of cuts of beef from the neck of the carcass as showing how cheaply a family may secure a meat supply, or who set forth dietary plans based wholly on the cheapest materials that can be selected. These devices are consistent with poverty, but do not meet the real needs of fairly well-to-do families.

B. Other Factors in the High Cost of Living

There come every now and then periods of popular discussion and even extensive complaint over what is believed to be the excessive cost of food products. Various causes are suggested as the real explanation of what, for a time at least, is regarded as an oppressive condition. Tariff

laws, trusts, excessive profits to transportation companies
and the retail trade are all points of attack by those who
seek to place the responsibility entirely outside of the business and domestic management of the consumer.   These
complaints come largely from those families that are sup-
ported by daily wages earned in manufacturing and commercial establishments.   It is often asserted by these wage
earners that their compensation is insufficient to meet
reasonable living expenses.   Whatever may be the facts as
to this claim, a generous share of the cost of food is due to
factors for which the family is itself responsible.   It is
fully as important for families of moderate means to understand how to expend money for life's necessities as to be
able to increase their earnings.   The relation of the cost
of foods to their nutritive value has been discussed elsewhere (pp. 226–231).   There is much unwise buying of
foods that, nutritively speaking, are very expensive, as has
been shown.

225. Cost of distribution of foods. — Another consideration of importance is what may be called the business
management of the food supply.   The cost of prepared
food as it reaches the table includes two general items:
viz., the money paid for the raw materials and the value
of the time and fuel used in preparing and cooking them.
Raw food materials may be purchased in two general ways:
in supplies sufficient for weeks or months, or in daily or
weekly small quantities.   The latter method, which is
the one generally adopted, and perhaps necessarily by
some families, imposes upon the consumer a heavy expense
for distribution.   The cost to the groceryman for deliver-
ing potatoes and apples by the four quarts or peck, beets

by the dozen, cabbages by the head, flour and sugar in lots of a few pounds, is heavy, and the consumer pays the bill.

In his report for 1910 the Secretary of Agriculture says that " the distribution of farm products from the farm to the consumer is elaborately organized, considerably involved and complicated, and burdened with costly features." On the basis of elaborate inquiry by his Department and by the Industrial Commission, the following increases in prices from the producer to the consumer were found to exist : —

TABLE XXXIX

COST OF DISTRIBUTING FOOD PRODUCTS TO THE CONSUMER

	PAID THE PRODUCER	PAID BY THE CONSUMER
Apples	100	190.5 by barrel
Beef [1]	100	138.0
Butter	100	115.8 prints
Cabbage	100	235.3 by head
Milk	100	200.8 by quart
Onions	100	183.4 by pound
Oranges	100	500.4 by dozen
Potatoes	100	180.5 by bushel
Poultry	100	188.8 by pound

	Apples	Cattle	Butter	Grains	Milk	Potatoes
Freight charges [2]	13.6%	2.5%	.9%	7.7%	18%	14.8%

It is clear that there is a good opportunity through the application of good business methods to lessen these differences.

[1] Price paid slaughter houses.   [2] Per cent of price paid producer.

226. Economy in buying food. — A large proportion of homes have storage space where it is possible to hold flour, sugar, vegetables, and fruits in good condition. When this is the case, the families of large villages and small cities, even of large cities, may safely arrange to buy directly from the producer in barrel or bushel lots a winter's supply of potatoes, apples, beets, carrots, and turnips. Flour may be bought by the barrel. Canned goods are cheaper by the case than when sold in single packages. Certain perishable articles like milk are necessarily taken in daily supply. Where refrigerator space is available, a two weeks' supply of butter will keep in good condition. Several families might unite to great advantage in buying supplies. No money can be invested at a higher rate of interest than purchasing certain food materials in considerable bulk.

227. Outside preparation expensive. — Again, the cash expense of supporting a family is greatly increased through the transfer to outside hands of much of the cooking that was formerly done in the home. Breakfast foods ready for the table instead of the cheaper corn meal, oatmeal, and hominy, that were cooked at home, bread, cake, and other pastry at more than twice the cost of the raw materials, prepared meats and other articles requiring the minimum of home labor, greatly increase the cash expense. It may be argued that cooked food is cheaper than hired help and is even a necessity where help cannot be obtained. Certainly the groceryman and the baker contribute to the ease and comfort of housekeeping, but these purveyors of prepared food must be paid for their services, and heavy cash payments are in this way substituted for home labor.

Many families do not realize how much is paid for the distribution and preparation of food before it comes into the house. One remedy is to buy more largely from the producer. It cannot justly be claimed that the prices he now receives yield him an undue profit. The other remedy is home preparation of food, when this is reasonably possible.

C. The Cost of Preparing and Serving Food

228. Elaborate meals burdensome. — All housewives recognize that cooking and serving three meals a day, with the accompanying dish washing, is a heavy household burden. In the homes of the wealthy where elaborate menus of several courses are served, for luncheon and dinner at least, additional service is a necessity, and the attendant expense is large, to say nothing of the increase of troubles and perplexities that surround the servant problem. In the homes of working people, where the limited income will not permit hired help, the wife and mother often regards it as necessary to spend many weary hours in cooking and serving a great variety of dishes, especially cakes, pies, and puddings.

229. A simple diet abundantly nutritious. — It is not claimed, and it is not true, that the nutritive value of a given amount of food materials is increased by serving them in a great variety of forms. This is done merely to offer to the sense of taste preparations that are delectable. It cannot reasonably be claimed, either, that beyond a certain limit the purchase of many kinds of raw food materials promotes nutritive efficiency. A simple diet involving a minimum of time and expense for preparation

R

and serving may be just as nutritious as a complex one, and is likely to be more healthful (see pp. 231–236). A noon lunch of a rich vegetable soup containing milk or meat products, with bread, butter, and fruit is abundantly nutritious and much less expensive than a series of dishes beginning with bouillon and ending with pastry and other delicacies. The writer recalls a luncheon in the home of a gentleman of wealth and prominence that consisted solely of a large peach pudding, with cream. A dinner of a meat course, not over one vegetable, possibly a salad, potatoes, bread and butter, and a simple dessert, meets all the requirements of health and imposes much less burden on the family than a meal with the approved sequence of courses. Indeed, the usual dessert could be omitted with no loss to the physical welfare of the family, for desserts are dictated by habit rather than by physiological demands. As a matter of fact, breakfasts, luncheons, and suppers often may advantageously consist of not over two or three articles of food.

230. Examples of simple living. — Examples may be cited in great number where, in newly settled countries, the kinds of raw food materials being very limited in number, families have been well nourished and children have developed into fine physical types of men and women. It is known on good authority that in the early days a New England family, whose children became men and women of long lives and great endurance, was limited many times during the winter months to as few foods as bean samp, corn bread, and salt pork. Such narrow limitations may not be wholly desirable, but they show the possibilities of a simple diet. Wood choppers and river

drivers have endured severe labor from October 1 to May 1
chiefly on baked beans and flour biscuit, the beans carrying a generous proportion of fat from salt pork. When it
is possible for one or two articles of diet to supply the nutrients essential to the needs of the human body, it is not necessary to add others, excepting as a variety of food promotes
a continuance of good appetite. The apparent demand for
an elaborate diet is the result of education, and if simpler
living were the fashion, there would be no loss of good
appetite, and there would be a certain decrease in household
expenses with a probable gain in good health. It is unfortunate, to say the least, that with so many opportunities for useful activity and real enjoyment, the lives of
men and women should be burdened with the unnecessary
labor caused by irrational dietetic habits.

D. THE RELATION OF FOOD ECONOMICS TO SOCIAL WELFARE

The continued existence of a strong and highly civilized
people is insured only when certain fundamental conditions prevail. A virile nation is one whose citizens are of
a good physical type, which means that they are well
nourished. A well-fed people, other conditions being
favorable, is a strong people. Food is the physical basis,
not only of individual activity, but also of social energy.
Any causes, therefore, which limit the food supply or increase the burden of securing adequate nourishment
strike a blow at a nation's vital powers. It is for these
reasons that thoughtful men are solicitous concerning the
conservation of the fertility of our soil. By just so much

as the crop-producing capacity of this nation is diminished
will its endurance and power be lessened.   But the conservation of the food supply involves, not only the preservation of the means of producing it, but also the economical
use of that which is produced.

231. Enormous food waste. — In recent times there
has been a widespread discussion over the cost of living,
and many have attributed the advance in the prices of
food materials to their wasteful use.   While doubtless
several factors are involved in the situation, the enormous
waste of food in the United States is not to be doubted.
This comes about through careless servants, ignorant
methods of preparation in the family kitchen, unskillful
cooking, and especially from the very large proportion of
refuse, originating in high-class raw material, that goes
out from boarding houses and hotels.   It is probably not
an exaggeration to claim that the people of this nation
waste enough raw food materials to properly feed half
their number.   If our raw foods were economically utilized
and this waste was stopped, we could export more wheat
and meat or other products, and the means saved could be
turned to useful ends.

232. Expensive service and equipment. — Moreover,
a generous part of our population lives under certain conditions at an expense that is a great drain upon individual
and social energy.   A simple breakfast, at a high-class
hotel, of fruit, cereal, eggs, potato, and bread and butter,
together with a ten-cent fee to the waiter, costs the par-
taker not less than $1.25, — a sum that would pay family
board for five meals, or would buy the raw material necessary to feed one person for at least three days.   The price

of this hotel meal is made up only in small part of the cost of the raw food materials, but comes largely from the absorption of capital in an expensive building and in elaborate equipment and service. The habitués of hotel tables pay more for their environment and manner of life than they do for what they eat. Now, if our living was more simple, and our flour, meats, vegetables, and fruits were used with maximum economy, the saving would support public utilities, extend charities, pay the national debt, and in other ways contribute to the higher aims of social life, besides promoting good health. In fact, the people of this nation, with a given amount of energy to apply in one direction or another, is expending an undue proportion of its activities in paying for expensively compounded and expensively served foods, with a corresponding limitation of the means which might secure larger individual and social values.

CHAPTER XIII

SPECIAL DIETETIC METHODS

. THERE are a few people who advocate, and claim to follow, special dietetic methods such as vegetarianism and uncooked (raw) foods. The advocates of these dietetic practices, which are followed in some countries at least by a few persons, profess to find in scientific facts and daily experience a justification of their position. It appears to the writer that arguments advanced in favor of these unusual eating habits are generally presented in a manner that is far from judicial. Certain well-established facts are assumed to support the contentions made, when a connection has not been established by proof, antagonistic facts are ignored, and the long-continued experience of the human family on a mixed diet of cooked meats and vegetables is given less weight than it deserves. It is the method of argument adopted by those persons who have come to see a single set of facts in exaggerated perspective.

A. VEGETARIANISM

Vegetarians are those persons who, while in some instances admitting and defending the use of eggs and milk, hold, in theory at least, that the eating of meats is deleterious to the physical welfare of the human family. Their position is based on the following grounds : —

246

1. Man is anatomically not a carnivorous animal.

2. Meat is an unnecessary article of diet.

3. The use of meat is a menace to the health of man mainly for the following reasons : —

a It causes an overconsumption of protein, which promotes certain diseases.

b It greatly promotes the growth of bacteria in the intestinal tract.

c It is a fruitful source of toxins that are dangerous to health or even life.

d Vegetarians are healthier and have greater physical endurance than meat eaters.

233. Anatomical considerations. — Does the structure of the human animal indicate that he should not eat flesh? This question seems somewhat absurd in view of the fact that man has been eating flesh for centuries, and that on a partially flesh diet men of great vigor and endurance have been grown. Facts overshadow theories. The earliest recorded history tells us of flesh eating. In a savage state man eats flesh freely. The Norsemen, the mighty men of the north, were flesh eaters. To be sure, man has not now prehensile teeth, but he succeeds fairly well in masticating cooked flesh. It is not surprising that in view of his intelligent methods of securing food, other means than teeth are used for capturing and holding his prey. So far as internal structure is concerned, the length of man's intestines is shorter than that of animals eating no meat, and longer than that of carnivorous animals, — a fact that may have little significance, however. Anyway, man successfully digests meat.

Vegetarians can find little in man's structure to support

their position, so far as we can discover. Man has always eaten flesh, and to say that he should not, because of his anatomical structure, is not a convincing reason for declaring that, through countless generations, man has failed to discover the food that best serves his bodily needs, and for so long has followed abnormal eating habits. This would be about as rational as to declare that a squirrel should not eat nuts.

234. Is flesh protein necessary? — One of the main arguments of the advocates of a fleshless diet is that the physical welfare of man does not demand meat as a part of his food. It is asserted, and with truth, that human beings have been grown and maintained in activity on a vegetable diet. Surely this can be done if milk and eggs are admitted to be " vegetarian."

Apart from practical experience, it is now very evident from our knowledge of the compounds of plants and from our studies of metabolism, that a vegetable diet can and does perform the complete round of nutritive functions. The larger part of food is used for energy production, and no source of energy is physiologically more efficient than starch and its allies. The proteins of plants and animals are closely alike in constitution, if we may judge from their cleavage products, and certainly perform similar functions. It is true, however, that the meat proteins correspond more closely to the constructive demands of the human body than do the plant proteins, and, consequently, in rearranging the " building stones " for the construction of animal tissue, it seems almost certain that there would be less waste from flesh proteins than from those having a vegetable source. But, after all, the protein tissue of many forms of brute life is constructed wholly from vegetable protein, and we may safely reason that the same may occur with the human species.

But while plant and flesh proteins are on a par as to kind of functions, is a purely vegetable diet likely to supply protein in a quantity essential to the most effective nutritive results, unless vegetable foods are reënforced by milk and eggs,—a practice which some vegetarians (?) admit to be good? The quantity of ingested protein that a vegetarian diet supplies is generally below the accepted dietary standards. Whether or not this minimum protein diet is desirable, is discussed elsewhere in this volume (pp. 195–199).

The real question is not whether flesh proteins are a necessary part of the human diet, but whether meat eating in a reasonable way is harmful, or may not have its advantages.

235. The harmfulness of a mixed flesh and vegetable diet. — Vegetarians allege not only that eating flesh is not necessary, but that it is harmful. This is a universal condemnation without reference to the extent to which flesh foods are incorporated in the diet, whether moderately or in excessive proportions.

The main grounds on which flesh eating is condemned are the following : —

1. Intestinal bacteria are thereby greatly increased.

2. Certain compounds in flesh are the progenitors of uric acid, and therefore flesh eating tends to rheumatic troubles.

3. Cases of toxic poisoning are caused by eating flesh foods that have undergone certain fermentations.

236. Bacteria in foods. — Figures are given in the arguments for vegetarianism showing that uncooked flesh carries with it very great numbers of bacteria, which is undoubtedly true, although, as little flesh is eaten the outside of which is not cooked, counts of surface bacteria unduly magnify the fact. No comparisons are made between the number of bacteria conveyed by meat and those in market milk, or in uncooked vegetables that have been exposed in the markets, neither is any direct proof furnished that the meat inhabiting bacteria are a cause of intestinal troubles in a normal, healthy individual.

237. Bacteria abundant in intestines. — The intestinal tract of man, chiefly the colon or large intestine, normally contains countless numbers of bacteria that are developed mostly in the intestine, although a minor part may be introduced with the food.

Competent investigators agree that quite a portion of the fecal residue consists of dead or living bacteria that have accumulated in the large intestine, but it is not affirmed that this fact is an indication of harm. Some able authorities hold that the presence of these organisms is essential to digestion. Their action on proteins is in some respects similar to that of the digestive enzymes, and the resulting products may have the same value to the body. The digestion of cellulose is accomplished wholly by bacteria, and these organisms cause acid formation from carbohydrates. Their action on fats is regarded as slight.

238. Relation of foods to intestinal bacteria. — It is argued that flesh foods are favorable to the growth of intestinal bacteria. They are present, however, in the large intestines in very great numbers with any diet. The fact is, vegetable foods are known to be very favorable media in which to develop micro-organisms, as is shown in laboratory processes and in the rapid fermentations which such foods undergo. It is significant that herbivorous animals are the subjects of acute intestinal fermentations. Doubtless the nature of the diet greatly influences the type of bacteria that is dominant in the intestinal tract at any given time. A heavy meat diet would favor the increase of the putrefactive forms, while a vegetable diet or one containing sugar, or sugar-forming bodies, would favor acid-producing forms. No proof is yet forthcoming that a reasonable mixed diet of flesh and vegetables is any more dangerous to health through the kind or extent of bacterial development than is a purely vegetable diet. Doubtless heavy meat eating, especially when excretion is imperfect, may result in toxic disturbances through putrefactive fermentations in the intestines, but while "auto intoxication" may be promoted under abnormal conditions by an abundance of meat proteins in the intestinal tract, there is no evidence that reasonable flesh eating is more dangerous in this particular than a vegetable diet. Inferential conclusions based on bacterial counts are not safe. That is, it is not proved that, under normal conditions, a possible excess of intestinal bacteria with a mixed diet does any harm. It seems probable that the acute indigestions sometimes attendant upon generous consumption of vegetables, fruits, and various "sweets," and which may be due to bacterial action, are fully as serious as any similar disturbances that may be caused by flesh eating.

239. Flesh foods contain uric acid formers. — Vegetarians urge that flesh should be excluded from the diet of man because such foods cause, or aggravate, rheumatic troubles. Physicians advise their patients afflicted with rheumatism to avoid certain meats or cut down to a minimum the amount eaten. While this advice is often, not consistent in its details, the reasons lying behind it are that flesh, and especially certain glands like liver, contain a small proportion of compounds known as purins which are progenitors of uric acid, and that an accumulation of uric acid in the body is regarded as the exciting cause of various forms of rheumatism. Vegetable foods, milk products, and eggs are allowed on the ground that, with such a diet, the minimum of uric acid is formed. As a matter of fact, it has been shown that the addition of flesh to a vegetable diet increases the output of uric acid, and it is rational that persons with a uric acid diathesis (tendency) should eat flesh sparingly, including the flesh of fish, or not at all.

240. Purins in vegetable foods. — At the same time, it is not yet fully determined whether uric acid may not result from synthesis in the human body, besides which vegetable foods are not free from purins, as the following table shows.

These figures make it evident that even on a vegetable diet, uric acid forming compounds are not escaped, only minimized. It is a question, too, whether rheumatism is not promoted fully as much by habits of life as by special articles of diet. It is certain that the great majority of persons who do not abuse themselves with overindulgence in eating or drinking, who take sufficient exercise and who

TABLE XL

THE PURIN CONTENT OF CERTAIN FOODS [1]

	GRAMS PER KILOGRAM		GRAMS PER KILOGRAM
Fish		*Special foods*	
Cod	0.50	Milk	——
Salmon	1.10	Butter	——
Halibut	1.00	Eggs	——
Meats		Cheese	——
Beef	1.10 to 2.00	*Beverages*	
Mutton	0.96	Lager beer . . .	0.12
Veal	1.10	Ale . . .	0.14
Pork (lean) . . .	1.20	Porter	0.15
Ham	1.10	Tea (per cup) . .	1.20
Chicken	1.20	Cocoa . . .	1.00
Vegetables		Chocolate . . .	0.70
Potatoes	0.02	Coffee	1.70
Rice	——	Claret	——
Flour	——	Sherry	——
Bread	——	Brandy	——
Oat meal	0.53		
Peas	0.39		
Lentils	0.38		
Beans	0.63		
Asparagus . . .	0.21		
Cabbage	——		
Lettuce	——		

do not submit themselves to extreme conditions of inactivity or exposure, generally are not afflicted with rheumatic troubles, even if generous meat eaters. Persons with

[1] "Metabolism and Practical Medicine." Von Noorden, Vol. III, p. 1297.

a pronounced uric acid tendency should avoid flesh eating, perhaps, just as some persons should avoid strawberries, sweets, milk, cheese, cabbage, or some other food that proves to be harmful because of constitutional peculiarities. It does not follow when one person cannot safely indulge in a mixed diet of flesh and vegetable food that every one else should exclude the flesh.

241. Danger from toxins. — It is pointed out that toxins (poisons), are developed in meats under certain conditions, the effect of which sometimes menaces human life. Occasionally cases of serious illness, sometimes fatal, are reported from this cause, but when we consider the immense quantities of flesh consumed by millions of people, such occurrences must be considered as infinitesimal in their proportions. Ice cream poisoning, probably due to badly fermented cream, and toxic cheese, the condition of which is not at present fully explained, cause illness fully as frequently as meat, fish, or poultry. It is safe to assert that acute indigestions due to overeating of sweets, unripe fruits and vegetables, cause fully as much human suffering and as many deaths as do unsound flesh foods. It is unfair to charge against any class of foods the harm which it does through bad conditions of holding and preparation, or through overindulgence on the part of the victim.

In normal digestion, it cannot be maintained on any ground whatever that the resulting products from flesh proteins and fats differ in their relations to good health from similar compounds that the digestive enzyms or the intestinal bacteria produce from plant substance. The digestive cleavage products of animal proteins and plant proteins are greatly alike in kind, though differing in proportion, and there is not the slightest evidence that those from one source have deleterious physiological reactions not possessed by those from the other source. What may happen with overindulgence with any class of foods is not to the point.

242. The physical quality of flesh eaters as compared with vegetarians. — Those who advocate a vegetable diet, with the exclusion of flesh products, claim that persons grown and maintained on foods of plant origin have greater physical stamina than those who have developed and subsist on a mixed diet. This appears to be an unwarranted assumption. In the first place, it is exceedingly difficult to produce conclusive proof by which to settle this question. A comparison of the endurance of a few individuals means but little, because it is almost impossible to select persons that represent the average of a race or a type. Conclusions, so far as they are justified, must be based on racial or regional data where it is possible to compare the physical quality associated with characteristic food supply.

Certain savage tribes exist at times on an almost exclusive meat diet, and the people of the United States, England, and European states, consume immense quantities of flesh. On the other hand, the inhabitants of China and Japan are, to a large extent, vegetarians. In the early history of this country, especially in the day of buffalo meat on the Western plains, the Indians, as well as the hardy trappers and early settlers, subsisted at times on a very heavy flesh diet. This has been true during the conquering of any new country where game has been a prominent article of food. It is within the facts to say that men and women of splendid physical physique have been produced and nourished under these primitive dietetic conditions, and it is equally certain that the meat-eating people have produced individual types of men, especially if we base our judgment on athletic contests, than which there have been no finer or more enduring. The athletes of the United States and England are the peers of any. It is fair to inquire, too, whether the small stature of the Chinese and Japanese is not related in some measure to their diet. And we should give full weight to the fact that the Romance peoples, into whose diet flesh enters very sparingly, cannot claim physical superiority. It is safe to assert that there are no facts or principles in nutrition, and no large experience of the human species, which justify the assertion that reasonable flesh eating is a cause of inferior physical quality. Physical quality is, of course, dependent on many factors, and, to analyze these in their relation to an individual or a group of individuals and assign to one a dominating influence, would be extremely difficult, if not impossible.

243. General considerations as to meat eating. — The apostles of the vegetarian doctrine are rendering a useful service in calling attention to the abuses of flesh eating. As has been pointed out, meat and fish are by far the most expensive part of the family food supply. Many families, even those of moderate means, burden their resources by the purchase of flesh food to an extent that is not essential to the very best dietetic conditions. The common belief, especially among laboring people, that a family is not well fed unless meats are eaten freely three times a day, is a tradition, and has no justification in fact. The energy used in manual labor comes very largely and most efficiently from carbohydrates, that is, from the grain foods. Moreover, the excessive use of meats places upon the human organism unnecessary burdens and promotes any tendency that may exist towards those ailments associated with the by-products of protein metabolism. Undoubtedly, if the American people would cut down its consumption of flesh foods, it would result in an advantage to health and would lighten the cost of living. On the other hand, the ease and completeness with which meats are digested by most persons, the efficiency for constructive purposes of meat proteins, and the absence of any conclusive proof that moderate meat eating is harmful, are good arguments for the reasonable use of meat in families of comfortable circumstances.

B. EATING RAW FOODS

One of the modern food fads that is occasionally advocated is the eating of all foods in a raw condition. The arguments in favor of this practice appear to be based wholly on a real or fancied personal experience; indeed, this must be so, because there are no well-established scientific facts that in fairness can be used to support the claim that foods in a raw state are, in general, more healthful or more efficient than when cooked.

If cooked foods are inferior to raw in healthfulness or efficiency, the explanation must lie largely in one or more of the following factors : —

1 Poorer mastication of the cooked food.

2 A lower ratio of digestibility.

3 A less nutritive efficiency or different function of the food compounds in a cooked state.

S

244. Mastication. — It is undoubtedly true that much more time would be consumed in masticating raw cereals and vegetables than is required after these foods are cooked. This would result in a more complete admixture of the saliva with the masticated food. It is probable, however, that the uncooked cereal, being much harder and more tenacious than the cooked, would not be reduced to as fine a mechanical condition as after being disintegrated by either wet or dry heat.

245. Digestibility. — In any case, there is every reason for asserting that cooking vegetable foods makes possible a prompter and more complete digestion because of a rupture of the cells containing the effective nutrients, which is certainly a desirable result. The less complete the digestion, the larger the fecal residue, and, for this reason, uncooked foods may possibly have some advantage for persons to whom constipation is a constant menace, although the use of coarse bread containing wheat or bran, or a free use of fruit and vegetables, is probably as efficient a bowel regulator as any uncooked materials could possibly be.

246. Influence of cooking on function. — No advantage can be claimed for uncooked foods because of any difference in function, or greater efficiency, of raw proteins or carbohydrates over those that have been submitted to heat, excepting that cooked animal proteins like those in meat and eggs more slowly digest after coagulation, but do not seem to be less completely digested. Function is not changed by cooking. Raw proteins and raw starch when digested will do no more work, or no different work, in the animal organism than coagulated protein or hydrolyzed starch. A real disadvantage attending the consumption of raw foods, fruits excepted, is the absence of the flavors that are developed by cooking. These flavors are a real nutritive asset as excitants of the secretion of the digestive fluids. On the whole, the proposition to eat all foods raw is not only irrational, but even absurd, when regarded in the light of well-established facts.

CHAPTER XIV

THE NUTRITION OF THE CHILD

THE nutrition of the child is a matter of supreme importance to the physical welfare of the race. It is during the time of active growth that the physical status of the adult is established, and the errors of nutrition committed during this period are likely to handicap the individual during his entire life. The development of a human being begins with the embryo and passes in succession through the fetal stage, the infantile period, when, under natural conditions, milk is the only food, and the later and longer period of growth, when the diet is similar in a general way to that of adults. No one of these periods is unimportant in its relation to the ultimate product, — the full-grown man or woman.

A. THE NOURISHMENT OF THE FETUS

247. Growth of fetus. — The growth of the human young begins with the development of the fertilized ovum in the uterus. During the succeeding nine months of *in utero* existence, the embryo and fetus increase in substance by the deposition of compounds the same in kind as those which are applied to constructive purposes subsequent to birth. The following analysis of the human fetus partially developed, and at time of birth, illustrates the truth of the above statement:—

TABLE XLI

COMPOSITION OF THE EMBRYO AND FULLY GROWN FETUS[1]

	WEIGHT	DRY SUBSTANCE	NITROGEN	FAT	ASH
	Grams	Grams	Grams	Grams	Grams
Embryo (7 months) .	900–1000	150–160	16	26	26
Fully grown fetus . .	3200	850–1000	60–65	350	85–100
Addition in about 100 days	2250	700–850	45–50	350	60–75
Average addition per day last 100 days .	22.5	7.0–8.5	.45–.50 3 grams albumin	3.5	0.6–.75

TABLE XLII

OTHER ANALYSES OF THE EMBRYO AND FULLY GROWN FETUS[2]

AGE	TOTAL WEIGHT	DRY MATTER	WATER	DRY MATTER CONTAINS		
				Ash	Protein	Fat
	Grams	Grams	Grams	Grams	Grams	Grams
4 mo.	36.5	3.00	33.5	0.33	1.77	0.20
6 mo.	361.8	39.10	322.7	7.01	24.13	2.60
Full grown . .	3294.0	855.52	2440.8	83.00	388.69	299.7

The figures in Table XLII confirm those of the previous table in a general way in showing that the growth of the fetus is mostly during the last three or four months of *in utero* life.

[1] " Metabolism and Practical Medicine," Von Noorden. Vol. I, p. 377.
[2] "Des Kindes Ernährung," Czerny-Keller, p. 87.

TABLE XLII1 [1]

COMPOSITION OF THE ASH OF A NEW-BORN CHILD [1]

	IN TOTAL ASH	IN 1000 GRAMS BODY WEIGHT
	Grams	Grams
Potassium oxid (potash) . .	1.64	0.88
Sodium oxid (soda)	6.20	3.35
Calcium oxid (lime)	25.40	13.73
Magnesium oxid (magnesia) .	0.67	0.36
Ferric oxid	1.15	0.61
Phosphorus pentoxid	22.81	12.25
Chlorine	3.50	1.89
	61.37	33.07

These tables set forth other facts than that the body of the fetus and new-born infant consists of ash, protein, and fat. It is evident that at least 75 per cent of the dry substance of the former is added during the last three months of intra-uterine life, and that the daily addition is small, amounting on the average, during the period of rapid growth, to about 3 grams of protein, 3.5 grams of fat, and 0.6 to 0.7 gram of ash elements.

248. Sources of fetal growth. — Fetal growth may be derived from either of two sources, the food of the mother, or the material already deposited in her body. If her food is sufficient to supply both her own needs and those of the growing fetus, then she will sustain no body loss; but with food insufficient to meet the demands in these two directions, the body substance of the mother will be transferred to the child. Doubtless both conditions occur, as is indi-

[1] "Des Kindes Ernährung," Czerny-Keller, p. 90.

cated by the facts that many mothers during pregnancy do not increase in weight, while others become as many pounds heavier, at least, as the weight of the fetus with its surrounding liquids and membranes. If the mother does not increase in weight, her own substance must have diminished.

249. Food demands during pregnancy. — The important question is, what are the special food needs, if any, of the gravid woman?

It is clear that in the kinds of nutrients utilized, the food needs of the pregnant woman do not differ from the ordinary needs of the human organism. If these needs are special, it is in the amount of nutrients required rather than in their kind. There is certainly a tendency to overestimate the demands made upon the parent organism for the growth of the unborn child. For the first two hundred days, the fetal growth does not call for over 1 gram of dry matter per day, and probably not even that. This demand is hardly appreciable when the food eaten each day ordinarily carries over 500 grams of dry matter. During the last three months of pregnancy, in which period three-fourths of the fetal growth occurs, the daily deposition of dry matter does not reach ten grams per day, which certainly does not call for a large increase in the food eaten by the mother.

250. Energy use. — But while the early demands for constructive purposes during pregnancy are small, are there not increased metabolic activities on the part of the parent organism that require an increased use of energy, that is, an increased oxidation of food compounds? There are several reasons why we would expect this to be the case.

First of all, there is the work of blood circulation in the body of the unborn child, which is accomplished by the muscular contractions of the fetal heart, and this requires an expenditure of energy from some source. Besides this, the weight of the pregnant woman is increased, except in cases of insufficient nutrition, and energy needs are in general in proportion to weight. The assimilative processes are intensified also. In one case, at least, the rate of the heart beats of the pregnant woman has been found to increase beyond the rate previous to conception, thus adding to the internal work performed. In the same investigation by Magnus-Levy, the rate of respiration increased, adding still further to muscular activity. To offset these factors it often happens that the mother is less active, especially during the last two or three months of pregnancy, at the time when the increased demand of food would appear to be greatest.

Accurate observations on the energy exchange (oxidation) during pregnancy are somewhat meager in number where women have been the experimental subjects. Magnus-Levy [1] followed the use of oxygen through the entire period of pregnancy of a woman, beginning with the third month. Observations were also made in the non-pregnant period. A quite constant and fairly uniform increased use of oxygen occurred, being greatest in the ninth month, when it amounted to 80 cubic centimeters per minute, or 25 per cent above the normal. Experimental data with two other women gave no such increase, and so our conclusions must be inferential rather than based upon scientific proof. It is certainly true, nevertheless, that

[1] " Metabolism and Practical Medicine," Von Noorden, Vol. I, p. 379.

fetal growth makes demands, though not large, on the nutrition of the mother, if her body substance is to be defended from loss; and it seems more than probable that the internal work of the parent organism is somewhat increased, requiring the expenditure of more energy.

251. Diet for pregnant woman. — At the same time, it should not be assumed that the diet of a pregnant woman should be largely increased, or that her needs require a diet unusual in kind. An ordinary mixed diet that is adapted to sustain a woman doing moderate work is certainly sufficient for the gravid mother. The diet should be judiciously selected, however. The extensive use of such foods as pastry, cakes, sweets, and all similar materials, largely carbohydrates, with a marked deficiency in protein and the ash elements, should be avoided. Reference to the tables on p. 261 shows that the body of the new-born child weighing about 7 pounds contains over 300 grams protein and 60 to 80 grams of ash, more than three-fourths of the latter being phosphoric acid and lime. A simple diet made up of meats, milk, and eggs in moderate proportions, and grain, vegetable, and fruit preparations which carry as nearly as possible the unmodified composition of the natural products, will be found sufficient for all the needs of the prospective mother. Several authors publish dietary standards for pregnant women, which vary greatly; but except in the case of institutions, where a general regulation of the food supply is possible, such standards will be applied to only a small extent. If a woman reasonably satisfies a normal appetite from food selected as indicated above, all real requirements will be met. The caution is that an appetite abnormal in its desires should be controlled, and that both excessive eating and overindulgence in foods markedly deficient in the ash elements and protein be kept in check. Abnormal conditions require the advice of a physician.

B. Feeding of the Child after Birth with Mother's Milk

252. Mother's milk best. — After birth, the natural food of the human young, and that which is best adapted to its physical welfare under normal conditions, is its mother's milk. Physicians, nurses, and modern science unite in declaring that this is the food which best insures the health, development, and good physical quality of the young child. Statistics confirm this conclusion. In 1890 there were born in Berlin alone 49,362 children. Before the end of a year, 12,623 died, of which 1588 had been breast-fed and 8008 fed on cow's milk. Further statistics show of these fed on mother's milk one in thirteen died, while of those brought up by hand one out of every two died. These figures require no comment. Notwithstanding such ominous facts, thousands of infants are fed from a bottle on some other food when circumstances do not render it necessary. A mother who selfishly refuses to feed her child from the fountains of her own life, merely because of the confinement or inconvenience it occasions, fails to meet one of her highest obligations, jeopardizes the life of her offspring, and hazards her right to be called " mother." The case is different when imperative demands of another kind or abnormal conditions of milk secretion or of health render artificial feeding necessary.

253. The composition of human milk. — In discussing

infant nutrition from the natural source, a logical consideration of the subject requires that we first learn what is the composition of human milk. A study of the records reveals the fact that the milk secreted by different individuals varies greatly, and there is by no means an agreement among the average figures that have been compiled by different authorities. There follows the average composition of human milk as presented by various compilers : —

TABLE XLIV

AVERAGE COMPOSITION OF WOMAN'S MILK [1]

	PFEIFFER	HEUBNER HOFFMAN	ADRIANCE	GURARD	JOHANNESEN
	Per Cent	Per Cent	Per Cent	Per Cent	Per Cent
Dry matter	11.78	12.34	12.04	——	——
Ash	0.19	0.21	0.17	0.19	——
Protein	1.94	1.03	1.17	1.18	1.10
Sugar	6.30	7.03	6.80	7.18	4.67
Fat	3.10	4.07	3.90	3.90	3.21

	CAMERER & SÄLDNER	SCHLOSSMAN	CARTER & RICHMANS	LEHMAN	LUFF
	Per Cent	Per Cent	Per Cent	Per Cent	Per Cent
Dry matter	11.95	——	11.96	11.7	11.49
Ash	0.21	——	0.26	0.2	0.34
Protein	1.03	1.56	1.96	1.7	2.35
Sugar	6.56	6.95	6.59	6.0	6.39
Fat	3.38	4.83	3.07	3.8	2.41

The preceding figures fail to show the great range of variation. This may be illustrated by a statement of the

[1] Mostly from " Des Kindes Ernährung," Czerny-Keller, pp. 417–418.

maximum and minimum percentages compiled by Pfeiffer, the samples being only those taken more than eleven days after parturition.

TABLE XLV

	PER CENT
Dry substance	8.23–15.56
Ash	0.10– 0.45
Protein	1.05– 3.04
Sugar	4.22– 7.65
Fat	0.76– 9.05

Analyses of mother's milk are occasionally made in the laboratory of New York Agricultural Experiment Station at the request of physicians and others. The table which follows shows the results of eleven such analyses.

TABLE XLVI

ANALYSES OF HUMAN MILK MADE AT THE LABORATORY OF THE NEW YORK AGRICULTURAL EXPERIMENT STATION

	TOTAL SOLIDS	ASH [1]	PROTEIN	SUGAR [2]	FAT
	Per Cent	Per Cent	Per Cent	Per Cent	Per Cent
(1)	10.89	0.20	1.20	7.20	2.29
(2)	10.51	0.20	1.48	7.07	1.76
(3)	10.63	0.20	1.45	7.98	2.00
(4)	12.58	0.20	1.34	7.84	3.20
(5)	——	——	1.01	——	1.21
(6)	11.12	0.20	1.20	7.62	2.10
(7)	12.18	0.20	1.26	6.72	4.00
(8)	12.24	0.20	1.53	6.68	3.83
(9)	10.67	0.20	1.64	6.90	1.93
(10)	13.15	0.20	1.44	8.46	3.05
(11)	13.08	0.20	1.69	7.69	2.50
	11.70	0.20	1.42	7.42	2.66

[1] Assumed.   [2] Determined by difference.

These figures showing such wide departure from what may be regarded as normal milk are an abundant justification for the recommendation that in any instance where a nursing child is not physically prosperous the mother's milk should be investigated both as to quantity and quality.

254. Conditions affecting mother's milk. — Certain causes which are to be noticed and that may operate to modify the mother's milk such as food, medication, exposure, and nervous condition, are those which are under control. Other possible causes are those that are not under control; and which may be termed " natural."

255. Period of lactation. — Among the latter it is very definitely shown that as the period of lactation progresses the proportions of ash and protein in the milk diminish, especially during the first few weeks.

Several authorities give figures that substantiate this statement.[1]

TABLE XLVII

EFFECT OF PERIOD OF LACTATION

PERIOD OF LACTATION	PFEIFFER		ADRIANCE	
	Protein	Ash	Protein	Ash
	Per Cent	Per Cent	Per Cent	Per Cent
1st month	2.97	0.237	1.55	0.21
2d month	2.04	0.184	1.54	0.17
3d month	1.99	0.184	1.49	0.19
11th month	1.47	0.145	0.64	0.18
12th month	1.73	0.160	1.18	0.14
13th month	1.65	0.155	1.02	0.16

[1] " Des Kindes Ernährung," Czerny-Keller, p. 419.

A gradual rise in the percentage of fat occurs in the progressive portions of milk that are drawn; that is, the more nearly the mammary gland is emptied, the richer the milk is in fat.   Account should be taken of this fact in selecting a sample for analysis, that is, a full breast should be entirely emptied by artificial means and a sample taken of the whole quantity after thorough mixing.   It may also be said that, as a rule, the richness of human milk in fat is inversely as the total amount of milk secreted.

256. Individuality. — There is also the effect of individuality, as shown by the tables on p. 268, which will be considered more fully later.

257. Demands on food for milk secretion. — As the secretion of milk is wholly dependent upon the mother's food, unless she is underfed and contributes from her body substance, her nutrition is a matter of fundamental importance.   All considerations of this phase of the nourishment of the child must be based upon the amount and composition of the milk which it consumes.   Authorities who have investigated this matter are somewhat at variance in the figures which they give for the milk secretion of the human mother.   If it is measured by what the infant takes, and there is no unused surplus artificially drawn, an average amount is probably 300 grams (10.6 oz.) daily for the first week and at the end of the fifth month not far from 1000 grams (35.5 oz.) daily.[1]   If this milk is of average composition, it would contain in each day's production at the two periods approximately the dry matter and ingredients stated as follows: —

[1] See " Des Kindes Ernährung," pp. 351–353.

TABLE XLVIII

SOLIDS IN MOTHER'S MILK

	FIRST WEEK	TWENTY-SECOND WEEK
	Grams	Grams
Dry matter	35.4	118.0
Ash	0.6	2.0
Proteins	4.6	15.4
Sugar	19.8	66.0
Fat	10.2	34.5
Energy (calories)	189.1	636.1

The increase of milk secretion seems to correspond to the increased demands of the child, and proceeds with a fair degree of regularity. In those cases where more than one child is suckled, the daily production sometimes becomes much greater than when only one child is at breast, rising in observed instances to 1750 grams (62.5 oz.) or more daily. Under ordinary circumstances with one child the mother is likely to be called upon to supply on the average about 800 grams of milk daily from the fourth to the twentieth week. This milk, if of average composition, would contain 94.6 grams dry matter, 1.6 grams ash, 12 grams protein, 54.4 grams sugar, and 26.4 grams fat, the combined energy of these nutrients being 518 calories. These facts are convincing evidence that the demands on the mother during the nursing period are much greater than during the period of pregnancy, indeed, they are demands that should receive adequate recognition in the mother's diet, especially after the first few weeks.

258. Necessary dietary. — The American dietary standard for women doing light muscular work is 2400 calories, and with women doing moderate work it is 2700 calories. If the food equivalents of these energy expenditures are necessary to maintain ordinary household activity without gain or loss of body substance, the additional demands of the nursing child require that the food consumed shall be increased one-fifth, or even more, as the child increases in size. It is often noticed that nursing mothers grow "thin," which is undoubtedly due to insufficient nutrition, especially when the milk secretion reaches 1000 grams or above that quantity, the dry matter of which represents not less than one-fourth the daily ration of a housewife doing light work.

259. Effect of insufficient diet. — The physical welfare, not only of the nursing mother, but also of her child, is dependent upon her proper nourishment. Observation indicates that when the mother's diet is insufficient, the milk is less in quantity and possibly poorer in quality. The failure of an infant at breast to grow as it should may sometimes be due to lack of sufficient food, and this possibility should receive careful attention. It should not be assumed, however, that in all cases the necessary milk secretion can be secured through abundant diet. Certain mothers seem to have constitutional limitations of capacity to secrete milk that cannot be overcome by a generous diet, or by the kind of diet.

260. Effect of foods on milk secretion. — There are many "old wives' sayings" concerning the relation of food to the mother's milk that have no foundation in fact. It is believed by some that copious drinking, or the free use of watery foods like soups or porridges, promotes the milk flow. Nothing could be more erroneous. The free use of milk is recommended, on the ground that " milk makes milk." While it is true that a reasonable amount of milk forms a very useful part of the diet of a nursing mother, and supplies all the needed materials for the secretion of human milk, it is also true that other foods, such as meat, eggs, grain foods, and vegetables, sustain milk secretion in a very satisfactory way when they are wisely combined. The constituents of milk are a secretion of the mammary glands in which the casein and milk fats are elaborated out of the raw materials supplied by the food or the mother's tissues. These bodies are not filtered out of the blood as such from the digested food compounds. If this were so, then the food would have a very direct and extensive influence on the quality of the milk, which is not the case. With species and breeds of animals the amount and kind of milk are determined by the specific activity of the secreting glands, and no variations of food will cause a Holstein cow to give Jersey milk or will cause any individual animal to abandon her constitutional habit of milk secretion, and the same is true of individuals of the human species.

261. Procedure when milk is abnormal. — It sometimes happens that a mother's milk is abnormal in its quality, that is, it may be unusually poor or unusually rich, or may have one constituent in unusual proportions. When this is true, and the child is unfavorably affected, the remedy lies in resorting to artificial feeding, and not in trying to modify the milk through the food supply. The attempt to change the richness of human milk or the

T

relative proportions of its constituents by giving the mother watery food, or food especially rich in one constituent such as protein or fat, is bound to fail in its purpose. All that is required is that the food shall be sufficient in quantity and not markedly insufficient in any needed constituent. A diet made up of meats and fish in reasonable proportions, eggs, milk, bread, breakfast foods in which the constituents of the whole grain are practically all retained, fruits in moderate quantity, and vegetables of such kinds and in such quantities as do not cause digestive disturbances, furnishes an adequate basis for abundant milk secretion.

262. Effect of mother's food upon child. — The assertion is often heard that a child has been harmfully affected by some food substance that entered into the mother's diet, or by some medicine she took. There are two ways in which it is conceivable that the food of the mother may work injury to the child: (1) the diet affecting the mother's health, with an accompanying reaction on the milk secretion, and (2) by the direct transfer to the milk of substances in the mother's food. Overeating, sudden changes in the diet, and the use of foods that, with a particular person are known to cause a disturbance of the digestion, may react on the milk secretion, and these causes should be avoided. Concerning the influence of particular foods on the child through the direct transference to the mother's milk of certain compounds, there is much tradition and little exact knowledge. Doubtless some foods are regarded as undesirable for the nursing mother without good reason, their bad reputation arising either from the results of eating an excessive quantity, or because the illness of some child has been coincident with the use of a certain food when it was not the disturbing factor. Tradition teaches that acid materials such as fruits and pickles, and condiments such as the spices and peppers, dangerously affect the mother's milk. Doubtless popular notions greatly exaggerate the real facts. There are no well established facts which justify the conclusion that a nursing mother may not eat acid fruits in moderation if under ordinary conditions she is accustomed to do so with comfort. It has been stated to the writer that beans, boiled cabbage, and other vegetables likely to cause intestinal fermentations should be excluded from the diet of a nursing mother; but this assertion seems to rest on hearsay, and not on demonstrative experience. It is hard to understand how these common foods, when eaten in reasonable quantities and with regularity as to kind and quantity, can cause the mother's milk to be harmful. A significant fact is that cow's milk produced from a ration of which acid silage forms a generous part may be safely fed to infants, as the writer knows from observation. Milk from a general milk supply, or even that known as " sanitary " or " certified," is produced from a great variety of foods, including silage, roots, and by-product feeding stuffs, and yet when such milk is sound, it seems to be a safe food for infants in hundreds of cases.

263. Effect of food upon cow's milk. — It is hardly to be expected that the human and the bovine mother are subject to greatly unlike laws in the relation of food to milk secretion, and consequently the outcome of experiments with cows to determine the effect of feeding various substances on the composition of milk is of importance in this connection. It has been found, as stated, that sudden and pronounced changes in the food of the cow may have a temporary effect on the proportions of milk constituents, an effect only temporary, however. The bovine mammary glands have a constitutional gauge not easily changed, if changed at all. It also appears that heavy feeding with certain vegetable oils, like cottonseed, linseed, and sesame oils, may appreciably modify the relative proportion of individual fats in the milk fat, and that the physical condition of the butter fat is modified to a small degree because of a change in the relative proportion of the harder to the softer fats in the food. Various investigators, after feeding a vegetable oil heavily, have discovered its characteristic fats in the milk of the experimental animal, but only in very small proportions.

But granting all these facts, and also that the milk of the human mother would be similarly affected by the food constituents, especially the fats, there is nothing in this to indicate that the milk thus becomes harmful, because the changes brought about are simply a slightly different proportion of food compounds of known value. We are justified in concluding, then, that the foods which the nursing mother may eat include practically the whole list, provided the diet is kept up on a fairly uniform basis as to kind and quality of material, involving no sudden changes, and that from it is excluded those foods which in particular cases cause discomfort.

264. Effect of medicines taken by mother. — When we come to consider the effect on her milk of administering medicinal substances to the mother, the evidence at hand is more definite. It has been conclusively shown that iodin and salicylic acid, or their compounds, antipyrin, mercury, and other substances may pass into the milk, though in very minute quantities, but probably in sufficient amounts to affect the child. For this reason a nursing mother should take medicine only under the advice and direction of a physician.

265. Effect of psychic condition. — The psychic or " nervous " condition of the mother may have a profound influence upon the physical welfare of the nursing infant. There is abundant evidence that continued grief, melancholia, or great anxiety may seriously affect the child, causing a loss of weight and sometimes bowel disturbances. From such causes, as well as by severe chill or some other unusual physical experience, the secretion of milk may suddenly cease. There is evidence, too, that from these causes the milk may be so modified as to become harmful, though just what occurs is not known. It is a strange and unexplained fact. To suggest that some toxic body is developed through nerve reaction is simply to advance an hypothesis. It is important, therefore, that.the mother avoid as far as possible all forms of disagreeable mental experience and maintain mentally and physically a condition of repose and comfort. If severe experiences are unavoidable, it may be wise or even necessary to transfer the child to artificial feeding or to a wet nurse.

266. Precautions in feeding. — There are certain precautions which should be observed in feeding infants, whether they receive mother's milk or are given artificial food. The feeding should be regular and, with a very young infant, once in two hours is probably good practice, although a single rule cannot be rigidly followed in all cases. It is a serious mistake for a mother to nurse her child too frequently as a means of quieting it whenever it is fretful. Such a practice may result in overloading the child's stomach. As the child grows older the frequency of feeding may be diminished.

The infant should be weighed frequently to determine its rate of gain. It should be said, however, that plumpness or the laying on of fat is not necessarily an indication of physical prosperity; indeed, a child may become too fat for its physical good. The real essential is the growth of the basal tissues, and the character of the food has much to do with this. Artificially fed children are often more fleshy than those fed at the breast, whereas the latter may in reality be making the more desirable growth.

C. ARTIFICIAL FEEDING OF INFANTS

There is no question but that in general the development and physical well being of the young child is most fully insured when its food is mother's milk. Sometimes, however, the necessities of the case require a resort to some other food. Under such circumstances use may be made of the milk of some other mammal, such as the cow or the goat, or one of the so-called infant foods prepared wholly or in part from one or more of the cereal grains may be fed, but as will be seen, these artificial preparations should be avoided with children in the nursing period, whenever possible.

TABLE XLIX
COMPARISON OF COW'S AND MOTHER'S MILK

	AVERAGE COW'S MILK	AVERAGE MOTHER'S MILK
	Per Cent	Per Cent
Total solids	12.90	11.80
Ash	0.70	0.20
Proteins	3.20	1.54
Sugar	5.10	6.61
Fat	3.90	3.45

Because the ash constituents are important as constructive material, there is also good reason for comparing the two kinds of milk on this basis.

	IN 100 PARTS MILK DRY SUBSTANCE	
	Cow's Milk	Human Milk
	Per Cent	Per Cent
Potassium oxid	1.67	0.58
Sodium oxid	1.05	0.17
Calcium oxid	1.54	0.24
Magnesium oxid	0.20	0.05
Iron oxid	0.003	0.004
Phosphorus oxid	1.86	0.35
Chlorine	1.60	0.32

	100 PARTS MILK CONTAINS IN GRAINS	
	Cow's Milk	Human Milk
	Per Cent	Per Cent
Potassium oxid	0.1776	0.0795
Sodium oxid	0.6972	0.0253
Calcium oxid	0.1671	0.0489
Magnesium oxid	0.0231	0.0065
Iron oxid	0.0021	0.0008
Phosphorus oxid	0.1911	0.0585
Chlorine	0.1368	0.0486

267. Unlike composition of human and cow's milk. —
Experience has demonstrated that if cow's milk is to be
fed successfully to infants it should be modified or " hu-
manized." In order to understand why and how this is
done, it is necessary to consider the chemical and physical
differences between mother's milk and cow's milk. The
chemical differences are well illustrated when we place side
by side the average composition of the two kinds of milk.

The preceding figures show that while cow's milk and
mother's milk are in general alike in the kind of compounds
they contain, they show marked differences in their percentage composition. The cow's milk is richer in solids,
that is, has less water; and these solids are made up in
much larger proportion of ash and protein than is the case
with mother's milk, while in the solids of the latter the
proportion of sugar is greater. The ash compounds,
while alike in kind, are not far from three times as abundant
in the cow's milk as in the mother's. These comparisons
are based on the average composition of the two kinds of
milk. The differences named are still greater when the
cow's milk is from one of the butter-making breeds such
as the Jersey or Guernsey, for in this case the percentage
of solids may be over 15 per cent or even 16 per cent, and
the protein between 4 and 5 per cent, especially if the cows
are fairly well advanced in the period of lactation.

268. Are the compounds similar? — We have seen that
the classes of compounds and the ash constituents are alike
in mother's and cow's milk, but the question naturally
arises whether the compounds themselves are similar.
Are the protein bodies and the fats alike in the two milks?
A negative answer must be given to this question. There

are several differences. As we know, the protein of milk is a mixture of several nitrogen compounds, casein, albumin, globulin, and others. These bodies do not exist in the same proportions in the two milks under discussion, the proportion of casein in the protein of cow's milk being 80 per cent, which is nearly twice as large as in human milk, the soluble bodies like albumin and globulin being proportionately larger in the latter milk.[1] The significance of this fact lies in the unlike behavior of casein and albumin toward acids and coagulating ferments. Casein is coagulated at ordinary temperatures by the combined action of acid and pepsin, while albumin is not, and partly for this reason the milks under comparison must behave quite differently in the human stomach when they come in contact with the gastric juice. It appears, too, that the casein of cow's milk is not quite the same compound as in mother's milk. This is shown by a difference in the proportions of the several elements in the casein from the two sources, especially of the phosphorus and sulfur.[2]

As with protein, the fat of milk is not a single body, but is a mixture of several individual fats, and these exist in the fat of the two milks in quite different proportions. As previously explained, the fats consist of fatty acids united with glycerine. When freed from the glycerine, some are solid, and some are liquids, at ordinary temperatures; some are volatile and gradually pass into the air, especially when heated; and some are non-volatile, or fixed. Cow's milk contains more than ten times as large

[1] " Handbuch der Milchkunde," Sommerfield, pp. 782–784.
[2] *Loc. cit.*, p. 787.

a proportion of the volatile acids as does human milk, while the percentage of oleic acid, an oil at room temperature, is much greater in the latter. The combined effect of these differences is that mother's milk fat melts at the lower temperature, a fact that is doubtless of some importance as related to the ease of digestion.[1]

269. Comparison of physical condition. — Certain other differences should be noted that show a marked difference in the physical character of the two milks. It is well understood that the casein of milk is not in solution therein, but is held in suspension as colloidal particles. When cow's milk is examined with the ultra microscope, it is possible to see these particles, which either by their constitution or their abundance completely hide the fat globules. When a similar examination is made of mother's milk, no casein particles are visible, and the fat globules show in a dark and apparently otherwise empty space. This difference can scarcely be due to the less amount of casein in the mother's milk, but shows rather that the constitution of the particles is unlike in the two cases. The fat globules of the mother's milk are much smaller than in the other.

270. The unlike curdling of the two milks. — The practical bearing of all these facts on the feeding of children is apparent when we come to observe the unlike curdling of the two milks. When a baby rejects cow's milk from its stomach, it is easily seen that the curds that have formed are of some size and show more or less solidity, that is, they look decidedly cheesy. On the contrary, when the food is the mother's milk, the curds are not nearly as evident, and are much more light and flaky. The same difference is observed in the laboratory when acid is added

[1] Loc. cit., p. 796.

to the two milks. That from the cow permits the prompt and complete separation of the casein by coagulation, which is not the case with woman's milk, the coagulation being quite different. The greater adaptability of mother's milk to infant feeding seems to be due to the difference in the proportion of the various compounds and to their unlike physical condition rather than to any inferiority of the casein, sugar, and fats of cow's milk in performing the functions of growth and maintenance when once digested. It appears to be a matter of ease of digestion, rather than nutritive function. One writer [1] advances the view that the difference, as infant's food, between cow's milk and mother's milk is mostly due to the larger proportion and consequent irritating influence of mineral salts in the former rather than to the differences in kind and quantity of the proteins and fat, but the facts cited can hardly be ignored in favor of this theory. It is not strange that the milk of the human mother is better suited to her young than that of any other species, otherwise Nature would seem to be a bungler.

271. The humanizing of cow's milk. — There are many cases where it is out of the question for the mother to feed her child with her own milk. Unless a " wet nurse " can be substituted, resort must be had to some artificial food, the one most commonly used being cow's milk. We have seen that cow's milk differs from human milk in the following particulars : —

1. A larger proportion of solids, especially when it is from either Jersey or Guernsey animals.

2. Twice as large an average proportion of protein, four-fifths of which is casein, whereas in human milk only

[1] The *Lancet*, Jan. 8, 1910.

two-fifths of the protein is casein, the soluble proteins like albumin being proportionately more in the human milk protein.

3. A much smaller proportion of milk sugar in the solids.

4. A different combination of fats, the mixture melting at a lower temperature in mother's milk.

When cow's milk is to be fed to the infant, it would seem wise to eliminate these differences as fully as possible, although a complete similarity to mother's milk can hardly be reached. If cow's milk is diluted with an equal volume of water, the proportion of casein in the mixture becomes approximately like that in human milk. But this gives a proportion of solids altogether too low for satisfactory results, and besides, the solids are too poor in sugar and fat. The sugar and fat not only aid in nourishing the child, but a greater proportion so divides the particles of casein that its coagulation approaches more nearly that of mother's milk. The desired result may be practically accomplished by a combination of cow's milk, cream, milk sugar and barley water, the latter adding more or less albumin and other soluble matter that still further modifies the coagulation.

272. Illustrative formulæ.—The two following formulæ may serve to illustrate this method of modifying cow's milk.

As the barley water carries some solid matter, it may be well to make up the foregoing mixtures to twenty ounces for the first two or three weeks. Following this more dilute preparation, a change may be made to the 16-ounce volume. The proportion of solids in the modified milk may safely be allowed to increase progressively as the child grows older. This may be accomplished by using the same

TABLE L

FORMULÆ FOR MODIFYING COW'S MILK

No. 1

	FORMULA FOR AVERAGE MILK				
	Solids	Ash	Protein	Sugar	Fat
	Oz.	Oz.	Oz.	Oz.	Oz.
7 oz. average milk	.903	.049	.224	.357	.273
1 oz. 18 per cent cream (average)	.26	.005	.025	.045	.185
½ oz. milk sugar	.50	——	——	.50	——
Dilute with barley water to 16 oz.					
	1.663	.054	.249	.912	.458
16 oz. average mother's milk .	1.888	.032	.246	1.057	.552
	%	%	%	%	%
Composition modified milk .	10.4	.34	1.55	5.70	2.86

No. 2

	FORMULA FOR AVERAGE JERSEY OR GUERNSEY MILK				
	Solids	Ash	Protein	Sugar	Fat
	Oz.	Oz.	Oz.	Oz.	Oz.
7 oz. milk	1.05	.56	.273	.350	.371
½ oz. 18 per cent cream . .	.13	.002	.012	.022	.090
½ oz. milk sugar	.50	——	——	.50	——
Dilute with barley water to 16 oz.					
	1.68	.058	.285	.872	.461
	%	%	%	%	%
Composition modified milk .	10.5	.40	1.80	5.45	2.87

amounts of milk, cream, and milk sugar, and making up the mixture to a less volume. At the end of ten or twelve weeks, the volume could safely be reduced to 14 ounces, and at five or six months to 12 ounces.

It is very commonly recommended that a certain proportion of lime water be used in diluting cow's milk. If the object of this is to cause a more desirable coagulation of the casein, it seems to be more rational to reach this result by the use of barley water or by adding a thoroughly soluble cereal preparation. It is questionable whether it is wise to neutralize the essential acidity of the gastric juice by adding to the food a free base like calcium hydrate.

273. Accuracy desirable. — Accuracy in modifying milk requires that the composition of the milk and cream be known. On a commercial scale or in a pediatric hospital where large numbers of children are fed, this is possible, but in the home it is not, although where a Babcock tester is available a determination of the fat and solids may be quickly made. If the milk is from Holstein or other thin milk cows, it will in general be safe to use 8 ounces with $1\frac{1}{2}$ ounces of cream and $\frac{1}{2}$ ounce milk sugar, the whole to be made up to 16 ounces. With Jersey or Guernsey milk the formula given above for that class of milk may be used. When the family is provided with high-priced certified milk, the composition is generally known and the formula may be varied accordingly. It is sometimes recommended to take a certain quantity of " top milk " and dilute it to a given volume; but this method is not to be commended, because top milk is a very uncertain composition. It will vary to a marked degree with the temperature at which the milk is kept; while the cream is rising, the higher the temperature the richer the cream.

It will also vary with the original quality of the milk, cream from thin milk containing less fat than cream from rich milk, other conditions being the same. If top milk is to be used, it should be from milk of a fairly uniform quality and kept at practically the same temperature from day to day.

274. Precautions. — A general supply of mixed milk should not be used if it can be avoided. Unless milk known to be sanitary and of fairly uniform composition can be procured, the milk of a single cow, known to be healthy, should be used. This cow should not be too far advanced in the period of lactation, should be rationally fed, and neither the cow nor her milk and utensils should come in contact with a person having an infectious disease or recovering from such. The milk should be drawn under cleanly conditions, cooled at once, and kept cold in a sanitary refrigerator until used. Such precautions are often difficult and sometimes impossible in large cities, except for the wealthy, a fact which greatly enhances the dangers from feeding children on cow's milk, especially during the summer months.

The use of all the knowledge and skill we now possess does not yet make it possible to perfectly simulate mother's milk by the use of other materials. We cannot yet attain nature's art in providing food for the human young.

275. Goat's milk as infant food. — Within a few years much attention has been given to goat's milk as a food for infants. The points urged in its favor are that one or more goats may be kept by a family having only a small area of land, thus insuring fresh milk, that the milk is economically produced, that this species is practically free from tuberculosis, though not entirely immune, and, what is most important, satisfactory results seem to attend the use of the milk.   It is objected that because of the long hair of the goat the milk is more likely to be contaminated, and the offensive odor from the animal's skin is liable to cause an undesirable flavor in the milk.   Both these objections may be obviated by thoroughly cleaning the hair and skin of the animal and by drawing the milk in some yard or room outside the living quarters of the animals.

The composition of goat's milk appears to vary widely, as is shown by the following figures.   Average analyses presented by several authors show a variation of the per cent of solid matter from 7 to 18.   Analyses of the milk of several goats have recently been made at the New York Agricultural Experiment Station with results as shown in Table LI

It appears that the quality of the milk bears quite a marked relation to the amount of the yield, the smaller the yield the larger the per cent of solids.   This is true of other mammals.

Goat's milk is seen to be greatly unlike human milk in its composition.   It contains in many instances not far from the same percentage of solid matter, but the proportion of protein in the solids is much higher and of sugar much lower.   The percentage of fat varies greatly.

As compared with cow's milk, certain differences exist. The fat globules of the goat's milk are smaller, and when it is coagulated, the particles of curd are finer.   It is also more viscous (sticky).   These physical conditions are such that cream does not rise on raw goat's milk even on long standing, but after boiling, a separation of the cream occurs. The reasons are not quite clear why goat's milk is to be preferred to properly modified cow's milk for feeding children. The proteins have about the same relative proportions of casein and albumin, and there is much similarity in other respects. The most probable reason for superiority, if such exists, is in the different manner of coagulation. It would seem that goat's milk of a high percentage of solids would be improved by modification in the manner recommended for cow's milk.

TABLE LI

ANALYSES OF THE MILK OF ELEVEN INDIVIDUAL GOATS, AUGUST 9, 1910

WEIGHT, MILK	TOTAL SOLIDS	ASH	TOTAL PROTEIN	CASEIN	ALBUMIN, ETC.	FAT
Pounds	Per Cent	Per Cent	Per Cent	Per Cent	Per Cent	Per Cent
2.8	11.47	0.49	2.88	2.12	0.76	3.7
3.3	10.49	0.48	2.48	1.64	0.84	2.7
0.6	11.80	0.57	2.56	1.71	0.85	3.9
5.3	10.73	0.49	2.48	1.66	0.82	3.0
1.4	11.11	0.51	2.77	1.83	0.94	3.4
4.4	9.66	0.43	2.34	1.58	0.66	2.4
0.7	15.18	0.53	4.16	3.27	0.89	5.6
2.1	10.23	0.53	2.88	2.13	0.75	3.0
2.1	11.79	0.61	3.33	2.47	0.86	3.4
0.6	18.55	0.80	4.81	3.84	0.97	8.4
0.6	16.13	0.68	3.92	3.07	0.85	6.5

D. INFANT FOODS

The markets are abundantly supplied with preparations known as infant foods, which, if the statements of the manufacturers are to be taken at their face value, are

U

remarkably efficient for feeding young children. Without question, these preparations have been widely used, and in many cases with apparently satisfactory results. An extended examination of their sources, *i.e.*, the raw materials out of which they are made, and their chemical condition abundantly justifies a recommendation of caution in their use.

276. Composition of infant foods. — As a means of setting forth the real facts as regards this class of foods, reference is made to the report of an exhaustive examination in 1908 of twenty-three brands.[1]

TABLE LII

Composition of Certain Infant Foods

	Water	Ash	Protein	Fiber	Carbo-hydrates	Fat	Lactose	Soluble in Water	Starch
Milk and Cereals	Per Cent	Per Cent	Per Cent	Per Cent	Per Cent	Per Cent	Per Cent	Per Cent	Per Cent
Allenbury's Milk Food No. 2	4.98	3.69	9.00	0.28	68.33	13.72	27.14	82.27	——
Horlick's Malted Milk	3.63	3.70	12.94	——	71.37	8.36	0.39	88.58	——
Lactated Food . . .	7.12	1.19	8.13	——	82.84	0.72	9.67	34.54	41.94
Malted Cereals									
Fessenden's Food . .	5.95	1.60	6.00	0.08	85.97	0.40	0.36	48.80	35.69
Mellin's Infant Food .	5.07	3.79	10.50	0.25	79.24	1.15	0.37	83.97	——
Sunbright's California Baby Food . . .	9.00	1.09	7.94	0.22	81.05	0.70	0.19	6.84	63.25
Ridges' Food . . .	9.24	0.60	11.81	0.05	77.26	1.04	0.12	3.90	69.46
Miscellaneous									
Peptogenic Milk Powder	3.02	1.40	0.81	——	94.67	0.10	90.53	95.40	——
Eskay's Albumenized Food	3.06	1.34	6.56	0.04	87.80	1.20	36.98	51.10	28.41

[1] Conn. Agric. Exp. Station, Rep., 1908, p. 599.

TABLE LIII

Sources and Ingredients of Certain Infant Foods

	What the Manufacturers Claim	What was Found
Allenbury's Milk Food No. 2	Made from pasteurized milk and malted wheat, no unaltered starch. Containing all elements of human milk in natural proportions.	No starch. Does not contain elements of human milk in natural proportions. Proportion of protein and fat too low.
Horlick's Malted Milk	Made from full cream milk and malted grains.	No starch.
Lactated Food	Contains the most important elements of mother's milk, with the nutritive principles of the cereal grains.	About two-fifths unaltered starch. Only about one-third dry matter soluble in water.
Fessenden's Food	Made from wheat, rye, arrowroot, and malted barley. No cane sugar or unaltered starch.	Raw arrowroot starch; over one-third dry matter is unchanged starch. Less than half dry matter soluble in water.
Mellin's Infant Food	Extract from wheat and malt. No cane sugar or starch.	No starch. Largely soluble in water.
Sunbright's California Baby Food	A perfect modifier of cow's milk.	Nearly two-thirds dry matter is unaltered starch. Only about one-seventh soluble in water.
Ridges' Food . .	Baked flour.	Largely raw wheat starch.
Peptogenic Milk Powder	Chiefly milk sugar.	No starch. Mostly milk sugar.
Eskays' Albumenized Food	Made from egg albumin and cereal.	Raw arrowroot starch. Cooked cereal starch. Very little soluble protein.

277. Important facts about infant foods. — The analyses quoted above reveal some facts that deserve careful consideration, which may be summarized in the following statements : —

1. In some brands the proportions of nutrients are greatly unlike what are found in human milk, the protein and fat, and sometimes the ash, being deficient, and the carbohydrates greatly in excess.

2. In most cases the carbohydrates are not present as lactose, but in part as sugar resulting from the hydrolysis of starch (probably glucose) and in part as untransformed starch.

3. In many of the foods, a large part of the solids is insoluble in water, this being true of both protein and carbohydrates.

278. Danger from unmodified starch. — It is clear that the commercial infant foods are decidedly unlike the natural food of the young child, in one respect very undesirably so. Reference is made to the presence of starch. When the infant receives its natural food, there is no occasion for the exercise of the diastatic function in digestion (hydrolysis of starch to sugar), as sugar is the only carbohydrate in milk. It was formerly held that the very young infant is not able to digest starch at all, but recent investigations throw doubt on the accuracy of this conclusion. Even if starch is more or less acted upon by the young child, it is an unnatural demand in the earliest stage of development, and the presence in the digestive tract of so much insoluble material, not only starch but proteins, is likely to be attended with disorders of the stomach and intestines. This would be especially true of the heated season. German statistics, previously cited as to the use of cow's milk, show a still greater per cent of mortality among infants fed with these artificial preparations. In addition to the unnatural substitution of starch for the milk sugar that is in the child's natural food, there is also the deficiency in the proportions of ash and fat to be considered, a condition which may easily have a serious influence upon the child's nutrition and the character of its growth. Such a defiance of the natural methods is excusable only in cases of necessity.

279. Standard for infant foods. — The following standard for infant foods quoted by Wiley from the *British Food Journal* is worthy of attention:

Definition : Infant's food is food described or sold as an article of food especially suitable for infants of twelve (12) months of age or under.

Standard : Infant's food shall contain no woody fiber, no preservative substance, and no mineral substance insoluble in acid; and, unless described or sold specifically as food suitable only for infants over the age of six (6) months, shall, when prepared as directed by any accompanying label, contain no starch, and shall contain the essential constituents of, and conform approximately in proportional composition to, normal mother's milk.

E. FEEDING THE CHILD AFTER IT HAS PASSED THE PERIOD OF INFANCY

280. Introduction of solid food into diet. — The child's nutrition gradually passes from an exclusive milk diet to one that is in part solid food. It is well for the development of the capacity for digestion that the admission of solid food be not too long delayed. Following weaning the food will, for some time, continue to be largely liquid, preferably cow's or goat's milk, or if necessary an infant food. The latter should be selected at first somewhat with reference to its composition and solubility, the presence of a desirable proportion of ash and protein and the absence of a large proportion of unmodified starch being essential points to consider. At eight to ten months a beginning may be made with solid food, and for this purpose there is nothing better than properly cooked egg (without leathery coagulation of the white), especially if a cereal food is the main part of the diet. As the child develops, milk should be eaten freely, and there may be added thoroughly cooked cereal preparations, crackers, stale bread, and so on gradually to the same plain foods that are eaten by adults.

281. Simple diet best. — For a few years, mothers should rigidly adhere to the policy of a simple diet from which is excluded pastry, cakes, sweets, condiments, indeed all desserts that generally are nutritively one-sided preparations which tempt the palate to the exclusion of simpler and better balanced materials. No more serious mistake can be made than to allow a child to acquire a distaste for plain food because of indulgence in desserts that are usually highly flavored and attractive to the taste. The result is that unless controlled, the child discards the simpler foods best calculated to promote vigorous growth, and substitutes preparations that carry large proportions of starch, sugar, and fat. There is much to commend the practice of a separate table for the children in the nursery, where temptation is out of reach.

This habit of simple living on meats in very moderate proportion, eggs, milk, cereal foods (from the whole grain), vegetables, and fruits, with a very small minimum of the usual desserts, may well continue through all the growing period and become a life habit.

282. Mixed diet desirable. — A fairly well mixed diet should be encouraged. While individual tastes cannot always be overcome by education, an exclusiveness of diet on the part of a boy or girl, such as relative excess of meat or bread and butter, or even milk, should be discouraged, and every effort made to include in the menu a reasonable proportion of vegetables and well ripened fruits, without neglecting the more substantial foods.

283. The candy habit. — One parental weakness cannot be too strongly condemned, *i.e.*, permitting a child to acquire the candy habit. It is true that pure candy is made of sugar, which, under right conditions, may play an important part in the animal economy. But sugar of itself exercises no constructive function, and when the free use of sweetmeats is permitted, generally at all times of the day, a desire for wholesome food is much lessened, and the child is robbed, sometimes disastrously and always unfortunately, of the nutrition to which it is entitled. The eating habits of some children are nothing short of abominable, and for these habits parents are responsible. It is a trite saying, but a true one, that the intelligent farmer's calves and pigs are fed more rationally than many children.

284. Suggestions for children's dietaries. — The following is a summary of a recent excellent pamphlet on the feeding of children issued by Columbia University.[1]

[1] " The Feeding of Young Children," Mary Swartz Rose, Ph.D.

The meals suggested for children of different ages illustrate rational food combinations.

1. The cultivation of a rational appetite is part of the training of a child.

2. Children should be fed regularly and not too often. The stomach should have a chance to rest.

3. Children from two to five years of age need four meals a day, older ones three, at fixed hours.

4. Milk is the best food for children of all ages, either as such or cooked into cereals, vegetables, soup, junket, custard, and simple puddings.

5. Well-cooked cereal should be served every day, but without sugar, syrup, or butter. Use cereals that are made from whole grains.

6. Use eggs freely, soft-cooked and not fried, and in simple cooked dishes.

7. "Children cannot thrive without fruit." Give only ripe fresh fruit in perfect condition, or that which is stewed or baked.

8. Fresh vegetables should be a part of the diet, as these are rich in the needed mineral elements. A great variety of well-cooked vegetables may be served.

9. In general, provide a plain fare of which bread and butter, cereals and milk should form a generous part.

10. Do not give meat to children under eight years of age when milk and eggs are available. When meat is allowed, it should be fairly free from fat.

11. For desserts provide simple puddings such as junket, rice, tapioca, or other cereal puddings. Do not allow candy, except a small piece at meal time.

12. Cultivate the habit in the child of drinking a liberal amount of water.

285. Illustrative meals for children. — The following meals are suggested for children of different ages as illustrating rational combinations of food :—

CHILD 2-4 YEARS OLD

Breakfast :
   7.30 A.M. Oatmeal Mush
               Milk
               Stale Bread
               Orange Juice

Lunch :
   11 A.M.   Milk
               Stale Bread
               Butter

   1.00 P.M. Baked Potato
               Boiled Onions
                 (Mashed)
               Bread and Butter
               Milk to Drink
               Baked Apple

Supper :
   5.30 P.M. Boiled Rice
               Milk
               Bread and Butter

PROTEIN Grams	FUEL VALUE Calories	COST Cents
47.80	1313	0.1377

Substitutes or additions : —

For rolled oats or rice : other cereals, such as rolled wheat, wheaten grits, farina, hominy, and corn meal.

For orange juice and baked apple : prune pulp or apple sauce.

For onions: spinach, strained peas, stewed celery, carrots, or cauliflower tips.

An egg may be added every day, and should be included at least two or three times a week.

These changes will alter the cost somewhat.

CHILD 4–8 YEARS OLD

Breakfast: Oatmeal Mush
Top Milk
Stewed Prunes
Toast
Milk to Drink

Dinner: Pea Soup
Croutons
Boiled Onions
Baked Potato
Molasses Cookies

Supper: Cream Toast
Rice Pudding with
Milk and Sugar
Milk to Drink

PROTEIN Grams	FUEL VALUE Calories	COST Cents
65.4	1892	0.1496

Substitutes or additions: —

For rolled oats: other cereals, as suggested on previous page.

For onions and peas: strained dried beans; other vegetables carefully cooked; fresh lettuce.

For prunes: fresh ripe apples, baked bananas, other mild fruits well cooked.

For rice pudding: junkets, custards, blanc manges, bread puddings, and other very simple desserts.

For cookies: gingerbread, sponge cake, or very plain cookies.

CHILD 8–12 YEARS OLD

Breakfast: Oatmeal Mush
Top Milk
Stewed Prunes
Toast
Milk to Drink

Luncheon: Pea Soup
Boiled Onions
Baked Potato
Bread and Butter
Molasses Cookies

Dinner: Baked Haddock
Creamed Hashed Potato
Spinach
Bread and Butter
Rice Pudding — Milk
and Sugar

PROTEIN Grams	FUEL VALUE Calories	COST Cents
86.44	2420	0.1875

Substitutes or additions: —

For rolled oats: other cereals thoroughly cooked.

For haddock: rare beefsteak, roast beef or mutton chops; other fish, especially white varieties.

For prunes: any mild ripe fruit uncooked or cooked.

For onions: string beans, stewed celery, beets, squash.

Peas or spinach: turnips or cauliflower.

SUGGESTIVE DIETARY FOR CHILD WHO WILL NOT DRINK MILK,
AGE 5 YEARS

(1 quart of milk concealed in the menu)

Breakfast:
    7 A.M.   Oatmeal
               Creamy Egg on Toast
               Cocoa

   10 A.M.   Zwieback and Cream

  1.30 P.M.   Spinach Soup
               Baked Potato with Cream
               Bread and Butter
               Caramel Junket

  5.30 P.M.   Rice and Prunes
               Zwieback

PROTEIN Grams	FUEL VALUE Calories	COST Cents
51.9	1431	0.1570

CHAPTER XV

THE CHARACTER AND FOOD VALUE OF CERTAIN COMMERCIAL ARTICLES

WITHIN the last three or four decades proprietary articles, either real or so-called foods, have been offered to the public in greatly increasing numbers. These have very properly received special consideration for two reasons, (1) in many instances remarkable but utterly unfounded claims have been made for their nutritive value, thereby deceiving an undiscriminating public, and (2) the general high cost of a unit of nutritive value in them as compared with home preparations of equal or greater nutritive efficiency. No more striking examples of deceptive or even utterly false statements and of bad business ethics are to be found than are shown in the exploitation of some of these articles.

A. MEAT PREPARATIONS, EXTRACTS, FLUID EXTRACTS, MEAT JUICES

286. True meat extract. — In order to judge intelligently the commercial meat extracts as they actually are, we should first consider what a real meat extract is. The manufacture of these preparations was greatly promoted by Baron von Liebig's researches on the chemistry of meat, although something similar had been used for many years before. The original Liebig method of making the extract is to treat finely chopped beef with eight times its weight of cold water, thus dissolving only a very small part of the beef, the substances taken into solution being ash compounds, chiefly potassium phosphate, some albumin and the extractive creatin and its anhydride creatinin. The liquid, after being strained from the beef, is heated sufficiently to coagulate the albumin, this coagulum is filtered off, and the remaining extract, containing the ash compounds and extractives, is evaporated to a paste. While popularly regarded as such, this preparation can hardly be considered as a food, for, as previously stated, the beef extractives creatin and creatinin furnish to the body neither constructive material nor energy, but are largely eliminated in the urine unchanged (see p. 61). These bodies impart a flavor to cooked beef, and besides have the important function of vigorously exciting the secretion of gastric juice (see Chap. V, p. 100). One author (Hutchinson) truly says of them that, " They are thus eminently calculated to rouse appetite and aid the digestion of any food with which they may be taken. This, indeed, is their true function both in health and disease. They are flavoring agents, and their proper place is in the kitchen and not by the bedside." [1]

287. Commercial meat extracts. — The foregoing are the specifications of a true beef extract as defined by Liebig. It is interesting to note what is the real character of the extracts now in the market, for which surprising claims are made. In 1908, the Connecticut Agricultural

[1] " Food and Dietetics," Hutchinson, p. 93.

Experiment Station[1] made an exhaustive examination of twenty-two brands of meat extracts, twenty-three brands of fluid and semi-fluid preparations, and four brands of meat juices. Of these 47 preparations 10 were found to be properly branded and up to the standards, 17 were found to be misbranded and varying from the standards, and the others were, in general, not up to the standards, though not misbranded. The standards with which the preparations were compared are those based on analyses of genuine beef extracts. The misbranding consisted in such misleading or false statements as the following: " no foreign matter," " absolutely unadulterated," when a large quantity of salt had been added, " the nutritious portion of beef in concentrated form," " a concentrated food that represents the nourishing constituents of fresh beef," " all that is nourishing, sustaining and palatable in fresh beef," " a combination of all the strengthening and stimulating properties of prime lean beef," " the most perfect form of concentrated food known," " pure essence " of beef, statements that deceive the uninformed, because these materials are not concentrated foods and can by no possibility contain more than a very small part of the nutriment of beef. There is no such thing as concentrating the nutritive constituents of beef, except by drying out the water, for practically all the dry matter of clear lean beef is digested, and all of it is nutritious. When beef extract is made, the major portion of the beef, indeed, nearly all its nutritive value, is rejected. Attention should be called to the very high cost of the dry organic matter in these extracts. It was found that the 22 meat extracts

[1] Rep., 1908, pp. 606–664.

contained from 14.8 to 40.4 per cent of water, from 17.6 to 35 per cent of ash, largely common salt, and 37.3 to 67.6 per cent of organic matter. The prices of packages varying in weight from 1.4 to 3.4 ounces ranged from 15 to 50 cents. The least cost per pound of dry matter was $1, and the greatest $5.70, the dry organic matter costing from $2.68 to $10.18 per pound. Beef tea and beef juice made at home are as good as or better than these preparations, and cost greatly less. The trade in some of these extracts is a fraud on the consumer.

B. BREAKFAST FOODS

288. Sources and kinds. — The so-called breakfast foods are sold under a great and steadily increasing variety of names and forms. They are extensively used, being now found on the table of nearly every family of well-to-do communities. The sources from which they are derived are the cereal grains, corn, oats, wheat. There are three general methods of preparation: (1) grinding the decorticated grain, (2) steaming or otherwise cooking with subsequent grinding or rolling, and (3) malting, that is, the production of materials in which the starch has been partially changed to a soluble form by the action of heat or diastase. It should be stated that these foods do not receive special mention because of inferior quality. They appear to be prepared in a hygienic manner, are not adulterated, are so thoroughly dried as to keep well, and, in general, may be considered to be among the very best of the foods carrying a high proportion of carbohydrates. It is the claims that are made for such extensively used materials, and the wide differences in their cost, that render it advisable to consider the real facts touching their nutritive value.

289. Composition. — The composition of these foods is found to be similar to that of the grains from which they are made. The following table will bear careful study on this point.

TABLE LIV

AVERAGE COMPOSITION OF CEREAL BREAKFAST PREPARATIONS COMPARED WITH WHEAT FLOUR VARIOUSLY MILLED [1]

NUMBER OF ANALYSES		WATER	PROTEIN	FAT	CARBOHYDRATES	ASH	HEAT OF COMBUSTION
		Per Cent	Per Cent	Per Cent	Per Cent	Per Cent	Calories per Gram
14	Corn meal and hominy (uncooked) . . .	10.7	8.6	0.7	79.7	0.3	3.854
28	Rolled oats (cooked) .	8.4	15.6	7.5	66.6	1.9	4.323
35	Rolled wheat (cooked)	9.9	12.0	1.9	74.8	1.4	3.966
1	Malted oats (cooked).	6.4	16.7	5.4	69.7	1.8	4.318
4	Malted wheat (cooked)	6.9	13.3	1.2	77.0	1.6	4.017
4	Graham flour . . .	10.7	14.8	2.3	70.3	1.9	4.029
4	Entire wheat flour .	11.4	14.1	2.0	71.5	1.0	3.967
4	Standard patent flour	11.4	13.9	1.4	72.8	0.5	3.959

290. Changes in preparation. — In the cooked and malted foods, the starch has been more or less changed to other carbohydrates, mostly dextrin (see Table LV).

291. Digestibility. — As the processes of manufacture have not rendered these preparations greatly unlike the cereal grains in which they have their source, except in some of them to dextrinize part of the starch, we must look to their digestibility for any increased nutritive efficiency which they may possess. The most reliable

[1] Maine Agric. Exp. Station, Bul. 118, p. 121.

x

TABLE LV

RELATIVE PERCENTAGES OF STARCH AND DEXTRIN IN CERTAIN CEREAL BREAKFAST FOODS [1]

	STARCH	DEXTRIN	EXTENT OF DEXTRINIZATION
	Per Cent	Per Cent	Per Cent
Corn meal	69.5	——	——
Oat meal	63.8	——	——
Rolled oats	60.5	3.6	5.6
Ralston breakfast food .	67.9	2.6	3.7
Malt breakfast food . .	71.7	3.2	4.3
Malta vita	62.4	9.3	13.0
Force	55.4	14.5	20.7
Grape Nuts	49.5	24.9	33.5

TABLE LVI

COMPARATIVE DIGESTIBILITY OF CEREAL FOODS

	DRY MATTER	TOTAL ORGANIC MATTER	PROTEIN	CARBOHY-DRATES	FATS	AVAILABLE ENERGY
	Per Ct.	Per Ct.	Per C .	Per Ct.	Per Ct.	Per Ct.
Rolled oats (simple diet) . .	——	95.4	84.7	——	——	94.2
Rolled wheat (simple diet) .	——	95.2	91.6	——	——	94.6
Force (simple diet) . .	——	94.6	89.6	——	——	91.1
Grape nuts (simple diet) .	——	94.0	87.6	——	——	93.1
Shredded whole wheat (simple diet)	——	92.8	84.1	——	——	91.4
Hecker's hominy (simple diet)	——	97.3	83.6	——	——	96.4
Granulated corn meal (simple diet)	——	97.2	82.3	——	——	95.9
Hulled corn (eaten alone) .	——	——	81.7	97.3	——	91.8
Wheat bread (eaten alone) .	——	——	93.9	99.1	——	97.3
Johnny cake (simple diet) .	——	——	93.2	98.9	——	93.5
Brown bread (simple diet) .	——	——	92.8	98.6	——	93.4

[1] Maine Agric. Exp. Station, Bul. 118, p. 126.

figures available do not show that breakfast foods differ essentially in digestibility from cereal flours and meals, and certain home-made preparations. The figures given in Table LVI, as well as those in the two previous tables are largely the result of work done at the Maine Agricultural Experiment Station, with others quoted by Atwater.

The digestibility of breakfast foods is proved to be in no respect superior to that of granulated corn meal, johnny cake, brown bread, or white bread.

292. Unwarranted claims. — It is clear that the claims made for certain breakfast foods, such as the nourishing of more persons for a given time than other foods do, " the most natural food for mankind," " the great brain and muscle food," " a condensed food," " the system will absorb a greater amount of nourishment from one pound of than from ten pounds of meat, wheat, oats or bread," are false, and the manufacturers making these claims either intend to deceive the public or are grossly ignorant of the real nutritive value of their products. The fact is, it is not possible so to transform the nutrients in meats and cereal grains as materially to enhance their nutritive efficiency, nor can such foods be " condensed," excepting as water is dried out. Cooking and malting may increase the ease and rapidity of digestion, but for persons normal in health and function there is nothing in the processes applied to breakfast foods superior in any respect to home cooking.

293. Money cost. — We can now consider intelligently the cost of breakfast foods, for this is practically the only question the housewife needs to raise. The pound cost of such foods varies greatly, ranging from four cents to

approximately 25 cents. In 1908 the average cost in a
New England market for the various classes was as follows, when purchased in packages: —

TABLE LVII

MAXIMUM, MINIMUM, AND AVERAGE COST PER POUND OF
WHEAT, OAT, AND CORN BREAKFAST FOODS PURCHASED IN
PACKAGES [1]

NUMBER OF SAMPLES	KIND OF CEREAL	PRICE PER POUND		
		Maximum	Minimum	Average
		Cents	Cents	Cents
24	Wheat . .	11.4	4.9	7.8
17	Oats . . .	7.8	4.1	6.0
10	Corn . . .	9.2	4.1	5.5

By use of the foregoing figures it is easy to calculate
the nutrition that could be bought for one dollar.[2]

TABLE LVIII

NUTRITION PURCHASED FOR ONE DOLLAR

	AVERAGE COST PER POUND	NUMBER OF POUNDS FOR ONE DOLLAR	PROTEIN	FAT	CARBOHY-DRATES	ASH	HEAT OF COMBUSTION
	Cents		Lb.	Lb.	Lb.	Lb.	Cal.
Rolled wheat . . .	7.8	12.8	1.54	0.24	9.57	0.18	40.3
Rolled oats	6.0	16.7	2.79	0.90	11.64	0.30	72.0
Hominy	5.5	18.2	1.56	0.13	14.50	0.05	70.2
Patent flour . . .	3.5	28.6	3.98	0.40	20.82	0.14	113.2

[1] Including only the hominies.
[2] Maine Agric. Exp. Station, Bul. 118, pp. 132, 133.

It should be noted that when some of these foods are bought in bulk, the cost is less than the above averages, not exceeding four cents per pound. In view of their ease of preparation, with the saving of fuel and labor, they may be economical when so purchased, as compared with the common raw materials, such as flour and the meals, which can be bought at from two to three cents per pound.

C. ALCOHOL IN NUTRITION

Immense quantities of alcohol are consumed by the human family in such beverages as koumis, kephir, beers, wines, and the strong drinks, whiskey, brandy, gin, and rum, the intemperate drinking of many of which has caused untold degradation and misery. The sentimental and moral considerations that relate to the use of alcohol in all forms have led to absurd and grossly inaccurate teachings concerning its real physiological functions and reactions.

294. Alcohol is oxidized in body. — Until the application of exact measurements, it was held that alcohol is largely excreted from the body as such, and performs no useful physiological service. It is now definitely proven that with the moderate use of alcohol only a very small proportion is given off in the breath and urine, perhaps not more than 2 per cent. More than this, it is demonstrated beyond question that alcohol, when taken up to $2\frac{1}{2}$ ounces per day, at least, is almost wholly oxidized, and serves the human organism as a source of energy. Moreover, up to a limited extent, it will replace such nutrients as sugar and starch. When in experiments by Atwater and Benedict 72 grams (about $2\frac{1}{2}$ oz.) of alcohol was substituted for an isodynamic (equivalent in energy) amount of sugar, the results in heat production and body storage were exactly the same.

The figures of the following table[1] showing the results of five-day periods of observation of a man in a respiration calorimeter are a convincing demonstration of the foregoing statements : —

TABLE LIX

USE OF ALCOHOL

SERIES	INTAKE		METAB-OLISM CAL-ORIES	BALANCE		RETEN-TION IN CAL-ORIES
	Diet	Gross Calories		Proteid	Fat	
				Grams	Grams	
23	Fixed diet	=2546	2176	−1.6	+ 9.0	77
22	Fixed diet + 72 grams alcohol (= 500 calories)	=3044	2258	+1.4	+62.7	589
24	Fixed diet + 130 grams sugar (= 515 calories	=3061	2272	+1.7	+59.7	56
22–23	Difference	= 498	+82	+3.0	+53.7	=512
24–23	Difference	= 515	+96	+3.3	+50.7	=485
24–22	Difference	= 15	+14	+0.3	− 3.0	= −27

It appears not only that 72 grams of alcohol took the place of 130 grams of sugar, but that the use of protein was not unfavorably affected.

295. Relation to muscular effort. — It should not be assumed from the above data that alcohol may serve as a direct source of muscular effort. It is true, however, that when in the diet of men at work fat has been replaced

---

[1] "Metabolism and Practical Medicine," Von Noorden, Vol. 1, p. 350.

by its energy equivalent of alcohol, and the work performed has not changed, the total output of heat has been no greater than on an alcohol-free diet. This may be explained on the ground that the alcohol spared the use of the carbohydrates in some other direction than muscular effort. It should be understood that these conclusions do not apply to the use of alcohol in quantities that are toxic and disturb the normal physiological processes. Nor is it argued that it is desirable or necessary to use alcoholic beverages. Indeed, the advice is rather to let these drinks alone.

296. Alcohol not a necessary food. — It is sometimes ignorantly asserted by individuals who have acquired an alcohol habit that it is a physiological necessity for them. Alcohol is never physiologically necessary for any normal human organism, and in health there is no advantage in its use. The exhilaration due to taking beer and wine or stronger drinks is not an evidence of physiological benefit. Another foolish belief is that alcoholic liquors are a defense against cold. The sensation of warmth following a drink of whiskey is due to an increased flow of blood to the surface of the body. This does not conserve body heat, but rather the reverse. Patent medicines containing alcohol often get a reputation for curative properties when the alleged benefits are nothing more than a temporary exhilaration. Notwithstanding all these errors that are believed, nothing is gained in the way of physiological welfare and temperance by ungrounded assertions as to the dire results of taking a little alcohol into the stomach.

CHAPTER XVI

THE PREPARATION OF FOOD

THE variety of food preparations that are served on the
tables of well-to-do families is almost endless in number,
and human ingenuity seems to be exercised to the limit in
devising new ones. It is no exaggeration to declare that
we are now living in a period of gastronomic luxury that
makes heavy demands on both our financial and physical
resources. It is not possible to deal with the recipe
phase of cookery, excepting within the limits of a " cook
book." There are, however, general principles pertaining
to all cookery that may properly be discussed in this connection. The preparation of food may be considered from
several points of view, viz. the chemical reactions produced
by certain combinations, the effects of cooking, special
considerations pertaining to classes of foods, and mechanical display.

A. CHEMICAL REACTIONS OR CHANGES DUE TO SPE-CIFIC CAUSES

The chemical reactions that need to be considered under
this head are the evolution of carbonic acid for lightening
bread and cake, and the action of acids upon coagulable
proteins.

297. The evolution of carbonic acid. — This is done in
order to lighten the texture of bread and cake, and is

brought about, excepting in yeast fermentation, by the reaction of some acid or acid salt on a bicarbonate of either sodium or potassium, generally the former. In old-fashioned cooking, sour milk and " saleratus " (potassium bicarbonate) were used in making " saleratus biscuit." In this case, the carbonic acid was displaced in the saleratus by the action of the acids or acid salts in the milk, forming little vesicles of gas all through the dough, thus greatly lightening its texture. When soda (sodium bicarbonate) is added to dough sweetened with molasses, the same result is reached because of the acid substances in the molasses. In order that there may be no excess of soda or acid, it is necessary that they be combined in definite proportions. In home cookery, where sour milk and molasses are used, the combination is more or less " hit or miss " for the acidity of these materials is not always the same. When the acids are in excess rather than the soda, the results are not serious, as is the case when too much soda is used. At the present time " baking powders " are in the market, in which the combinations are chemically correct.

298. The coagulation of proteins. — The housewife of experience does not need to be reminded that vinegar and milk do not always constitute a compatible mixture, as the casein of the milk sometimes precipitates or forms a curd. The same change sometimes takes place when milk is improperly added to tomato soup. The results with vinegar and milk, that is, acetic acid and the calcium casein, depend upon the proportion of acid to casein. The curdling of the milk is due to the fact that the acid of the vinegar removes the lime from its combination with the casein; but precipitation of the casein does not begin until the amount of acid passes a certain proportion. Probably one half ounce of 4 per cent vinegar could be added to one quart of milk without causing curdling when the milk is heated to boiling, but much beyond this proportion would precipitate the casein.   At ordinary temperatures much more vinegar would be used, perhaps two ounces.   The proportion of vinegar would depend on its strength, of which the housewife is not generally informed, an example of the inexact way in which much cooking is necessarily done.   The same considerations apply to the use of milk with acid materials, such as fruits containing citric, tartaric, or malic acids.   The condition of the milk is to be considered, too.   Fresh milk will bear more acid than milk in which more or less lactic acid has developed and combined with part of the lime in the casein compounds.

When meat proteins and the white of egg are cooked, coagulation occurs, with a hardening of the meat tissue and of the egg albumin.   This is discussed more fully in what follows.

B. THE EFFECT OF COOKING, OR THE ACTION OF HEAT UPON FOODS IN ROASTING, FRYING, BAKING, AND BOILING

299. Effect of cooking on tissues. — All methods of applying heat, whether dry or wet, modify the mechanical condition of raw foods.   Both dry and wet heat harden the tissues of meat, and wet heat, or boiling, disintegrates the fibers, softens the connective tissue, and renders the meat more easily masticated. In the case of cereals, whether with dry or wet heat, the starch grains that are confined in the vegetable cells are expanded, and the cellulose covering of the cells is burst, liberating the cell contents. In the case of boiled vegetables their fiber is disintegrated, the contents of the cells are more or less liberated, and the tissue is rendered much more tender. Cooking foods at boiling temperature by any process whatever coagulates and hardens certain of the proteins such as the albumin and myosin of meat and the white of egg. Boiling milk causes a coagulum. The same thing occurs to a limited extent in vegetable foods, but the result is not so evident. Dry heat converts starch into dextrin, a soluble carbohydrate, as in the brown crust of corn and wheat breads, the surface of toasted bread and of baked potatoes. When apples or other fruits are baked, their tissue is gelatinized through the conversion by hydrolysis of pectin into pectose. In cooking food of whatever class by steaming or boiling, more or less of the soluble matter is extracted.

300. Losses in cooking meats. — The various meats contain from five to eight per cent of soluble constituents, including ash compounds, albumin, the extractives creatin and creatinin, organic acids, glycogen, inosite, and other organic bodies. When meat is cooked by any method whatever, a portion of these compounds, together with some of the fat, is taken into solution or is found in the drippings. At a boiling temperature, the collagen of the connective tissue is changed to gelatin, which is soluble in hot water, and assumes a semi-solid state when meat broth is cooled.

Extensive experiments by Grindley[1] revealed the following losses from the meat by the various methods of cooking: —

TABLE LX

Losses From Meat by Various Methods of Cooking

Kind of Meat	Method of Cooking	Temperature of Cooking At Beginning °C	Temperature of Cooking During Cooking °C	Time of Cooking Hrs.	Nutrients in Broth or Dripping in Percentage of Total Amounts in Uncooked Meat Water Per Cent	Nutrients in Broth or Dripping in Percentage of Total Amounts in Uncooked Meat Protein Per Cent	Nutrients in Broth or Dripping in Percentage of Total Amounts in Uncooked Meat Fat. Per Cent	Nutrients in Broth or Dripping in Percentage of Total Amounts in Uncooked Meat Ash Per Cent
Beef, round, lean .	Boiling	100	80–85	5	52.7	8.0	10.3	55.4
Beef, round, lean .	Boiling	100	80–85	2½	51.0	4.9	5.1	44.0
Beef, round, lean	Boiling	25–25	80–85	5	54.6	5.3	14.7	41.8
Beef, round, lean .	Boiling	20–25	81	2½	53.1	9.7	20.7	54.2
Beef, round, lean, large piece . . .	Boiling	100	80–85	2	45.8	6.3	6.2	41.5
Beef, round, lean, small piece . . .	Boiling	100	80–85	2	57.0	8.5	17.8	57.2
Beef, round, lean, ½-inch cubes . .	Boiling	100	80–85	2	60.7	11.9	13.4	61.0
Beef, round, rather fat	Boiling	100	80–85	3	53.5	7.4	22.5	49.3
Beef, round, lean .	Pan broiling	——	——	15–20 min.	30.5	0.16	0.1	0.06
Beef, round, lean .	Sautéing	——	——	15 min.	36.5	0.46	3.3[2]	0.04
Beef ribs	Roasting	249	193	¾ to 1½	33.7	1.2	24.7	15.1

301. Relative loss from meats by different methods of cooking. — These data are important because meats are the most costly part of the family diet. The results of Grindley's conclusions are summarized in the following statements: —

[1] Bul. 141, O.E.S.　　　[2] Apparent gain.

TABLE LXI

LOSSES FROM VEGETABLES WHEN COOKED IN VARIOUS WAYS

KIND OF VEGE- TABLE	MANNER OF TREATMENT	LOSS IN PER CENT OF TOTAL AMOUNTS IN UNCOOKED VEGETABLES				
		Dry Matter	Protein Ni- trogen	Total Ni- trogen	Starch or Sugar	Ash
		Per Cent	Per Cent	Per Cent	Per Cent	Per Cent
Potatoes	Skins removed, soaked in cold water before cooking. Cooking begun in cold water	6.5	25.0	51.8	——	38.3
Potatoes	Skins removed. Not soaked. Cooking begun in cold water.	3.1	7.3	15.8	1.0	18.8
Potatoes	Skins removed. Not soaked. Cooking begun in hot water.	3.4	3.2	8.2	1.0	18.0
Potatoes	Skins not removed. Cook- ing begun in cold water.	0.4	0.6	1.0	0.1	3.5
Potatoes	Skins not removed. Cook- ing begun in hot water.	0.4	0.4	1.0	0.1	3.3
Carrots	Small pieces	29.9	10.3	42.5	26.0	47.3
Carrots	Medium sized pieces	23.5	6.4	27.5	26.5	37.0
Cabbage	Cooking begun in cold water.	39.3	6.7	39.6	38.2	47.06
Cabbage	Cooking begun in hot water.	35.1	7.0	35.8	34.3	40.2

1. The chief loss in weight with any method of cooking is water, except that in roasting much fat goes into the drippings.

2. The smallest loss was in pan broiling, sautéing caus- ing but little more. Much the largest loss was by roasting and boiling, averaging the most for fat in roasting, and most for proteins (extractives and gelatin largely) and ash in boiling.

3. The temperature of the water into which the meat

was introduced, whether boiling heat or 68–77° F., seemed to have little influence upon the contents of the broth.

4. Large pieces of meat lost less relatively than small pieces.

5. The loss increased with the time of cooking.

302. Losses in cooking vegetables. — In cooking vegetables in water, a much greater loss by solution occurs than is generally realized. The extraction of ash ingredients is especially large, and in throwing away the water in which potatoes and other vegetables are cooked a considerable waste of nutritive material occurs. The method of preparing vegetable food determines the proportion of loss. Peeling potatoes, carrots, beets, and turnips greatly increases the loss as the experimental results given in Table LXI show.[1]

303. Relative loss from vegetables by different methods of cooking. — Several conclusions are clearly warranted by the foregoing figures.

1. When potatoes with their skins removed are boiled, beginning with cold water, after previous soaking, the loss is large. Omitting the soaking greatly diminishes the loss, as also does placing the potatoes immediately in hot water.

2. When potatoes are boiled without removing the skins, the loss is small, almost negligible.

3. The loss in boiling carrots is large, one-quarter or more of the dry matter, but is greatest when they are cut in small pieces.

4. The loss in cooking cabbage is still larger, amounting to more than one-third of the dry matter. The loss is

[1] Bul. 43, O.E.S.

not very much diminished by using hot water at the start. It was found that making the water alkaline increased the loss of protein nitrogen.

304. Influence of cooking upon nutritive efficiency. — The effect of these complex changes upon the nutritive efficiency of foods it is not easy to measure. There is no reason for supposing that the various nutrient compounds are, in any case, so modified as to change the office they perform in building and maintaining the human body. The only factor to consider, then, is the influence of cooking upon digestibility. Such observations as have been made with raw and cooked meats indicate that the digestion of the latter may be no less complete, but is slower. Doubtless the same is true of eggs. On the other hand, the cooking of cereals and vegetables can but greatly increase the ease and rapidity of digestion. Unless the cells were previously ruptured, the digestive juices would slowly reach and act upon the starch granules and other bodies inclosed in the cellulose covering. With many foods cooking may be said with truth to be the preliminary step to rapid and the completest possible digestion.

CHAPTER XVII

FOOD SANITATION

FOOD sanitation is now a subject of the highest importance. Either because of their source or condition, human foods may be the direct cause of disease, sometimes because they communicate to the human subject pathogenic germ life, and sometimes because of the physiological effect of compounds that they contain naturally, or that have developed in them by holding them under undesirable conditions. With the changes in commercial conditions caused by the increasing spread and density of our population, the defense of the public against dangerous food materials has become an exceedingly complex and difficult matter.

There are several reasons for this, among which are the following : —

1. The collection of raw food materials over wide areas from sources it is not easy to supervise or even know much about.

2. The transportation of foods over long distances, with the attendant danger of fermentative changes and contamination.

3. The exposure of foods to dust and flies, especially in city markets.

4. The storage of foods during long periods of time with consequent changes in their composition.

5. The introduction into foods, especially meats and canned goods, of compounds known as preservatives, that, when introduced into the digestive tract, may be deleterious to health.

In order to control these conditions, national, state, and municipal regulations have been adopted which have done much to improve the quality and healthfulness of commercial human foods. Such control is more or less imperfect, however. The best defense against unhealthful foods is such an understanding on the part of the purchaser of the sources of danger as to permit a wise discrimination in the selection of foods and in the conditions to which they are submitted.

A. Cow's Milk

There is no food which has been the subject of more investigation as to its sanitary relations, or concerning which there has been more regulative legislation in order to insure healthful quality, than is the case with cow's milk. This is justified by the importance of this milk as human food. Not only is it quite generally consumed by adults, but it constitutes the entire food of many infants, and forms a generous share of the diet of thousands of young children. The fact that this article of food may exert a determinative influence upon the health of the young, and therefore upon the physical status of the adult, raises it to a position of supreme importance. It is essential, therefore, that those who control the milk supply for the family and for institutions shall be able to exercise an intelligent judgment concerning its quality.

Y

305. Ways in which quality of milk is modified. — There are several ways in which the sanitary or other qualities of normal milk may be modified, of which the following are the principal : —

1. Adulteration by the addition of water, causing a reduction of food value.

2. The removal of a portion of the milk solids.

3. The introduction of non-pathogenic germ life after it is drawn from the cow, causing, under certain conditions, undesirable fermentations.

4. The introduction of pathogenic germ life after the milk is drawn from the cow, rendering the milk a means of communicating infectious diseases.

5. The introduction of disease germs through the udder of the cow.

6. The introduction of compounds known as preservatives, having for their purpose the prevention of fermentations in milk that must be kept a long time before consumption.

306. What is normal milk? — Before discussing the various ways in which milk may be harmed for human consumption, it is well to form a clear idea of what normal milk is. It is, in brief, such milk as the child draws from the breast of a perfectly healthy mother, or the calf from the udder of the healthy cow. It is fresh milk from a healthy mammal, to which nothing whatever has been added, even of invisible germ life, from which nothing has been taken, and in which no changes have occurred. It is milk that would keep sound for a long time, and which might be given to infants with the assurance that it is wholesome and free from any form of infectious disease.

It is such milk as is found in the village or city supply only when it is drawn and handled by expensive and elaborate methods that are rigidly controlled. Only a minute percentage of commercial milk can be considered as normal when it reaches the consumer. Even that which is found on the tables of farm homes is far from normal, for it must be confessed that much milk used for home consumption is badly managed.

307. The adulteration of milk with water. — As will be seen elsewhere in this volume, the normal milk of all species of animals contains a large percentage of water, that of the cow varying from 84 to 89 per cent as nearly extreme limits. It is evident, therefore, that cow's milk has no standard composition; for it varies with breed, period of lactation, and from other less definite causes. Because milk intended for domestic consumption has been mostly sold by volume without much opportunity on the part of the purchaser to know its composition, producers and middlemen have not always resisted the temptation to increase their profits by adding water. The milkman and the pump handle have long been associated in the minds of consumers of "blue" milk. It is possible to add a certain proportion of water to the milk of one breed of cows without reducing its quality below that of some other breed, and even the thinnest normal milk may be rendered more dilute without the consumer being able to detect the fraud. Nothing short of an examination of the original milk in comparison with the suspected sample is competent to detect all degrees of adulteration with water, though the grosser dilutions may be established on other grounds.

308. Effect of adulteration. — It cannot be claimed that the adulteration of milk with water renders it unsanitary or unhealthful, except that the food value may be reduced to a point that, in particular instances where milk is the chief article of diet, would cause undernourishment. Much market milk has not contained over 12.5 to 13 per cent solid matter, and when in sound condition it is considered a healthful article of food. It is absurd, therefore, to claim that the reduction of rich Jersey or Guernsey milk to as low a standard by the addition of pure water renders it unhealthful. The claim that the consumer may rightfully make is that he is defrauded when he pays for normal milk and gets a diluted article.

309. Milk standards. — In recent years the national government and some state governments have established food standards, including milk, have provided penalties for the sale of foods falling below the standards and the necessary machinery for enforcing such regulations. In the state of New York, the legal standard for cow's milk, below which it must not fall, is 11.5 per cent total solids, and 3 per cent of fat. It is provided, however, that if it can be shown that the normal milk of the cow or herd from which the milk is produced is below that standard, no penalty is attached to its sale. This law has accomplished much good; but, on the other hand, it is quite evident that this legislation has tended to reduce a large proportion of market milk to approximately the legal standard through the keeping of cows giving a large volume of thin milk. A much more sensible plan would be to permit the vender of milk to guarantee a standard for his goods and then hold him responsible for meeting it.

310. The removal of a portion of the milk solids. —
This is done by the removal of cream. The effect of this
is to decrease the proportion of solids in the milk, and to
decrease the proportion of fat in the solids that remain behind. Because cream bears a much higher price than whole
milk, some dealers have practiced removing the cream
from the top of the cans, the partially skimmed milk
being sold at the price of whole milk. The practice of partially creaming table milk has evidently been followed by
hotels and restaurants, if we may judge by the quality of
the milk that is furnished to guests to drink. In such cases,
the laws intended to maintain commercial milk up to a
certain standard fail to defend the actual consumer against
an inferior article, and really operate to increase the gains
of the dishonest purveyor. Just why the hotel keeper
should be protected against fraud and then be permitted
to offer illegal milk to his guest is not clear. It would
seem that the law should protect the individual who
actually uses the milk as food.

**311. The introduction into cow's milk of non-patho-
genic germ life. —** Normal cow's milk as it comes from the
udder is not entirely free from germ life, but the number of
germs present are few. With the procedure ordinarily
followed, milk almost immediately acquires bacteria, and
under some circumstances continues to do so. These
organisms have their source in the dust in the stable air,
dirty utensils, the surface of the cow, the hands and
clothes of the milker, and exposure to dirt and air in the
house or during transportation. The germ life included
in this class, that is, the non-pathogenic, cannot of itself
produce disease. Apart from its effect on the milk, it is

entirely harmless to the human subject. It is very undesirable to have milk heavily loaded with bacteria, however,
especially that which must be held for some time before
consumption, or is to be kept under conditions favorable for
the growth of germ life, for the fermentations which these
organisms cause render the milk unsound. Such milk is
inferior in taste, and is unfit for feeding infants, as with the
latter it induces diarrhea and cholera infantum, especially
during the heated season.

**312. The introduction of pathogenic (disease) germs
after the milk is drawn.** — It is well established that
epidemics of typhoid fever have been caused by the distribution of the germs of this disease in milk. There appears
to be good evidence that cases of scarlet fever and diphtheria have originated in the same way. These particular
germs are communicated to the milk after it leaves the
cow's udder, for the bovine species is not subject to the
diseases mentioned. The source of such disease germs in
milk is directly or indirectly some diseased person, perhaps
convalescent, who comes in contact with the milk or milk
utensils, or who inhabits the premises where the milk is
produced. Fresh infectious material having its source
in feces, the skin, or sputum, may find its way into milk,
especially where cleanly habits are not maintained on the
part of the infecting individual. The danger is augmented
in the case of typhoid fever by the fact that the disease
may exist for some time before being recognized, and the
so-called " walking " cases are even more to be feared,
where the disease germs may inhabit an individual for long
periods of time without discovery. Such cases, when
located on a farm, are a distinct menace to the sanitary

quality of milk and other foods. Outside of the diseases mentioned, it is possible for milk to be infected with the germs of tuberculosis when this disease exists in the family where the milk is produced or handled. This is a danger scarcely appreciated by the great majority of persons.

313. Infection of milk from diseased cows. — Tuberculosis, which is practically the only bovine disease that it is necessary to consider in this connection, is very prevalent among dairy cows. It is possible that one-tenth of the cows in New York are affected with this ailment, and perhaps more. Under certain conditions, the bacteria of tuberculosis are conveyed to milk through the udder. Milk so contaminated is a menace to human health. Fortunately only a small per cent of the diseased cows are dangerous in this way. Much investigation and discussion has been given to the relation between human and bovine tuberculosis, and it now seems more than probable that the danger to the human family from the bovine germ has been overestimated. The best authorities have come to hold that tuberculosis of the lungs will not be contracted from infected milk, or rarely, and that the chief danger is that such milk may be a source of glandular tuberculosis with children. In any case, tuberculous persons not under control are a vastly greater menace to humankind than are tuberculous cows.

314. The precautions necessary to secure pure milk. — Housewives, and especially persons responsible for the supply of milk to hospitals and other institutions, should understand the conditions necessary to the production and handling of milk in order to secure a pure and safe product. They are as follows : —

1. Clean premises where milk is produced, including the stable and its surroundings. An accumulation of filth in immediate contact with the stable should be avoided. If possible, the excreta from the cows should be at once removed to some distance from the stable.

2. Cows should not be milked while the air is heavily laden with dust from the moving of hay and litter. It is possible to so arrange the feeding and milking periods as to avoid this.

3. The cows should be kept as free as possible from dirt and dust by thorough brushing. The long hair around the udder should be clipped short, and especially before milking should the udder be thoroughly brushed and then rubbed with a moist cloth.

4. The hands and clothing of the milker should be clean.

5. The milking utensils should be cleaned and sterilized by heat in the most thorough manner.

6. Special forms of milking pails should be used that protect the milk as fully as possible while it is being drawn.

7. Persons afflicted with, or convalescent from, infectious diseases should be kept away from the stables, milk, and milk utensils. It is almost criminal for such persons to be allowed to infect milk and thereby cause epidemics of diseases dangerous to human life.

8. The herd should be inspected at intervals for the presence of tuberculosis, and if diseased cows are found, they should be isolated from the well animals, and their milk should neither be sold nor used in the home unless previously pasteurized. With the knowledge now possessed, no milk producer has any right, even unknowingly, to distribute milk from tuberculous animals. It is time

for a general demand from consumers that herds producing their milk supply shall be tested for affected animals.

315. Pasteurization of milk as a safeguard against the effects of pollution. — It has often been advocated that the consumers of milk in cities be safeguarded against the effects of polluted milk by requiring that the entire city supply be pasteurized. Legislation to this effect has been proposed, but it has been opposed by the rational argument that such a provision places clean and unclean milk on the same commercial level, and would greatly reduce the incentive for the production of milk of good sanitary quality. Pasteurization would simply "throw a blanket" over dirty and infected milk, and would check the campaign of education for a better milk supply. It is probable, too, that milk heated to 155°F., or higher, is not as well adapted to the stomachs of infants and invalids, as is clean raw milk. The requirement should rest on the producer to market a healthful article, and he should be given no excuse for doing otherwise.

B. WATER AS A SOURCE OF DISEASE

No article of food is used more constantly or in larger quantities than is water. At the same time, no food material is more dangerous as a carrier of disease. This is shown by the serious epidemics of typhoid fever and other maladies which infected water has caused. The dangers in this direction, at least for the inhabitants of large villages and cities, are augmented by the fact that their water supply comes in most instances from extensive watersheds, or from rivers or lakes, subject to pollution, and in any case, from sources not under the immediate control of the user and about the condition of which he generally has very little or no accurate knowledge.

316. Pure water. — Pure water, chemically speaking, consists entirely of the compound H_2O, without the presence of any other compound or foreign bodies. In this sense, there are no natural waters that are pure. Even the first rain water that falls brings down with it dust and gases from the air. The only waters that approximate to chemical purity are carefully distilled water and rain water, after the rain has been falling for a few hours. The term " pure," as popularly applied to water, as for instance to the water of springs, signifies that the water is free from undesirable compounds or bodies, that is, that it is of good sanitary quality. Natural waters from uninhabited regions and from carefully guarded sources in inhabited places are of this kind. Springs, streams, and lakes along which or near which there are no inhabitants, and the vicinity of which is not frequented by any number of people, or streams and storage reservoirs that are carefully policed, furnish the safest water supply, excepting, possibly, deeply driven wells where the water entering them is subject to effective ground filtration.

317. The impurities of water. — The various sources to water of compounds of bodies foreign to itself, some dangerous and some not, are as follows : —

1. Substances washed out of the air by falling rain. These consist mainly of nitrogen compounds, nitrates and nitrites of ammonia, carbon dioxid, and particles of dust. The latter contains germ life which is dangerous only in exceptional cases. Rain water, at least after ground filtration, and certainly that which falls after the first

hour or so, must be regarded as of excellent sanitary quality.

2. Water takes into solution substances from the soil. When the soil has not been polluted with animal matter, these impurities do not convey disease. They consist mostly of inorganic salts, carbonates, nitrates, sulfates, and chlorides, chiefly of the bases potassium, sodium, calcium, magnesium, and iron. Occasionally some of the less common metals are found, such as lithium. Ordinarily, these salts are not present in such quantities in natural water as to render them unfit for domestic use, although some springs are so charged with certain compounds, of which magnesium sulfate is an example, that their water has a pronounced medicinal effect.

Organic matter exists only in those natural waters that ooze out of or filter through, deposits of vegetable matter such as leaf mold and peat. While such material in solution may give water a dark color and make it look very impure, there is no evidence that the health of the user would thereby be affected.

3. The waters that menace human health are generally those that are contaminated by human excreta. Both private and public water supplies may become unfit for use, in this way. Numerous instances are on record where wells have become infected from nearby cases of typhoid fever, thereby causing a spread of this disease, or where public water systems polluted with infectious material have caused serious epidemics of various maladies.

318. Certain precautions are necessary to insure sanitary water for domestic use. — (1) No water should be used from a well which can, by any possibility, be contaminated from a nearby cesspool, or that is so built as to allow the direct entrance of surface wash. Farm wells remote from cesspools, with proper covers, and into which water can flow only after it filters through several feet of soil, are a fairly safe source of water, provided the excreta of diseased persons on the farm are properly disposed of. Even if a well is distant from a cesspool, care should be taken that the soil strata do not incline from the cesspool toward the well, especially where a sandy or gravelly surface stratum is underlaid by a stratum of dense clay. In villages and cities, wells should always be regarded with suspicion, because they are liable to contamination in ways that are not easily prevented.

(2) Public water supplies are safe only when the water is conveyed in pipes from an indisputably pure source, or where, if contamination is possible, the best modern devices are adopted to render the water sanitary. Water from a lake or stream into which sewage enters, or the borders of which are thickly populated, should always be regarded as dangerous to health, and the citizens of any village or city should protest against such a supply unless it is rendered sanitary by certain modern devices. The defense of the family against suspected water is thorough boiling, to kill any disease germs which it may contain.

C. Relation of Ice to Health

Ice is now very generally used for domestic purposes, especially in cities. As a means of maintaining low temperatures for the preservation of food materials it is extremely useful. Used in this way, it cannot possibly be a menace to health. If it is dangerous at all, it is only through the enormous quantities introduced into foods and drinks that it can by any possibility be a vehicle of disease.

319. Does ice ever carry disease germs? — A general opinion prevails that water purifies itself from foreign matter on freezing. This does not appear to be strictly true. Both natural and artificial ice are not always free from living bacteria or other micro-organisms. This is made clear by various observers. Epidemics of disease have been attributed to contaminated ice, or frozen snow, upon evidence that appears to be fairly reliable. Ice that comes from rivers or ponds which are a receptacle for sewage or human dejecta is to be regarded with suspicion. On the other hand, the freezing of water tends to purify it through exclusion of foreign matter. More than this, only a small proportion of individual bacteria survive a freezing temperature, especially when this temperature lasts for a considerable period of time; and those that survive are regarded as being less virulent.

However, ice pollution may have other sources than the pond or river, among which may be named filthy workmen, the droppings of horses used on the ice field, and the dirty materials in which the ice is packed. Of course the washing of ice by pure water, or by its own melting, cleanses it from superficially attached matter. When everything is considered, however, public ice supplies cannot be regarded as safely sanitary, even in the case of artificial ice, which may be subjected to some of the same sources of infection as natural ice, and, because it is promptly used, may be more dangerous. The only ice that is sure to be sanitary is that which is made from pure water and is handled in a cleanly manner. Housewives should be advised that there is more or less danger in the promiscuous use of ice in drinks unless its source guarantees its purity. When used for cooling water, danger can be averted by setting a receptacle containing the ice into the water to be cooled, rather than putting the ice directly into the water. Such a precaution is worth while, even though the chances of the conveyance of disease by ice are rather small.

D.   UNHEALTHY MEATS AND VEGETABLES

While water and milk are doubtless the most important food materials in their relation to disease, other foods should be considered in this connection. These include meats, raw oysters, milk products, fruits, vegetables, and certain commercially prepared foods, indeed, any material which is subject to injurious fermentation or to contamination in preparation and through handling in the market. It may be said in a general way that the causes of unhealthfulness in these foods may arise from two general causes, viz. (1) the acquisition of disease-producing forms of life from without, and (2) the development within of disease organisms or of toxic bodies through fermentative processes. Certain of these disease-producing conditions rarely occur. The danger from them is slight as experience shows, and all such dangers may usually be avoided by intelligent precautions.

The disease organisms that may be found in the tissues of animals used for food are trichina and the germs of tuberculosis.

320. Trichinosis. — Since 1860 it has been known that the muscular tissue of swine is sometimes infested, though perhaps rarely now, with a minute parasitic worm known as the *Trichina spiralis*. It is parasitic on other domestic animals, particularly cats, rabbits, rats, and mice. The young worms, after developing from the eggs, become imbedded by millions in the muscles of the hog, and are then invisible to the naked eye. After a time, they become encysted, and at the end of a year or so are visible to the naked eye as specks scattered through the muscular tissue or red meat. In this form, the worms are dormant, and may live a long time. When uncooked pork so infested is eaten by man, the worms are liberated, attach themselves to the lining of the stomach, and the females produce broods, sometimes of as many as a thousand young worms. These young find their way into the tissues of the intestines, and finally throughout the whole system. It seems that with the rarity of this disease in swine, and with present methods of inspection, pork infested in this way very seldom finds its way into the family larder. In any case, the thorough cooking of pork renders it a safe food.

321. Tuberculosis. — The widespread existence of this disease not only among dairy cows, but among animals slaughtered for meat, even those raised and fed on the western plains, has rendered the public solicitous concerning the healthfulness of beef, so much of which is eaten without thorough cooking. There is a not unnatural prejudice against eating the flesh of an animal known to have been affected with tuberculosis; and in dealing with this disease in the way of suppression, animals so affected have quite generally been killed and buried. The indiscriminate rejection of such animals for human consumption has undoubtedly caused the waste of a large amount of perfectly safe food material.   Experience has shown that the flesh of animals that are affected with tuberculosis within certain limits may be safely used as food for man. This is so because of the nature of the disease.   Its effect, at first at least, is not to diffuse diseased, toxic or infectious material throughout the entire mass of the animal's body, but to destroy the tissue of certain glands or organs in which it gains a foothold.   The regulations of the federal meat inspection that have been established in the large abattoirs permit the carcasses of animals to be sold as sound when the lesions (diseased tissues) are localized and are restricted to certain organs, and exist in the less dangerous forms.   It is not true, then, that the flesh of all tuberculous animals is unfit for human food, or that such meat is wholly excluded from the market, even under the most rigid inspection.   There is good reason for maintaining inspection, and consumers have a right to demand that this be of the most thorough kind.

322. Raw oysters as a source of disease. — There is no doubt but that at least one epidemic of typhoid has been caused by infectious material contained in uncooked oysters.   Reference is made to twenty-five cases of typhoid fever among the students of Wesleyan University, Middletown, Conn., in the fall of 1894.   It was shown that these oysters were " fattened " near the mouths of sewers, one of which led from a private house where two cases of typhoid had occurred.   It is necessary to conclude that when oysters are placed near the mouths of sewers they are a menace to human health when eaten raw. But there is danger of unduly magnifying this danger, for most oysters are not subject to such contamination, and the widespread use of raw oysters does not seem to be attended with bad results. At the same time, it is possible that the sporadic cases of typhoid fever, which so frequently occur, may be explained through the conveyance of infectious material in oysters. It is rational to demand, therefore, that no oysters shall be grown near the mouths of sewers.

323. Conveyance of infectious diseases by fruits and vegetables. — The chances of the contamination of fruit and vegetables with infectious material are not very remote. In the first place market gardeners who use a city supply of animal manure in contact with small fruits and vegetables are not unlikely to market a contaminated product. Moreover, the vegetables and fruits displayed on the streets and even in shops, in a majority of instances, are swarming with flies. When it is realized that these flies may have walked over cesspool deposits and are thus conveying infectious germs on their feet, as flies are known to do, confidence in such exposed food materials is shaken. These facts should lead the housewife to patronize groceries where the commodities are kept shielded from flies, and to give all fruits and vegetables a thorough cleansing before they are eaten, especially if they are to be eaten in the uncooked state.

324. Cooking as a safeguard against disease. — From the foregoing statements it is easy to see that there are good reasons outside the matter of palatableness for thoroughly cooking meats and vegetables. The eating in a

z

raw state of vegetables and fruits raised in the home
garden, and such fruits as oranges and bananas from
which the skin is removed, is generally not attended with
danger.

325. Toxic effect of fermented meats and milk products. — Numerous instances are on record where serious
and sometimes dangerous or even fatal illnesses have
resulted from eating poultry, cheese, and ice cream.
These are explained by the general statement that toxic
compounds have developed in these materials through
some form of fermentation, compounds that produce a
severe reaction on the digestive tract and result in vomiting and diarrhea. Neither these fermentations nor their
products are well understood. The practical fact for the
producer and consumer to consider is that fresh products
and those that have been produced and held under proper
conditions of cleanliness and temperature do not become
dangerous to human health. The question has been raised
whether poultry and other materials that have been held
in cold storage for a long time are a menace to health.
Certainly immense quantities of foods so treated have been
eaten during the past ten years, and very little evidence of
dangerous quality has been obtained. It is conceivable
that when the conditions of storage, such as temperature
regulation, are bad, an unhealthy and even dangerous
product might result.

E. Effect of Food Preservatives upon Health

A practice has developed on the part of manufacturers
and handlers of such food materials as meats, fish, canned
goods, and sauces, of applying to these, or introducing

into them, certain compounds known as preservatives. The most common of these compounds are boric acid, salicylic acid, and sodium salicylate, benzoic acid, sodium benzoate, and sulfurous acid and sulfites. Formaldehyde has also been used. The effect of these is to prevent the activity of the germ life that causes destructive changes in animal and vegetable products. Manufacturers of canned goods have sometimes found it difficult to " process " their goods so as to entirely prevent later fermentations and, at the same time, not develop undesirable flavors in the contents of the cans, and some canners have at times taken advantage of preservatives as an easy way of overcoming this difficulty. On the other hand, many manufacturers have withheld from this practice. Sauces such as tomato catsup have been found to contain benzoic acid. Preservatives have also been used in milk, and boric acid has been found on salt fish and meats. These are merely examples of the extensive use of preservatives.

326. Should the use of preservatives in food products be permitted? — This matter has received much attention in the way of scientific investigation and legislation. The most extended recent study of this question was conducted by Dr. H. W. Wiley, chief chemist of the U. S. Department of Agriculture, and his verdict is unfavorable to the use in foods of any of the common preservatives. He concludes from his data that benzoic acid as such or as sodium benzoate, administered in from 1 to 2 grams per day, causes disturbances of digestion attended by headache and nausea, loss of weight, and other results; that when $\frac{1}{2}$ gram of boric acid is taken daily, no marked effects are immediately produced, but that ultimately there is a loss of appetite, and the general health suffers, and that a daily dose of as high as 4 to 5 grams caused some subjects to become ill and unfit for duty; that formaldehyde in food " tends to derange metabolism, disturb the normal functions, and produce irritations, and undue stimulation of the secretory activities "; that salicylic acid in daily doses of .2 gram to 2 grams, while stimulating at first, ultimately loses its stimulating property and " becomes a depressant," "tending to break down tissues of the body more rapidly than they are built up," " disturbs the metabolic processes," has a tendency to diminish the weight of the body, and produces " a feeling of discomfort and *malaise* "; that sulfurous acid or sodium sulfite in daily quantities of .113 to .762 gram of the latter disturbs metabolism, retards the assimilation of organic phosphorous compounds, creates a " marked tendency to the production of albuminuria," and causes the " impoverishment of the blood with respect to the number of red and white corpuscles."

Protests against Dr. Wiley's conclusions caused the appointment of a commission consisting of three well-known biological chemists, to investigate the issues involved. This has been done in the case of sodium benzoate, and these scientists are unanimous in concluding that neither small (.3 gram) nor large (.6 gram to 6 grams) daily doses, continued for considerable periods of time, produced any appreciable effect upon the metabolism and health of the subjects under experiment.   If this latter conclusion is fully accepted, then there is no just ground for excluding sodium benzoate from human foods, provided the existing provisions of federal and state laws are obeyed, which require that each package of goods containing a preservative shall carry a statement of its kind and amount so present. The methods used by the Department of Agriculture are criticised as to the manner of administering the experimental substances on the ground that in concentrated forms (in capsules) these substances are an irritant, but that when taken in very dilute forms, evil effects are not observed.

327. Use of food preservatives a doubtful policy. — After the investigation and discussion of the past, there is not a general agreement that the policy of permitting the introduction of preservatives into human food is a wise one, even if food packages accurately state their contents. First of all, it is doubtful if the investigations so far carried on demonstrate conclusively that the long-continued introduction of the preservative compounds into the human system under all conditions of age and physical vigor is devoid of undesirable effects. It may be difficult to secure convincing testimony either way on this point. But the absence of appreciable effect with vigorous adults during comparatively brief periods is not convincing evidence to those who understand how subtle and difficult of detection are the nutritive factors that determine our bodily and mental states.

The various compounds classed as preservatives have a strongly repressive influence on the unicellular organisms or bacteria that are the direct cause of fermentations. These cells are essentially the same in structure and contents as those that compose the tissues of the more complex organisms, and it is unsafe to assume an absence of effect on any cellular tissue. The profound influence of the chemical environment of living cells upon their activities is coming to be more and more appreciated as we gain added insight into biological processes. The human organism, through centuries of development, has been brought into nutritive adjustment and harmony with the compounds present in plant and animal tissues, and it is unsafe to conclude that no deleterious influence will be exerted by the life-long use, even in minute proportions, of substances that exert so marked an effect on the simpler forms of life.

328. Use of food preservatives promotes careless methods. — It is also urged that the introduction of preservatives into food materials in order to prevent fermentations will permit careless methods of manufacture and the use of unsound materials. There is abundant evidence that all classes of vegetables and fruits may be held in a sound condition without the use of preservatives, and the presence of one of these in any food justifies the suspicion that the manufacturer is using materials or methods inferior to those of manufacturers who do not add preservatives to their goods. It is a very serious question whether indicating the presence of a preservative on a food package is an efficient defense of public welfare, because a very large proportion of consumers are neither enlightened nor warned by such printed statements. Buyers of food supplies will do well to give themselves the benefit of the doubt as to the healthfulness of preservatives and purchase goods not containing them.

CHAPTER XVIII

THE PRESERVATION OF FOOD

THE preservation of food materials may be considered from two points of view: (1) the holding in good condition for a sufficient length of time the current supply of food, and (2) the preservation for an indefinite period of such food products as canned goods and preserves.

Food preservation as a whole involves many methods and devices. It is not intended to discuss these in detail, but rather to set forth the principles that are generally applicable to the maintenance of food materials in a sound condition.

329. Factors involved. — A fundamental and main factor in causing undesirable changes in food is the presence and activity of micro-organisms such as the molds and many types of bacteria. The conditions related to the control of these minute and ever present organisms are cleanliness, moisture, temperature, heat, sunlight, various disinfectants, and preservatives. It is not proposed to treat each of these conditions or factors separately, but to show their relation to different classes of food materials.

330. Moist foods. — Many foods, such as milk, meats, certain kinds of pastry, puddings, and similar cooked preparations, and breads and cakes that are stored in a closed space to prevent evaporation, necessarily contain an amount of water that is favorable to the inroads of the low forms of life. With such foods two conditions determine the success with which they are held against fungus or bacterial action, viz., cleanliness and temperature. The receptacle of whatever kind in which moist foods are kept should be scrupulously clean, that is, no accumulation of dirt, however small, should be permitted as a breeding place for germ life. This is fundamental. The refrigerator is often neglected and does not receive the frequent thorough cleaning that is necessary to the best conditions. Jars, cake boxes and other receptacles in which bread and cake are stored, should receive no less careful attention. A low temperature is a safeguard against the growth of micro-organisms. In a refrigerator where meat and other perishable articles are kept the ice supply should be sufficient to hold the temperature down to 40° F. or less. This means a larger ice box in proportion to the rest of the space than is found in some refrigerators.

Jars or boxes in which bread and cake are kept should be located in as cool a place as possible.

331. Dry foods. — These are principally flours, meals, sugar, dried and preserved meats, and dried fruits. Some of these are immune to the action of germ life because of the presence of some substance like salt or sugar in sufficient concentration to act as a germicide. This may be true of preserved meats. The flours, meals, and dried fruits maintain a sound condition unless through dampness they absorb moisture beyond a safe proportion. Such materials should be kept in a dry place, well lighted and well ventilated, if possible. Fresh air and sunlight, even diffused light, are inimical to bacteria and similar organisms. Dark and unventilated storerooms are not desirable.

332. The cellar as a storage place. — The aim in holding vegetables and fruits is to maintain them in a fresh, crisp condition by preventing the evaporation of water from their tissues and also to defend them against the attacks of destructive forms of germ life. Here again we see the importance of cleanliness, the right temperature, and varying moisture conditions according to the kind of material.

The cellar is the usual storage place for vegetables and fruits. The first consideration is that it be properly built and drained, so that undue moisture may be avoided. This means a dry location, if possible, good cement walls, and effective drainage. As the cellar generally contains the heating apparatus, the portions used for food storage should be separated from the furnace and fuel room by well-built partitions.

The storage space should be well ventilated and in the main well lighted. An annual whitewashing is an effective method of cleansing the walls and ceiling.

For most fruits and vegetables the lower the temperature at which they are held, above freezing of course, the more completely are they defended against molds and rots and the better they retain their tissue water. If a cellar is quite dry, roots like carrots, parsnips, and turnips should be packed in earth and sand. Celery should be treated in the same way with the heads up. Fruits should be treated with especial care. Not only should they be kept cool, but all diseased and imperfect specimens should be culled out. Small lots of choice fruit, apples and pears, are held much longer when the individual fruits are wrapped in paper. Fruits thus separated are much less likely to decay, and evaporation of moisture is somewhat retarded. Cabbage may be packed in barrels or boxes. Potatoes keep best in a cool, dry, dark bin. Pumpkins and squashes are stored most successfully on shelves either in the cellar or in upstairs closets, where it is dry and warm. A dry and well-ventilated cellar may be used as a place for storing cured meats (smoked), which are best held in thin bags hung from the ceiling.

333. Canning and preserving. — The preservation of food materials by canning and preserving is effected in two general ways: (1) by the application of boiling heat for a sufficient length of time to kill all germ life with the subsequent sealing of the cooked material in air-tight vessels, and (2) by the introduction of some substance like sugar or certain chemical preservatives that render the vegetable or fruit immune to the attacks of germ life.

The home canning of some vegetables, for instance tomatoes, is successfully accomplished with no great difficulty by the mere application of heat. The operation with green corn and peas is more precarious, the difficulty being by home methods to render these sterile without carrying the cooking process so far as to injure their flavor. There has existed a tendency to remedy the defects of the home canning of vegetables by the use of some one of the chemical preservatives such as benzoic acid and its compounds, but this practice is not to be commended. As before stated, it is a debatable question whether the continued use of such substances in food is not ultimately injurious to health.

In the preserving of fruits where the sterilization is not affected by heat, sugar is used in sufficient proportions to prevent fermentation.

334. Insects. — There is more or less loss of food materials through the depredations of insects. Housewives have often found an insect infestation of foods a troublesome matter to deal with. Several species of weevils and beetles infest dry foods, especially the cereal preparations like flour, meal, and breakfast foods. " An ounce of prevention is worth a pound of cure," so the housekeeper should be careful not to accept from the grocer any food stuff containing insect life. In order to exercise great care in this matter, the presence of larva and beetles may be discovered by sifting flour or meal through a sieve with very fine meshes.

When an insect infestation of the pantry is discovered, then methods of getting rid of it must be considered. If the amount of infested material is small, then its destruction or the use of it as food for animals is the safest and most satisfactory course to pursue. If a barrel of flour or other large bulk of ground cereal is found to contain insect life, then the remedy is likely to depend somewhat upon the degree of fastidiousness of the family.

Flour or meal cannot with certainty be freed from insect life by the use of a sieve, as the eggs and young larva slip through the finest meshes. Heat and disinfection are the only sure means of killing the insects. Heating the infested material in an oven for a time at the temperature of 125° to 150° F. is fatal to eggs, larva, and perfect insects. Disinfection of a barrel of flour or other large quantity of prepared cereal may be accomplished by the use of a liquid chemical known as bi-sulfide of carbon. This liquid is volatile at ordinary temperatures, and, as a gas, it will fill any space, provided a sufficient quantity is used.

With a barrel of flour a cup full of bi-sulfide may be placed on top of the flour in a shallow dish, and the barrel tightly covered, to remain so for a day or more. Sometimes it is necessary to repeat the operation. An entire room may be freed from insects by placing in it in shallow dishes bi-sulfide at the rate of 1 pound to 1000 cubic feet of space, keeping the room tightly closed. The gas is inflammable and should not be exposed to a light or other means of ignition. Its odor is very disagreeable, but it all passes away from food without harming it, and a slight inhalation of the gas does no harm.

It is probable that many persons would object to eating food in which dead insects are retained, therefore the infestation of a large supply of food materials is a somewhat serious matter, and great care should be taken to prevent it.

Diagrams of Cuts of Meat from Various Animals

In the subsequent table of composition of food stuffs are given the analyses of a great variety of cuts of meat.

The diagrams[1] which follow show very clearly the parts of the animal from which the cuts are taken. These may serve to aid the housewife in dealing with the meat market.

[1] Reproduced from Bul. 28, O.E.S. (revised edition).

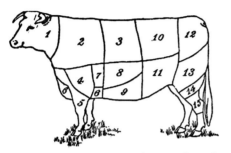
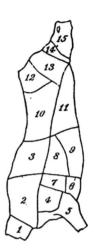

FIG. 13. — Diagrams of cuts of beef.

1. Neck.	6. Brisket.	11. Flank.
2. Chuck.	7. Cross ribs.	12. Rump.
3. Ribs.	8. Plate.	13. Round.
4. Shoulder clod.	9. Navel.	14. Second cut round.
5. Fore shank.	10. Loin.	15. Hind shank.

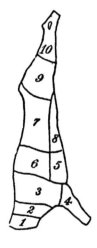
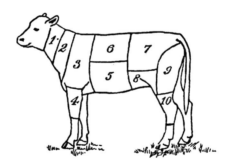

FIG. 14. — Diagrams of cuts of veal.

1. Neck.	5. Breast.	8. Flank.
2. Chuck.	6. Ribs.	9. Leg.
3. Shoulder.	7. Loin.	10. Hind shank.
4. Fore shank.		

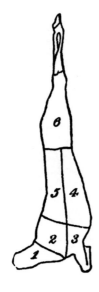

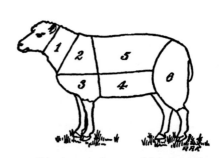

FIG. 15. — Diagrams of cuts of lamb and mutton.

1. Neck.	3. Shoulder.	5. Loin.
2. Chuck.	4. Flank.	6. Leg.

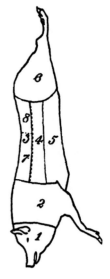

FIG. 16. — Diagrams of cuts of pork.

1. Head.	5. Belly.
2. Shoulder.	6. Ham.
3. Back.	7. Ribs.
4. Middle cut.	8. Loin.

CHEMICAL COMPOSITION OF AMERICAN FOOD MATERIALS[1]

The figures in black type are the averages of several analyses of the materials of the same definite character. The figures in Roman type represent single analyses or the averages of all analyses of several groups of materials. The estimated percentages of protein are also in Roman type.

Food Materials	Number of Analyses	Refuse	Water	Protein N × 6.25	Protein By Difference	Fat	Total Carbohydrates	Ash	Fuel Value per Pound
ANIMAL FOOD									
BEEF, FRESH									
Brisket, medium fat:		Per Cent	Per Cent	Per Cent	Per Cent	Per Cent	Per Cent	Per Cent	Cal- ories
Edible portion —									
Average	3	—	54.6	15.8	16.0	28.5		0.9	1495
As purchased —									
Average	3	23.3	41.6	12.0	12.2	22.3		0.6	1165
Chuck, including shoulder, very lean:									
Edible portion . . .	1	—	73.8	22.3	21.3	3.9		1.0	580
As purchased . . .	1	18.4	60.2	18.2	17.4	3.2		0.8	475
Chuck, including shoulder, lean:									
Edible portion —									
Average	2	—	71.3	20.2	19.5	8.2		1.0	720
As purchased —									
Average	2	19.5	57.4	16.3	15.7	6.6		0.8	580
Chuck, including shoulder, medium fat:									
Edible portion —									
Average	4	—	68.3	19.6	18.9	11.9		0.9	865
As purchased —									
Average	4	15.2	57.9	16.6	16.0	10.1		0.8	735
Chuck, including shoulder, fat:									
Edible portion —									
Average	4	—	62.3	18.5	18.0	18.8		0.9	1135
As purchased —									
Average	3	14.7	53.3	15.9	15.4	15.9		0.7	965
Chuck, including shoulder, very fat:									
Edible portion —									
Average . . .	2	—	53.2	17.2	16.9	29.0		0.9	1555
As purchased —									
Average .	2	22.8	40.8	13.3	13.0	22.7		0.7	1205

[1] From Bul. 28, O.E.S. (Revised edition).

351

CHEMICAL COMPOSITION OF AMERICAN FOOD MATERIALS —
Continued

Food Materials	Number of Analyses	Refuse	Water	Protein N × 6.25	Protein By Difference	Fat	Total Carbohydrates	Ash	Fuel Value per Pound
ANIMAL FOOD—*Continued*									
BEEF, FRESH—*Continued*									
Chuck, including shoulder, all analyses:		Per Cent	Per Cent	Per Cent	Per Cent	Per Cent	Per Cent	Per Cent	Calories
Edible portion . . .	13	——	65.0	19.2	*18.7*	15.4	——	0.9	1005
As purchased . . .	12	17.3	54.0	15.8	*15.5*	12.5	——	0.7	820
Chuck rib, very lean:									
Edible portion . . .	1	——	75.8	22.2	*21.7*	1.4	——	1.1	470
As purchased . . .	1	16.7	63.1	18.6	*18.1*	1.2	——	0.9	395
Chuck rib, lean:									
Edible portion —									
Average	11	——	71.3	19.5	*19.4*	8.3	——	1.0	715
As purchased —									
Average	11	22.7	55.1	15.1	*15.0*	6.4	——	0.8	550
Chuck rib, medium fat:									
Edible portion —									
Average	7	——	62.7	18.5	*18.3*	18.0	——	1.0	1105
As purchased —									
Average	7	16.3	52.6	15.5	*15.3*	15.0	——	0.8	920
Chuck rib, fat:									
Edible portion —									
Average	2	——	52.0	16.5	*16.1*	31.1	——	0.8	1620
As purchased —									
Average	2	10.2	46.8	14.8	*14.4*	27.9	——	0.7	1455
Chuck rib, all analyses:									
Edible portion . . .	21	——	66.8	19.0	*18.8*	13.4	——	1.0	920
As purchased . . .	21	19.1	53.8	15.3	*15.2*	11.1	——	0.8	755
Chuck, free from all visible fat	1	——	74.1	22.6	*22.0*	2.8	——	1.1	540
Flank, very lean:									
Edible portion —									
Average	3	——	70.7	25.9	*24.8*	3.3	——	1.2	620
As purchased —									
Average	3	3.5	68.2	24.9	*23.9*	3.3	——	1.1	605
Flank, lean:									
Edible portion —									
Average	3	——	67.8	20.8	*19.9*	11.3	——	1.0	865
As purchased —									
Average	3	1.4	66.9	20.5	*19.7*	11.0	——	1.0	845

CHEMICAL COMPOSITION OF AMERICAN FOOD MATERIALS — *Continued*

FOOD MATERIALS	NUMBER OF ANALYSES	REFUSE	WATER	PROTEIN N × 6.25	PROTEIN By Difference	FAT	TOTAL CARBO-HYDRATES	ASH	FUEL VALUE PER POUND
ANIMAL FOOD—*Continued*									
BEEF, FRESH—*Continued*									
Flank, medium fat:		Per Cent	Per Cent	Per Cent	Per Cent	Per Cent	Per Cent	Per Cent	Cal-ories
Edible portion —									
Average	5	——	60.2	18.9	*17.9*	21.0	——	0.9	1240
As purchased —									
Average	5	10.2	54.0	17.0	*16.1*	19.0	——	0.7	1115
Flank, fat:									
Edible portion —									
Average . . .	3	——	54.2	17.1	*16.6*	28.4	——	0.8	1515
As purchased —									
Average	3	3.3	52.4	16.5	*16.2*	27.3	——	0.8	1460
Flank, very fat:									
Edible portion —									
Average	2	——	34.7	14.0	*12.8*	51.8	——	0.7	2445
As purchased —									
Average	2	6.0	33.0	13.2	*12.0*	48.3	——	0.7	2275
Flank, all analyses:									
Edible portion . . .	16	——	59.3	19.6	*18.7*	21.1	——	0.9	1255
As purchased . . .	16	5.5	56.1	18.6	*17.7*	19.9	——	0.8	1185
Loin, very lean:									
Edible portion —									
Average	3	——	70.8	24.6	*24.2*	3.7	——	1.3	615
As purchased —									
Average	3	23.0	54.6	18.8	*18.5*	3.0	——	0.9	475
Loin, lean:									
Edible portion —									
Average	12	——	67.0	19.7	*19.3*	12.7	——	1.0	900
As purchased —									
Average	11	13.1	58.2	17.1	*16.7*	11.1	——	0.9	785
Loin, medium fat:									
Edible portion —									
Average	32	——	60.6	18.5	*18.2*	20.2	——	1.0	1190
As purchased —									
Average	32	13.3	52.5	16.1	*15.8*	17.5	——	0.9	1040
Loin, fat:									
Edible portion —									
Average	6	——	54.7	17.5	*16.8*	27.6	——	0.9	1490

CHEMICAL COMPOSITION OF AMERICAN FOOD MATERIALS — *Continued*

FOOD MATERIALS	NUMBER OF ANALYSES	REFUSE	WATER	PROTEIN N × 6.25	PROTEIN By Difference	FAT	TOTAL CARBO-HYDRATES	ASH	FUEL VALUE PER POUND
ANIMAL FOOD—*Continued*									
BEEF, FRESH—*Continued*									
Loin, fat — *Continued*		Per Cent	Per Cent	Per Cent	Per Cent	Per Cent	Per Cent	Per Cent	Cal-ories
As purchased —									
Average	6	10.2	49.2	15.7	*15.0*	24.8	——	0.8	1305
Loin, very fat:									
Edible portion —									
Average	3	——	49.7	17.8	*17.1*	32.3	——	0.9	1695
As purchased —									
Average	3	9.7	44.9	16.0	*15.5*	29.1	——	0.8	1525
Loin, all analyses:									
Edible portion . . .	56	——	61.3	19.0	*18.6*	19.1	——	1.0	1155
As purchased . . .	55	13.3	52.9	16.4	*16.0*	16.9	——	0.9	1020
Loin, boneless strip, as purchased: [1]									
Average . . .	6	——	66.3	17.8	*16.2*	16.7	——	0.8	1035
Loin, sirloin butt, as purchased: [1]									
Average	6	——	62.5	19.7	*18.9*	17.7	——	0.9	1115
Loin, porterhouse steak: [1]									
Edible portion . . .	7	——	60.0	21.9	*18.6*	20.4	——	1.0	1270
As purchased . . .	7	12.7	52.4	19.1	*16.2*	17.9	——	0.8	1110
Loin, sirloin steak: [1]									
Edible portion . . .	21	——	61.9	18.9	*18.6*	18.5	——	1.0	1130
As purchased . . .	21	12.8	54.0	16.5	*16.2*	16.1	——	0.9	985
Loin, top of sirloin: [1]									
Edible portion . . .	1	——	42.2	13.8	*13.3*	43.7	——	0.8	2100
As purchased . . .	1	3.2	40.9	13.3	*12.9*	42.3	——	0.7	2030
Loin, tenderloin, as purchased: [1]									
Average . . .	6	——	59.2	16.2	*15.6*	24.4	——	0.8	1330
Loin trimmings: [1]									
Edible portion . . .	6	——	55.0	16.9	*16.2*	28.0	——	0.8	1495
As purchased . . .	6	48.8	27.9	8.5	*8.2*	14.7	——	0.4	780
Loin, free from all visible fat . . .	2	——	74.0	22.1	*21.7*	3.1	——	1.2	540
Navel, very lean:									
Edible portion . .	1	——	68.6	30.7	*29.4*	0.6	——	1.4	595

[1] All loin parts are included under analyses of "loin."

CHEMICAL COMPOSITION OF AMERICAN FOOD MATERIALS —
Continued

Food Materials	Number of Analyses	Refuse	Water	Protein N × 6.25	Protein By Difference	Fat	Total Carbo-hydrates	Ash	Fuel Value per pound
ANIMAL FOOD—*Continued*									
BEEF, FRESH—*Continued*									
Navel, very lean — *Continued*		Per Cent	Per Cent	Per Cent	Per Cent	Per Cent	Per Cent	Per Cent	Calories
As purchased . . .	1	2.9	66.6	29.8	*28.5*	0.6	——	1.4	580
Navel, medium fat:									
Edible portion . . .	1	——	47.6	15.6	*15.1*	36.5	——	0.8	1830
As purchased . . .	1	11.4	42.2	13.8	*13.4*	32.3	——	0.7	1620
Neck, very lean:									
Edible portion —									
Average . . .	3	——	73.2	22.5	*22.5*	3.2	——	1.1	555
As purchased —									
Average	3	44.3	40.7	12.5	*12.2*	2.2	——	0.6	325
Neck, lean:									
Edible portion —									
Average	2	——	70.1	21.4	*20.5*	8.4	——	1.0	750
As purchased —									
Average	2	29.5	49.5	15.1	*14.4*	5.9	——	0.7	530
Neck, medium fat:									
Edible portion —									
Average	10	——	63.4	20.1	*19.2*	16.5	——	0.9	1070
As purchased —									
Average	10	27.6	45.9	14.5	*13.9*	11.9	——	0.7	770
Neck, all analyses:									
Edible portion . . .	15	——	66.3	20.7	*20.0*	12.7	——	1.0	920
As purchased . . .	15	31.2	45.3	14.2	*13.6*	9.2	——	0.7	650
Plate, very lean:									
Edible portion —									
Average	3	——	69.1	22.8	*22.1*	7.7	——	1.1	750
As purchased —									
Average . . .	3	37.4	43.0	13.6	*13.2*	5.7	——	0.7	495
Plate, lean:									
Edible portion —									
Average	3	——	65.9	15.6	*14.6*	18.8	——	0.7	1085
As purchased —									
Average	3	17.3	54.4	13.0	*12.2*	15.5	——	1.6	895
Plate, medium fat:									
Edible portion —									
Average	7	——	54.4	16.5	*15.7*	29.1	——	0.8	1535

CHEMICAL COMPOSITION OF AMERICAN FOOD MATERIALS —
Continued

FOOD MATERIALS	NUMBER OF ANALYSES	REFUSE	WATER	PROTEIN N × 6.25	PROTEIN By Difference	FAT	TOTAL CARBO-HYDRATES	ASH	FUEL VALUE PER POUND
ANIMAL FOOD—*Continued*									
BEEF, FRESH—*Continued*									
Plate, medium fat — *Continued* As purchased —		Per Cent	Per Cent	Per Cent	Per Cent	Per Cent	Per Cent	Per Cent	Cal-ories
Average	7	16.5	45.3	13.8	13.1	24.4	——	0.7	1285
Plate, fat:									
Edible portion — Average	3	——	45.2	14.6	14.2	39.8	——	0.8	1950
As purchased — Average . . .	3	16.0	38.0	12.2	11.9	33.5	——	0.6	1640
Plate, very fat:									
Edible portion . . .	1	——	34.6	10.6	9.8	55.1	——	0.5	2520
As purchased . . .	1	9.0	31.4	9.7	8.9	50.2	——	0.5	2300
Plate, all analyses:									
Edible portion . . .	17	——	56.3	16.8	16.0	26.9	——	0.8	1450
As purchased . . .	17	19.8	44.4	13.1	12.5	22.7	——	0.6	1200
Ribs, very lean:									
Edible portion — Average . . .	4	——	70.9	25.0	24.4	3.5	——	1.2	615
As purchased — Average	4	23.3	54.2	19.4	18.9	2.7	——	0.9	475
Ribs, lean:									
Edible portion — Average . . .	6	——	67.9	19.6	19.1	12.0	——	1.0	870
As purchased — Average	6	22.6	52.6	15.2	14.8	9.3	——	0.7	675
Ribs, medium fat:									
Edible portion — Average . . .	15	——	55.5	17.5	17.0	26.6	——	0.9	1450
As purchased — Average	15	20.8	43.8	13.9	13.5	21.2	——	0.7	1155
Ribs, fat:									
Edible portion — Average . . .	9	——	48.5	15.0	15.2	35.6	——	0.7	1780
As purchased — Average . . .	8	16.8	39.6	12.7	12.4	30.6	——	0.6	1525
Ribs, very fat:									
Edible portion . . .	1	——	45.9	14.6	14.8	38.7	——	0.6	1905
As purchased . . .	1	6.4	42.9	13.7	13.9	36.2	——	0.6	1780

CHEMICAL COMPOSITION OF AMERICAN FOOD MATERIALS —
Continued

FOOD MATERIALS	NUMBER OF ANALYSES	REFUSE	WATER	PROTEIN N × 6.25	PROTEIN By Difference	FAT	TOTAL CARBOHYDRATES	ASH	FUEL VALUE PER POUND
ANIMAL FOOD—*Continued*									
BEEF, FRESH—*Continued*		Per Cent	Per Cent	Per Cent	Per Cent	Per Cent	Per Cent	Per Cent	Cal-ories
Ribs, all analyses:									
Edible portion . .	35	——	57.0	17.8	*17.5*	24.6	——	0.9	1370
As purchased . . .	34	20.1	45.3	14.4	*13.9*	20.0	——	0.7	1110
Rib rolls, very lean, as purchased:									
Average	2	——	**73.7**	**20.8**	*20.3*	**5.0**	——	**1.0**	**600**
Rib rolls, lean, as purchased:									
Average	3	——	**69.0**	**20.2**	*19.5*	**10.5**	——	**1.0**	**820**
Rib rolls, medium fat, as purchased:									
Average	4	——	**63.9**	**19.3**	*18.5*	**16.7**	——	**0.9**	**1065**
Rib rolls, fat, as purchased:									
Average	2	——	**51.5**	**17.2**	*16.4*	**31.3**	——	**0.8**	**1640**
Rib rolls, all analyses, as purchased . . .	11	——	64.8	19.4	*18.8*	15.5	——	0.9	1015
Rib trimmings, all analyses:									
Edible portion —									
Average	11	——	**54.7**	**16.9**	*16.1*	**28.4**	——	**0.8**	**1515**
As purchased —									
Average	11	**34.1**	**35.7**	**11.0**	*10.5*	**19.2**	——	**0.5**	**1015**
Ribs, cross, very lean:									
Edible portion . . .	1	——	65.8	18.0	*18.4*	14.9	——	0.9	965
As purchased	1	12.8	57.4	15.6	*16.1*	13.0	——	0.7	840
Ribs, cross, medium fat:									
Edible portion . . .	1	——	43.9	13.8	*13.7*	41.6	——	0.8	2010
As purchased . . .	1	12.2	38.6	12.1	*12.0*	36.5	——	0.7	1765
Ribs, cross, all analyses:									
Edible portion . . .	2	——	54.9	15.9	*16.1*	28.2	——	0.8	1485
As purchased . . .	2	12.5	48.0	13.8	*14.0*	24.8	——	0.7	1305
Round, very lean:									
Edible portion —									
Average	6	——	**73.6**	**22.6**	*22.3*	**2.8**	——	**1.3**	**540**
As purchased —									
Average	6	10.6	**65.9**	**20.2**	*19.9*	**2.4**	——	**1.2**	**475**

CHEMICAL COMPOSITION OF AMERICAN FOOD MATERIALS —
Continued

FOOD MATERIALS	NUMBER OF ANALYSES	REFUSE	WATER	PROTEIN N × 6.25	PROTEIN By Difference	FAT	TOTAL CARBO-HYDRATES	ASH	FUEL VALUE PER POUND
ANIMAL FOOD—*Continued*									
BEEF, FRESH—*Continued*									
Round, lean :		Per Cent	Per Cent	Per Cent	Per Cent	Per Cent	Per Cent	Per Cent	Cal-ories
Edible portion —									
Average	31	——	70.0	21.3	*21.0*	7.9	——	1.1	730
As purchased —									
Average	29	8.1	64.4	19.5	*19.2*	7.3	——	1.0	670
Round, medium fat :									
Edible portion —									
Average	18	——	65.5	20.3	*19.8*	13.6	——	1.1	950
As purchased —									
Average	14	7.2	60.7	19.0	*18.3*	12.8	——	1.0	895
Round, fat :									
Edible portion —									
Average	5	——	60.4	19.5	*19.1*	19.5	——	1.0	1185
As purchased —									
Average	3	12.0	54.0	17.5	*17.1*	16.1	——	0.8	1005
Round, very fat :									
Edible portion —									
Average	2	——	55.9	18.2	*17.1*	26.2	——	0.8	1445
As purchased —									
Average	2	11.4	49.6	16.1	*15.2*	23.1	——	0.7	1275
Round, all analyses :									
Edible portion . .	62	——	67.8	20.9	*20.5*	10.6	——	1.1	835
As purchased . . .	54	8.5	62.5	19.2	*18.8*	9.2	——	1.0	745
Round, free from all vis-									
ible fat	4	——	73.5	23.2	*22.8*	2.5	——	1.2	535
Round, second cut :									
Edible portion —									
Average	2	——	69.8	20.4	*20.5*	8.6	——	1.1	740
As purchased —									
Average	2	19.5	56.2	16.4	*16.5*	6.9	——	0.9	595
Rump, very lean :									
Edible portion —									
Average	4	——	71.2	23.0	*22.5*	5.1	——	1.2	645
As purchased —									
Average	4	14.3	60.9	19.5	*19.1*	4.6	——	1.1	555
Rump, lean :									
Edible portion —									
Average	4	——	65.7	20.9	*19.6*	13.7	——	1.0	965

CHEMICAL COMPOSITION OF AMERICAN FOOD MATERIALS — *Continued*

FOOD MATERIALS	NUMBER OF ANALYSES	REFUSE	WATER	PROTEIN N×6.35	PROTEIN By Difference	FAT	TOTAL CARBO- HYDRATES	ASH	FUEL VALUE PER POUND
ANIMAL FOOD—*Continued*									
BEEF, FRESH—*Continued*									
Rump, lean—*Continued*		Per Cent	Per Cent	Per Cent	Per Cent	Per Cent	Per Cent	Per Cent	Cal- ories
As purchased —									
Average	3	14.0	56.6	19.1	*17.5*	11.0	——	0.9	820
Rump, medium fat:									
Edible portion —									
Average . . .	10	——	56.7	17.4	*16.9*	25.5	——	0.9	1400
As purchased —									
Average . . .	10	20.7	45.0	13.8	*13.4*	20.2	——	0.7	1110
Rump, fat:									
Edible portion —									
Average . . .	5	——	47.1	16.8	*16.4*	35.7	——	0.8	1820
As purchased —									
Average	5	23.0	36.2	12.9	*12.6*	27.6	——	0.6	1405
Rump, very fat:									
Edible portion . . .	1	——	40.2	15.0	*14.7*	44.3	——	0.8	2150
As purchased . .	1	16.2	33.7	12.6	*12.3*	37.2	——	0.6	1805
Rump, all analyses:									
Edible portion . . .	24	——	57.9	18.7	*18.1*	23.1	——	0.9	1325
As purchased . . .	23	19.0	46.9	15.2	*14.7*	18.6	——	0.8	1065
Rump, free from all vis- ible fat	1	——	73.9	21.2	*21.2*	3.8	——	1.1	555
Shank, fore, very lean:									
Edible portion —									
Average	4	——	74.4	22.1	*21.7*	2.8	——	1.1	530
As purchased —									
Average	4	44.1	41.6	12.3	*12.1*	1.6	——	0.6	295
Shank, fore, lean:									
Edible portion —									
Average	5	——	71.5	22.0	*21.4*	6.1	——	1.0	665
As purchased —									
Average	5	36.5	45.4	14.0	*13.6*	3.9	——	0.6	425
Shank, fore, medium fat:									
Edible portion —									
Average . . .	5	——	67.9	20.4	*19.6*	11.6	——	0.9	870
As purchased —									
Average . . .	5	36.9	42.9	12.8	*12.3*	7.3	——	0.6	545
Shank, fore, very fat:									
Edible portion . . .	1	——	59.0	20.1	*18.6*	21.6	——	0.8	1285

CHEMICAL COMPOSITION OF AMERICAN FOOD MATERIALS — *Continued*

FOOD MATERIALS	NUMBER OF ANALYSES	REFUSE	WATER	PROTEIN N × 6.25	PROTEIN By Difference	FAT	TOTAL CARBO-HYDRATES	ASH	FUEL VALUE PER POUND
ANIMAL FOOD—*Continued*									
BEEF, FRESH—*Continued*									
Shank, fore, very fat—		Per Cent	Per Cent	Per Cent	Per Cent	Per Cent	Per Cent	Per Cent	Cal-ories
Continued									
As purchased	1	30.9	40.7	13.9	*12.9*	14.9	——	0.6	890
Shank, fore, all analyses:									
Edible portion	15	——	70.3	21.4	*20.7*	8.1	——	0.9	740
As purchased	15	38.3	43.2	13.2	*12.7*	5.2	——	0.6	465
Shank, hind, very lean:									
Edible portion	1	——	71.2	26.6	*25.8*	1.7	——	1.3	565
As purchased	1	50.0	35.6	13.3	*12.9*	0.6	——	0.7	280
Shank, hind, lean:									
Edible portion —									
Average	6	——	72.5	21.9	*21.1*	5.4	——	1.0	635
As purchased —									
Average	6	58.5	30.1	9.1	*8.8*	2.2	——	0.4	260
Shank, hind, medium fat:									
Edible portion —									
Average	6	——	67.8	20.9	*19.8*	11.5	——	0.9	875
As purchased —									
Average	6	53.9	31.3	9.6	*9.1*	5.3	——	0.4	405
Shank, hind, fat:									
Edible portion	1	——	61.4	20.4	*18.9*	18.8	——	0.9	1170
As purchased	1	51.6	29.7	9.9	*9.2*	9.1	——	0.4	570
Shank, hind, all analyses:									
Edible portion	14	——	69.6	21.7	*20.7*	8.7	——	1.0	770
As purchased	14	55.4	31.0	9.7	*9.3*	3.9	——	0.4	345
Shoulder and clod, very lean: [1]									
Edible portion —									
Average	4	——	76.1	21.3	*21.5*	1.3	——	1.1	450
As purchased —									
Average	4	23.3	58.3	16.3	*16.5*	1.0	——	0.9	345
Shoulder and clod, lean:									
Edible portion —									
Average	5	——	73.1	20.4	*20.4*	5.4	——	1.1	605
As purchased —									
Average	4	18.8	59.4	16.4	*16.5*	4.4	——	0.9	490

[1] The "clod" usually contains no refuse.

CHEMICAL COMPOSITION OF AMERICAN FOOD MATERIALS —
Continued

FOOD MATERIALS	NUMBER OF ANALYSES	REFUSE	WATER	PROTEIN N × 6.25	PROTEIN By Difference	FAT	TOTAL CARBO-HYDRATES	ASH	FUEL VALUE PER POUND
		Per Cent	Per Cent	Per Cent	Per Cent	Per Cent	Per Cent	Per Cent	Cal-ories
ANIMAL FOOD—*Continued*									
BEEF, FRESH—*Continued*									
Shoulder and clod, medium fat:									
Edible portion —									
Average . .	14	—	68.3	19.6	*19.3*	11.3	—	1.1	840
As purchased —									
Average	12	16.4	56.8	16.4	*16.1*	9.8	—	0.9	720
Shoulder and clod, fat:									
Edible portion —									
Average	5	—	60.4	19.5	*18.8*	19.8	—	1.0	1200
As purchased —									
Average	3	11.9	52.8	17.7	*16.7*	17.7	—	0.9	1075
Shoulder and clod, all analyses:									
Edible portion . . .	28	—	68.9	20.0	*19.7*	10.3	—	1.1	805
As purchased . . .	23	17.4	57.0	16.5	*16.3*	8.4	—	0.9	660
Shoulder, free from all visible fat . . .	1	—	74.6	21.6	*21.5*	2.7	—	1.2	515
Socket:									
Edible portion . .	1	—	57.1	16.9	*16.7*	25.2	—	1.0	1380
As purchased . . .	1	35.7	36.7	10.8	*10.7*	16.2	—	0.6	885
Forequarter, very lean:									
Edible portion —									
Average	2	—	74.1	22.1	*21.3*	3.6	—	1.0	565
As purchased —									
Average	2	30.3	51.5	15.4	*14.8*	2.7	—	0.7	400
Forequarter, lean:									
Edible portion —									
Average	4	—	68.6	18.9	*18.4*	12.2	—	0.8	865
As purchased —									
Average	4	22.3	53.3	14.7	*14.3*	9.5	—	0.6	675
Forequarter, medium fat:									
Edible portion —									
Average . . .	10	—	60.4	17.9	*17.3*	21.4	—	0.9	1235
As purchased —									
Average	10	18.7	49.1	14.5	*14.0*	17.5	—	0.7	1010
Forequarter, fat:									
Edible portion . . .	1	—	53.5	15.9	*15.8*	30.0	—	0.7	1560
As purchased . . .	1	21.7	41.9	12.5	*12.4*	23.4	—	0.6	1220

CHEMICAL COMPOSITION OF AMERICAN FOOD MATERIALS —
Continued

FOOD MATERIALS	NUMBER OF ANALYSES	REFUSE	WATER	PROTEIN N × 6.25	PROTEIN By Difference	FAT	TOTAL CARBO-HYDRATES	ASH	FUEL VALUE PER POUND
ANIMAL FOOD—*Continued*									
BEEF, FRESH—*Continued*		Per Cent	Per Cent	Per Cent	Per Cent	Per Cent	Per Cent	Per Cent	Cal- ories
Forequarter, very fat:									
Edible portion . . .	1	——	44.6	15.0	*14.0*	40.7	——	0.7	1995
As purchased . . .	1	12.6	41.5	12.4	*13.6*	31.7	——	0.6	1570
Forequarter, all analyses:									
Edible portion . . .	18	——	62.5	18.3	*17.7*	18.9	——	0.9	1135
As purchased . .	18	20.6	49.5	14.4	*14.1*	15.1	——	0.7	905
Hind quarter, very lean:									
Edible portion —									
Average	2	——	72.0	24.0	*23.3*	3.5	——	1.2	595
As purchased —									
Average	2	21.0	56.9	19.0	*18.4*	2.8	——	0.9	470
Hind quarter, lean:									
Edible portion —									
Average	4	——	66.3	20.0	*19.3*	13.4	——	1.0	935
As purchased —									
Average	4	16.6	55.3	16.7	*16.1*	11.2	——	0.8	785
Hind quarter, medium fat:									
Edible portion —									
Average	11	——	59.8	18.3	*17.7*	21.6	——	0.9	1250
As purchased —									
Average	11	15.7	50.4	15.4	*14.9*	18.3	——	0.7	1060
Hind quarter, fat:									
Edible portion . . .	1	——	52.1	17.7	*16.4*	30.7	——	0.8	1625
As purchased . . .	1	12.4	45.6	15.5	*14.4*	26.9	——	0.7	1425
Hind quarter, all analyses:									
Edible portion . . .	18	——	62.2	19.3	*18.6*	18.3	——	0.9	1130
As purchased . . .	18	16.3	52.0	16.1	*15.5*	15.4	——	0.8	950
Sides, very lean:									
Edible portion —									
Average	2	——	73.1	23.0	*22.3*	3.5	——	1.1	575
As purchased —									
Average . . .	2	26.0	54.0	17.0	*16.5*	2.7	——	0.8	430
Sides, lean:									
Edible portion —									
Average	4	——	67.2	19.3	*18.7*	13.2	——	0.9	915
As purchased —									
Average	4	19.5	54.1	15.5	*15.1*	10.6	——	0.7	735

CHEMICAL COMPOSITION OF AMERICAN FOOD MATERIALS — *Continued*

FOOD MATERIALS	NUMBER OF ANALYSES	REFUSE	WATER	PROTEIN N × 6.25	PROTEIN By Difference	FAT	TOTAL CARBOHYDRATES	ASH	FUEL VALUE PER POUND
ANIMAL FOOD—*Continued*									
BEEF, FRESH—*Continued*									
Sides, medium fat:		Per Cent	Per Cent	Per Cent	Per Cent	Per Cent	Per Cent	Per Cent	Cal-ories
Edible portion —									
Average . . .	11	—	59.7	18.1	*17.4*	22.0	—	0.9	1265
As purchased —									
Average . . .	11	17.4	49.4	14.8	*14.4*	18.1	—	0.7	1040
Sides, very fat:									
Edible portion . . .	1	—	47.8	16.2	*15.1*	36.4	—	0.7	1835
As purchased . .	1	13.2	41.5	14.0	*13.1*	31.6	—	0.6	1595
Sides, all analyses:									
Edible portion . . .	18	—	62.2	18.8	*18.1*	18.8	—	0.9	1145
As purchased . . .	18	18.6	50.5	15.2	*14.7*	15.5	—	0.7	935
Miscellaneous cuts, free from all visible fat[1]	11	—	73.8	22.4	*22.1*	2.9	—	1.2	540
Clear fat	7	—	13.4	4.1	*4.1*	82.1	—	0.4	3540
Soup stock	1	—	89.1	—	*5.8*	1.5	—	3.6	170
BEEF ORGANS									
Brain, edible portion .	1	—	80.6	8.8	*9.0*	9.3	—	1.1	555
Heart:									
Edible portion —									
Average	2	—	62.6	16.0	*16.0*	20.4	—	1.0	160
As purchased . . .	1	5.9	53.2	14.8	*15.3*	24.7	—	0.9	1320
Kidney:									
Edible portion —									
Average	3	—	76.7	16.6	*16.9*	4.8	0.4	1.2	520
As purchased . .	1	19.9	63.1	13.7	*14.1*	1.9	—	1.0	335
Beef liver:									
Edible portion —									
Average	6	—	71.2	20.7	*21.2*	4.5	1.5	1.6	605
As purchased . . .	1	7.3	65.6	20.2	*20.2*	3.1	2.5	1.3	555
Lungs, as purchased . .	1	—	79.7	16.4	*16.1*	3.2	—	1.0	440
Marrow, as purchased .	1	—	3.3	2.2	*2.6*	92.8	—	1.3	3955
Sweetbreads, as purchased	1	—	70.9	16.8	*15.4*	12.1	—	1.6	825
Suet, as purchased:									
Average	6	—	13.7	4.7	*4.2*	81.8	—	0.3	3540

[1] Includes those given under "chuck," "round," "loin," etc.

CHEMICAL COMPOSITION OF AMERICAN FOOD MATERIALS —
Continued

FOOD MATERIALS	NUMBER OF ANALYSES	REFUSE	WATER	PROTEIN		FAT	TOTAL CARBOHYDRATES	ASH	FUEL VALUE PER POUND
				N × 6.25	By Difference				
ANIMAL FOOD—*Continued*									
BEEF ORGANS—*Continued*									
Tongue:		Per Cent	Per Cent	Per Cent	Per Cent	Per Cent	Per Cent	Per Cent	Calories
Edible portion —									
Average	3	——	70.8	18.9	*19.0*	9.2	——	1.0	740
As purchased —									
Average	3	26.5	51.8	14.1	*14.2*	6.7	——	0.8	545
BEEF, COOKED									
Cut not given, boiled, as purchased . . .	1	——	38.1	26.2	*26.1*	34.9	——	0.9	2805
Scraps, as purchased:									
Average	2	——	23.2	21.4	*21.6*	51.7	——	3.5	2580
Roast, as purchased:									
Average	7	——	43.2	22.3	*21.9*	28.6	——	1.3	1620
Pressed, as purchased .	1	——	44.1	23.6	*26.7*	27.7	——	1.5	1610
Round steak, fat removed, as purchased:									
Average	18	——	63.0	27.6	*27.5*	7.7	——	1.8	840
Sirloin steak, baked, as purchased . . .	1	——	63.7	23.9	*24.7*	10.2	——	1.4	875
Loin steak, tenderloin, broiled, edible portion:									
Average	6	——	54.8	23.5	*23.6*	20.4	——	1.2	1300
Sandwich meat, as purchased:									
Average	3	——	58.3	28.0	*27.9*	11.0	——	2.8	985
BEEF, CANNED									
Boiled beef, as purchased	1	——	51.8	25.5	*24.4*	22.5	——	1.3	1425
Cheek, ox, as purchased	1	——	66.1	22.2	*22.3*	8.4	——	3.2	765
Chili-con-carne, as purchased	1	——	75.4	13.3	*13.3*	4.6	4.0	2.7	515
Collops, minced, as purchased	1	——	72.3	17.8	*17.9*	6.8	1.1	1.9	640
Corned beef:									
Average	15	——	51.8	26.3	*25.5*	18.7	——	4.0	1280

CHEMICAL COMPOSITION OF AMERICAN FOOD MATERIALS —
Continued

FOOD MATERIALS	NUMBER OF ANALYSES	REFUSE	WATER	PROTEIN N × 6.25	PROTEIN By Difference	FAT	TOTAL CARBO- HYDRATES	ASH	FUEL VALUE PER POUND
ANIMAL FOOD—*Continued*									
BEEF, CANNED—*Continued*		Per Cent	Per Cent	Per Cent	Per Cent	Per Cent	Per Cent	Per Cent	Cal- ories
Dried beef, as purchased :									
Average	2	—	44.8	39.2	*38.6*	5.4	—	11.2	960
Kidneys, stewed, as pur- chased :									
Average	2	—	71.9	18.4	—	5.1	2.1	2.5	600
Luncheon beef, as pur- chased	1	—	52.9	27.6	*26.4*	15.9	—	4.8	1185
Palates, ox, as purchased :									
Average	2	—	71.4	17.8	*17.4*	10.0	—	1.2	755
Roast beef, as purchased :									
Average	4	—	58.9	25.9	*25.0*	14.8	—	1.3	1105
Rump steak, as pur- chased	1	—	56.3	24.3	*23.5*	18.7	—	1.5	1240
Sweetbreads, as pur- chased	1	—	69.0	20.2	*19.5*	9.5	—	2.0	775
Tails, ox :									
Edible portion . . .	1	—	67.9	26.3	*24.6*	6.3	—	1.2	755
As purchased . . .	1	29.7	47.7	18.5	*17.3*	4.5	—	0.8	535
Tongue, ground, as pur- chased :									
Average	6	—	49.9	21.4	*21.0*	25.1	—	4.0	1455
Tongue, whole, as pur- chased :									
Average	5	—	51.3	19.5	*21.5*	23.2	—	4.0	1340
Tripe, as purchased :									
Average	2	—	74.6	16.8	*16.4*	8.5	—	0.5	670
BEEF, CORNED AND PICKLED									
Brisket :									
Edible portion . . .	1	—	50.9	18.3	*18.7*	24.7	—	5.7	1385
As purchased . . .	1	21.4	40.0	14.4	*14.7*	19.4	—	4.5	1085
Flank :									
Edible portion —									
Average	2	—	49.9	14.6	*14.2*	33.0	—	2.9	1665
As purchased —									
Average	2	12.1	43.7	12.9	*12.4*	29.2	—	2.6	1470

CHEMICAL COMPOSITION OF AMERICAN FOOD MATERIALS —
Continued

Food Materials	Number of Analyses	Refuse	Water	Protein N × 6.25	Protein By Difference	Fat	Total Carbohydrates	Ash	Fuel Value Per Pound
ANIMAL FOOD—*Continued*									
BEEF, CORNED, ETC.—*Continued*		Per Cent	Per Cent	Per Cent	Per Cent	Per Cent	Per Cent	Per Cent	Cal-ories
Plate:									
Edible portion . . .	1	—	40.1	13.7	*13.3*	41.9	—	4.7	2025
As purchased . . .	1	14.5	34.3	11.7	*11.4*	35.8	—	4.0	1730
Rump:									
Edible portion —									
Average	3	—	58.1	15.3	*15.3*	23.3	—	3.3	1270
As purchased —									
Average . . .	3	6.0	54.5	14.3	*14.4*	22.0	—	3.1	1195
Extra family beef:									
Edible portion . . .	1	—	37.0	12.3	*11.8*	47.2	—	4.0	2220
As purchased . . .	1	10.4	33.1	11.1	*10.6*	42.3	—	3.6	1990
Mess beef, salted:									
Edible portion —									
Average	2	—	37.0	12.6	*12.0*	44.5	—	6.5	2110
As purchased —									
Average	2	10.5	33.0	11.2	*10.7*	39.9	—	5.9	1890
Corned beef, all analyses:									
Edible portion . . .	10	—	53.6	15.6	*15.3*	26.2	—	4.9	1395
As purchased	10	8.4	49.2	14.3	*14.0*	23.8	—	4.6	1271
Spiced beef, rolled, as purchased . . .	1	—	30.0	12.0	*11.8*	51.4	—	6.8	2390
Tongues, pickled:									
Edible portion —									
Average	2	—	62.3	12.8	*12.5*	20.5	—	4.7	1105
As purchased —									
Average	2	6.0	58.9	11.9	*11.6*	19.2	—	4.3	1030
Tripe, as purchased:									
Average	4	—	86.5	11.7	*11.8*	1.2	0.2	0.3	270
Dried, salted, and smoked									
Edible portion —									
Average	7	—	54.3	30.0	*29.7*	6.5	(²)0.4	9.1	840
As purchased —									
Average	2	4.7	53.7	26.4	*25.8*	6.9	—	8.9	780
VEAL, FRESH									
Breast, very lean:									
Edible portion . . .	1	—	73.2	23.1	*23.1*	2.5	—	1.2	535

CHEMICAL COMPOSITION OF AMERICAN FOOD MATERIALS —
Continued

Food Materials	Number of Analyses	Refuse	Water	Protein N × 6.25	Protein By Difference	Fat	Total Carbohydrates	Ash	Fuel Value per Pound
ANIMAL FOOD—*Continued*									
VEAL, FRESH—*Continued*									
Breast, very lean—*Continued*		Per Cent	Per Cent	Per Cent	Per Cent	Per Cent	Per Cent	Per Cent	Cal- ories
As purchased . . .	1	46.8	38.9	12.3	*12.3*	1.3	——	0.7	285
Breast, lean:									
Edible portion —									
Average	3	——	70.3	21.2	*20.7*	8.0	——	1.0	730
As purchased —									
Average	3	23.4	54.0	15.7	*16.1*	6.2	——	0.7	560
Breast, medium fat:									
Edible portion —									
Average	5	——	66.4	19.4	*18.8*	13.8	——	1.0	930
As purchased —									
Average	5	20.6	52.7	15.6	*14.9*	11.0	——	0.8	740
Breast, all analyses:									
Edible portion . . .	8	——	68.2	20.3	*19.8*	11.0	——	1.0	840
As purchased . . .	8	24.5	51.3	15.3	*14.8*	8.6	——	0.8	645
Chuck, lean:									
Edible portion . . .	1	——	76.3	——	*20.6*	1.9	——	1.2	465
As purchased .	1	19.0	61.8	——	*16.7*	1.6	——	0.9	380
Chuck, medium fat:									
Edible portion —									
Average	6	——	73.3	19.7	*19.2*	6.5	——	1.0	640
As purchased —									
Average	6	18.9	59.5	16.0	*15.6*	5.2	——	0.8	515
Chuck, all analyses:									
Edible portion . . .	7	——	73.8	19.7	*19.4*	5.8	——	1.0	610
As purchased . . .	7	19.0	59.8	16.0	*15.7*	4.7	——	0.8	495
Flank, medium fat, as purchased:									
Average	5	——	68.9	20.5	*19.7*	10.4	——	1.0	820
Flank, fat, as purchased	1	——	57.0	18.1	*18.0*	24.1	——	0.9	1355
Flank, all analyses, as purchased . . .	6	——	66.9	20.1	*19.4*	12.7	——	1.0	910
Leg, lean:									
Edible portion —									
Average	9	——	73.5	21.3	*21.2*	4.1	——	1.2	570
As purchased —									
Average	9	9.1	66.8	19.4	*19.3*	3.7	——	1.1	520

CHEMICAL COMPOSITION OF AMERICAN FOOD MATERIALS.—
Continued

FOOD MATERIALS	NUMBER OF ANALYSES	REFUSE	WATER	PROTEIN N × 6.25	PROTEIN By Difference	FAT	TOTAL CARBOHYDRATES	ASH	FUEL VALUE PER POUND
ANIMAL FOOD—*Continued*									
VEAL. FRESH—*Continued*									
Leg, medium fat:		Per Cent	Per Cent	Per Cent	Per Cent	Per Cent	Per Cent	Per Cent	Calories
Edible portion —									
Average	10	——	70.0	20.2	19.8	9.0	——	1.2	755
As purchased —									
Average	9	14.2	60.1	15.5	16.9	7.9	——	0.9	620
Leg, all analyses:									
Edible portion . . .	19	——	71.7	20.7	20.5	6.7	——	1.1	670
As purchased . .	18	11.7	63.4	18.3	18.1	5.8	——	1.0	585
Leg, cutlets:									
Edible portion —									
Average	3	——	70.7	20.3	20.5	7.7	——	1.1	705
As purchased —									
Average	3	3.4	68.3	20.1	19.8	7.5	——	1.0	690
Loin, lean:									
Edible portion —									
Average	5	——	73.3	20.4	19.9	5.6	——	1.2	615
As purchased —									
Average	5	22.0	57.1	15.9	15.6	4.4	——	0.9	480
Loin, medium fat:									
Edible portion —									
Average	6	——	69.0	19.9	19.2	10.8	——	1.0	825
As purchased —									
Average	6	16.5	57.6	16.6	16.0	9.0	——	0.9	690
Loin, fat:									
Edible portion —									
Average	2	——	61.6	18.7	18.5	18.9	——	1.0	1145
As purchased —									
Average	2	18.3	50.4	15.3	15.1	15.4	——	0.8	935
Loin, all analyses:									
Edible portion . . .	13	——	69.5	19.9	19.4	10.0	——	1.1	790
As purchased . .	13	18.9	56.3	16.1	15.7	8.2	——	0.9	645
Loin, with kidney:									
Edible portion . . .	1	——	73.3	14.7	14.1	11.8	——	0.8	770
As purchased . .	1	9.1	66.7	13.4	12.8	10.7	——	0.7	700
Neck:									
Edible portion —									
Average	6	——	72.6	20.3	19.5	6.9	——	1.0	670

CHEMICAL COMPOSITION OF AMERICAN FOOD MATERIALS —
Continued

FOOD MATERIALS	NUMBER OF ANALYSES	REFUSE	WATER	PROTEIN N × 6.25	PROTEIN By Difference	FAT	TOTAL CARBOHYDRATES	ASH	FUEL VALUE PER POUND
ANIMAL FOOD—*Continued*									
VEAL, FRESH—*Continued*									
Neck:—*Continued*		Per Cent	Per Cent	Per Cent	Per Cent	Per Cent	Per Cent	Per Cent	Calories
As purchased —									
Average	6	31.5	49.9	13.9	*13.3*	4.6	—	0.7	455
Rib, medium fat:									
Edible portion —									
Average	9	—	72.7	20.7	*20.1*	6.1	—	1.1	640
As purchased —									
Average	9	25.3	54.3	15.5	*15.0*	4.6	—	0.8	480
Rib, fat:									
Edible portion —									
Average	3	—	60.9	18.7	*18.8*	19.3	—	1.0	1160
As purchased —									
Average	3	24.3	46.2	14.2	*14.2*	14.5	—	0.8	875
Rib, all analyses:									
Edible portion . . .	12	—	69.8	20.2	*19.7*	9.4	—	1.1	775
As purchased . . .	12	25.0	52.3	15.2	*14.8*	7.1	—	0.8	580
Rump:									
Edible portion . . .	1	—	62.6	19.8	*20.1*	16.2	—	1.1	1050
As purchased . . .	1	30.2	43.7	13.8	*14.0*	11.3	—	0.8	735
Shank, fore:									
Edible portion —									
Average	6	—	74.0	20.7	*19.8*	5.2	—	1.0	605
As purchased —									
Average	6	40.4	44.1	12.2	*11.8*	3.1	—	0.6	360
Shank, hind, medium fat:									
Edible portion —									
Average	6	—	74.5	20.7	*19.9*	4.6	—	1.0	580
As purchased —									
Average	6	62.7	27.8	7.7	*7.4*	1.7	—	0.4	215
Shank, hind, fat:									
Edible portion . . .	1	—	68.1	20.5	*20.0*	10.7	—	1.2	835
As purchased . . .	1	51.4	33.1	10.0	*9.7*	5.2	—	0.6	405
Shank, hind, all analyses:									
Edible portion . . .	7	—	73.6	20.7	*19.9*	5.5	—	1.0	615
As purchased . . .	7	61.1	28.6	8.0	*7.7*	2.2	—	0.4	240
Shoulder, lean:									
Edible portion —									
Average	2	—	73.4	20.7	*20.7*	4.6	—	1.3	580

2 B

CHEMICAL COMPOSITION OF AMERICAN FOOD MATERIALS —
Continued

| FOOD MATERIALS | NUMBER OF ANALYSES | REFUSE | WATER | PROTEIN | | FAT | TOTAL CARBO-HYDRATES | ASH | FUEL VALUE PER POUND |
				N × 6.25	By Difference				
ANIMAL FOOD—*Continued* VEAL, FRESH—*Continued*									
Shoulder, lean : —*Continued* As purchased —		Per Cent	Per Cent	Per Cent	Per Cent	Per Cent	Per Cent	Per Cent	Cal-ories
Average . . .	2	18.3	59.9	16.9	*16.9*	3.9	——	1.0	480
Shoulder and flank, medium fat: Edible portion —									
Average . . .	2	——	65.2	19.7	*19.3*	14.4	——	1.1	975
As purchased —									
Average . . .	2	23.0	50.2	15.1	*14.9*	11.0	——	0.9	745
Forequarter: Edible portion —									
Average . .	6	——	71.7	20.0	*19.4*	8.0	——	0.9	710
As purchased —									
Average . . .	6	24.5	54.2	15.1	*14.6*	6.0	——	0.7	535
Hind quarter: Edible portion —									
Average . . .	6	——	70.9	20.7	*19.8*	8.3	——	1.0	735
As purchased —									
Average . . .	6	20.7	56.2	16.2	*15.7*	6.6	——	0.8	580
Side, with kidney, fat, and tallow: Edible portion —									
Average . .	6	——	71.3	20.2	*19.6*	8.1	——	1.0	715
As purchased —									
Average . . .	6	22.6	55.2	15.6	*15.1*	6.3	——	0.8	555
Leg, hind, medium fat: Edible portion —									
Average . . .	2	——	63.9	19.2	*18.5*	16.5	——	1.1	1055
As purchased —									
Average . . .	2	17.4	52.9	15.9	*15.2*	13.6	——	0.9	870
Leg, hind, fat:									
Edible portion . . .	1	——	54.6	18.3	*17.1*	27.4	——	0.9	1495
As purchased . . .	1	13.4	47.3	15.8	*14.8*	23.7	——	0.8	1295
Leg, hind, very fat:									
Edible portion . . .	1	——	51.8	17.6	*17.2*	30.1	——	0.9	1595
As purchased . . .	1	7.0	48.2	16.4	*16.0*	28.0	——	0.8	1485

CHEMICAL COMPOSITION OF AMERICAN FOOD MATERIALS —
Continued

FOOD MATERIALS	NUMBER OF ANALYSES	REFUSE	WATER	PROTEIN N × 6.25	PROTEIN By Difference	FAT	TOTAL CARBO-HYDRATES	ASH	FUEL VALUE PER POUND
ANIMAL FOOD—*Continued*									
VEAL, FRESH—*Continued*		Per Cent	Per Cent	Per Cent	Per Cent	Per Cent	Per Cent	Per Cent	Cal-ories
Leg, hind, all analyses:									
Edible portion . . .	4	——	58.6	18.6	*17.8*	22.6	——	1.0	1300
As purchased . . .	4	13.8	50.3	16.0	*15.3*	19.7	——	0.9	1130
Loin, without kidney and tallow:									
Edible portion —									
Average . . .	4	——	**53.1**	**18.7**	*17.6*	**28.3**	——	**1.0**	**1540**
As purchased —									
Average	4	**14.8**	**45.3**	**16.0**	*15.0*	**24.1**	——	**0.8**	**1315**
Neck.									
Edible portion . . .	1	——	56.7	17.7	*17.5*	24.8	——	1.0	1375
As purchased . . .	1	17.7	46.7	14.6	*14.4*	20.4	——	0.8	1135
Leg, free from all visible fat, as purchased	1	——	72.3	25.3	*23.6*	2.7	——	1.4	585
Shoulder:									
Edible portion . . .	1	——	51.8	18.1	*17.5*	29.7	——	1.0	1590
As purchased . . .	1	20.3	41.3	14.4	*14.0*	23.6	——	0.8	1265
Forequarter:									
Edible portion . . .	1	——	55.1	18.3	*18.1*	25.8	——	1.0	1430
As purchased . . .	1	18.8	44.7	14.9	*14.7*	21.0	——	0.8	1165
Hind quarter:									
Edible portion . . .	1	——	60.9	19.6	*19.0*	19.1	——	1.0	1170
As purchased . . .	1	15.7	51.3	16.5	*16.0*	16.1	——	0.9	985
Side, without tallow:									
Edible portion —									
Average	3	——	**58.2**	**17.6**	*17.6*	**23.1**	——	**1.1**	**1300**
As purchased —									
Average	3	**19.3**	**47.0**	**14.1**	*14.2*	**18.7**	——	**0.8**	**1055**
LAMB, COOKED									
Chops, broiled:									
Edible portion —									
Average	4	——	**47.6**	**21.7**	*21.2*	**29.9**	——	**1.3**	**1665**
As purchased . . .	1	13.5	40.1	18.4	*18.5*	26.7	——	1.2	1470
Cut not given, as purchased	1	——	47.1	23.7	*22.1*	29.4	——	1.4	1680
Leg, roast	1	——	67.1	19.7	*19.4*	12.7	——	0.8	900

CHEMICAL COMPOSITION OF AMERICAN FOOD MATERIALS —
Continued

FOOD MATERIALS	NUMBER OF ANALYSES	REFUSE	WATER	PROTEIN N × 6.25	PROTEIN By Difference	FAT	TOTAL CARBO-HYDRATES	ASH	FUEL VALUE PER POUND
ANIMAL FOOD—*Continued*									
LAMB, CANNED									
Tongue, spiced and cooked:		Per Cent	Per Cent	Per Cent	Per Cent	Per Cent	Per Cent	Per Cent	Cal- ories
Edible portion . . .	1	——	67.4	13.9	*14.3*	17.8	——	0.5	1010
As purchased . . .	1	2.6	65.7	13.5	*13.9*	17.3	——	0.5	980
MUTTON, FRESH									
Chuck, lean:									
Edible portion . . .	1	——	64.7	17.8	*18.1*	16.3	——	0.9	1020
As purchased . . .	1	19.5	52.1	14.3	*14.5*	13.1	——	0.8	820
Chuck, medium fat:									
Edible portion — Average	6	——	**50.9**	**15.1**	*14.6*	**33.6**	——	0.9	**1700**
As purchased — Average	6	21.3	**39.9**	**11.9**	*11.5*	**26.7**	——	0.6	**1350**
Chuck, fat:									
Edible portion — Average	2	——	**40.6**	**13.9**	*13.7*	**44.9**	——	0.8	**2155**
As purchased — Average	2	16.5	**33.8**	**11.6**	*11.5*	**37.5**	——	0.7	**1800**
Chuck, very fat:									
Edible portion . . .	1	——	29.9	9.6	*9.4*	60.1	——	0.6	2715
As purchased . . .	1	13.8	25.8	8.3	*8.1*	51.8	——	0.5	2340
Chuck, all analyses:									
Edible portion . . .	10	——	48.2	14.6	*14.2*	36.8	——	0.8	1825
As purchased . . .	10	19.4	38.5	11.7	*11.4*	30.0	——	0.7	1485
Flank, medium fat:									
Edible portion — Average	8	——	**46.2**	**15.2**	*14.8*	**38.3**	——	0.7	**1900**
As purchased — Average	2	9.9	**39.0**	**13.8**	*13.6*	**36.9**	——	0.6	**1815**
Flank, very fat, as purchased:									
Average	2	——	**28.9**	**10.7**	*10.7*	**59.8**	——	0.6	**2725**
Flank, all analyses:									
Edible portion . . .	10	——	42.7	14.3	*14.0*	42.6	——	0.7	2065
As purchased . . .	2	9.9	39.0	13.8	*13.6*	36.9	——	0.6	1815

CHEMICAL COMPOSITION OF AMERICAN FOOD MATERIALS —
Continued

FOOD MATERIALS	NUMBER OF ANALYSES	REFUSE	WATER	PROTEIN N × 6.25	PROTEIN By Difference	FAT	TOTAL CARBOHYDRATES	ASH	FUEL VALUE PER POUND
ANIMAL FOOD—*Continued*									
MUTTON, FRESH — *Continued*									
Leg, hind, lean:		Per Cent	Per Cent	Per Cent	Per Cent	Per Cent	Per Cent	Per Cent	Calories
Edible portion —									
Average	3	——	67.4	19.8	*19.1*	12.4	——	1.1	890
As purchased —									
Average	3	16.8	56.1	16.5	*15.9*	10.3	——	0.9	740
Leg, hind, medium fat:									
Edible portion —									
Average	11	——	62.8	18.5	*18.2*	18.0	——	1.0	1105
As purchased —									
Average	11	18.4	51.2	15.1	*14.9*	14.7	——	0.8	900
Leg, hind, fat:									
Edible portion . . .	1	——	55.0	17.3	*17.0*	27.1	——	0.9	1465
As purchased . . .	1	12.4	48.2	15.2	*14.8*	23.8	——	0.8	1290
Leg, hind, all analyses:									
Edible portion . . .	15	——	63.2	18.7	*18.3*	17.5	——	1.0	1085
As purchased . . .	15	17.7	51.9	15.4	*15.1*	14.5	——	0.8	900
Loin, without kidney or tallow, fat:									
Edible portion —									
Average	3	43.3	——	14.7	*14.2*	41.7	——	0.8	2035
As purchased —									
Average	3	11.7	38.3	13.0	*12.5*	36.8	——	0.7	1795
Loin, without kidney or tallow, very fat:									
Edible portion . . .	1	——	30.8	10.6	*10.0*	58.7	——	.5	2675
As purchased . . .	1	9.0	28.1	9.6	*9.1*	53.4	——	.4	2435
Loin, without kidney or tallow, all analyses									
Edible portion . . .	17	——	47.8	15.5	*15.2*	36.2	——	0.8	1815
As purchased . . .	16	14.8	40.4	13.1	*12.7*	31.5	——	0.6	1575
Loin, free fat removed .	1	——	56.5	23.7	*23.9*	18.5	——	1.1	1225
Neck, medium fat:									
Edible portion —									
Average	10	——	58.1	16.9	*16.3*	24.6	——	1.0	1355
As purchased —									
Average	10	27.4	42.1	12.3	*11.9*	17.9	——	0.7	985

CHEMICAL COMPOSITION OF AMERICAN FOOD MATERIALS — *Continued*

FOOD MATERIALS	NUMBER OF ANALYSES	REFUSE	WATER	PROTEIN N × 6.25	PROTEIN By Difference	FAT	TOTAL CARBO-HYDRATES	ASH	FUEL VALUE PER POUND
ANIMAL FOOD—*Continued*									
MUTTON, FRESH—*Continued*		Per Cent	Per Cent	Per Cent	Per Cent	Per Cent	Per Cent	Per Cent	Calories
Neck, very fat:									
Edible portion . . .	1	—	42.1	13.9	*13.6*	43.5	—	0.8	2095
As purchased . . .	1	16.1	35.3	11.7	*11.4*	36.5	—	0.7	1760
Neck, all analyses:									
Edible portion . . .	11	—	56.6	16.7	*16.1*	26.3	—	1.0	1420
As purchased . . .	11	26.4	41.5	12.2	*11.8*	19.6	—	0.7	1055
Shoulder, lean:									
Edible portion . . .	1	—	67.2	19.5	*18.9*	12.9	—	1.0	905
As purchased . . .	1	25.3	50.2	14.6	*14.2*	9.6	—	0.7	675
Shoulder, medium fat:									
Edible portion —									
Average	7	—	61.9	17.7	*17.3*	19.9	—	0.9	1170
As purchased —									
Average	7	22.5	47.9	13.7	*13.4*	15.5	—	0.7	910
Shoulder, fat:									
Edible portion . . .	1	—	53.0	16.2	*15.9*	30.3	—	0.8	1580
As purchased . . .	1	19.5	42.7	13.0	*12.8*	24.4	—	0.6	1270
Shoulder, very fat:									
Edible portion . . .	1	—	48.4	15.6	*15.2*	35.6	—	0.8	1790
As purchased . . .	1	18.7	39.3	12.7	*12.4*	28.9	—	0.7	1455
Shoulder, all analyses:									
Edible portion . . .	10	—	60.2	17.5	*17.1*	21.8	—	0.9	1245
As purchased . . .	10	22.1	46.8	13.7	*13.3*	17.1	—	0.7	975
Forequarter:									
Edible portion —									
Average	10	—	52.9	15.6	*15.3*	30.9	—	0.9	1595
As purchased —									
Average	10	21.2	41.6	12.3	*12.0*	24.5	—	0.7	1265
Hind quarter:									
Edible portion —									
Average	10	—	54.8	16.7	*16.3*	28.1	—	0.8	1495
As purchased —									
Average	10	17.2	45.4	13.8	*13.5*	23.2	—	0.7	1235
Side, including tallow:									
Edible portion —									
Average	25	—	54.2	16.3	*16.0*	28.9	—	0.9	1520

CHEMICAL COMPOSITION OF AMERICAN FOOD MATERIALS — *Continued*

Food Materials	Number of Analyses	Refuse	Water	Protein N × 6.25	Protein By Difference	Fat	Total Carbohydrates	Ash	Fuel Value per Pound
ANIMAL FOOD—*Continued* MUTTON, FRESH—*Continued*									
Side, including tallow — *Continued* As purchased —		Per Cent	Per Cent	Per Cent	Per Cent	Per Cent	Per Cent	Per Cent	Calories
Average	25	18.1	45.4	13.0	*12.7*	23.1	——	0.7	1215
Side, not including tallow : Edible portion —									
Average	10	——	53.6	16.2	*15.8*	29.8	——	0.8	1560
As purchased —									
Average	10	19.3	43.3	13.0	*12.7*	24.0	——	0.7	1255
MUTTON, COOKED									
Mutton, leg roast, edible portion:									
Average	2	——	50.9	25.0	*25.3*	22.6	——	1.2	1420
MUTTON, ORGANS									
Heart, as purchased:									
Average	2	——	69.5	16.9	*17.0*	12.6	——	0.9	845
Kidneys, as purchased .	1	——	78.7	16.5	*16.8*	3.2	——	1.3	440
Kidney and kidney fat, as purchased . .	1	——	18.8	6.2	*4.3*	76.5	——	0.4	3345
Kidney fat, as purchased:									
Average	2	——	3.4	1.8	*1.1*	95.4	——	0.1	4060
Liver, as purchased:									
Average	2	——	61.2	23.1	——	9.0	5.0	1.7	905
Lungs, as purchased:									
Average	2	——	75.9	20.2	*20.1*	2.8	——	1.2	495
MUTTON, CANNED									
Corned, as purchased .	1	——	45.8	28.8	*27.2*	22.8	——	4.2	1500
Tongue, as purchased .	1	——	47.6	24.4	*23.6*	24.0	——	4.8	1465
PORK, FRESH									
Chuck ribs and shoulder : Edible portion —									
Average . .	2	——	51.1	17.3	*16.9*	31.1	——	0.9	1635
As purchased —									
Average	2	18.1	41.8	14.1	*13.8*	25.5	——	0.8	1340

CHEMICAL COMPOSITION OF AMERICAN FOOD MATERIALS —
Continued

FOOD MATERIALS	NUMBER OF ANALYSES	REFUSE	WATER	PROTEIN N × 6.25	PROTEIN By Difference	FAT	TOTAL CARBO-HYDRATES	ASH	FUEL VALUE PER POUND
ANIMAL FOOD—*Continued*									
PORK, FRESH—*Continued*									
Flank:		Per Cent	Per Cent	Per Cent	Per Cent	Per Cent	Per Cent	Per Cent	Cal-ories
Edible portion —									
Average	3	—	59.0	18.5	*17.8*	22.2	—	1.0	1280
As purchased —									
Average	3	18.0	48.5	15.1	*14.2*	18.6	—	0.7	1065
Ham, fresh, lean:									
Edible portion —									
Average	2	—	60.0	25.0	*24.3*	14.4	—	1.3	1075
As purchased —									
Average	2	0.9	59.4	24.8	*24.2*	14.2	—	1.3	1060
Ham, fresh, medium fat: [1]									
Edible portion —									
Average	10	—	53.9	15.3	*16.4*	28.9	—	0.8	1505
As purchased —									
Average	10	10.7	48.0	13.5	*14.6*	25.9	—	0.8	1345
Ham, fresh, fat [2]									
Edible portion —									
Average	5	—	38.7	12.4	*10.6*	50.0	—	0.7	2345
As purchased —									
Average	5	13.2	33.6	10.7	*9.2*	43.5	—	0.5	2035
Ham, fresh, average all analyses:									
Edible portion . . .	17	—	50.1	15.7	*15.6*	33.4	—	0.9	1700
As purchased . . .	17	10.3	45.1	14.3	*14.1*	29.7	—	0.8	1520
Ham, fresh, visible fat largely removed .	3	—	64.5	19.2	*18.4*	16.2	—	0.9	1040
Head:									
Edible portion —									
Average . .	3	—	45.3	13.4	*12.7*	41.3	—	0.7	1990
As purchased —									
Average	3	68.4	13.8	4.1	*3.8*	13.8	—	0.2	660

[1] Seven samples contained an average of lecithin 0.32, gelatinoids 0.8, and "flesh bases" 1.28 per cent.

[2] One sample contained lecithin 0.45, gelatinoids 0.9, and "flesh bases" 0.8 per cent.

CHEMICAL COMPOSITION OF AMERICAN FOOD MATERIALS —
Continued

Food Materials	Number of Analyses	Refuse	Water	Protein N × 6.25	Protein By Difference	Fat	Total Carbohydrates	Ash	Fuel Value per Pound
ANIMAL FOOD—*Continued*									
PORK, FRESH—*Continued*									
Head cheese:		Per Cent	Per Cent	Per Cent	Per Cent	Per Cent	Per Cent	Per Cent	Calories
Edible portion —									
Average	3	—	43.3	19.5	*16.9*	33.8	—	3.3	1790
As purchased . . .	1	12.1	42.3	18.9	*18.6*	24.0	—	3.0	1365
Loin (chops), lean:									
Edible portion . . .	1	—	60.3	20.3	*19.7*	19.0	—	1.0	1180
As purchased . . .	1	23.5	46.1	15.5	*15.1*	14.5	—	0.8	900
Loin (chops), medium fat:									
Edible portion [1] —									
Average	19	—	52.0	16.6	*16.9*	30.1	—	1.0	1580
As purchased —									
Average	19	19.7	41.8	13.4	*13.5*	24.2	—	0.8	1270
Loin (chops), fat:									
Edible portion —									
Average	4	—	41.8	14.5	*13.1*	44.4	—	0.7	2145
As purchased —									
Average	4	16.5	34.8	11.9	*10.9*	37.2	—	0.6	1790
Loin (chops), average all analyses:									
Edible portion . . .	24	—	50.7	16.4	*16.4*	32.0	—	0.9	1655
As purchased . . .	24	19.3	40.8	13.2	*13.1*	26.0	—	0.8	1340
Loin, tenderloin, as purchased: [2]									
Average	11	—	66.5	18.9	*19.5*	13.0	—	1.0	900
Middle cuts:									
Edible portion —									
Average	3	—	48.2	15.7	*14.8*	36.3	—	0.7	1825
As purchased —									
Average	3	19.7	38.6	12.7	*12.1*	28.9	—	0.7	1455
Shoulder:									
Edible portion [3] —									
Average	19	—	51.2	13.3	*13.8*	34.2	—	0.8	1690

[1] Eight samples contained an average of lecithin 0.35, gelatinoids 1.0, and "flesh bases" 1.5 per cent.

[2] Eight samples contained an average of lecithin 0.51, gelatinoids 0.6, and "flesh bases" 0.9 per cent.

[3] Eight samples contained an average of lecithin 0.25, gelatinoids 0.8, and "flesh bases" 1.1 per cent.

Chemical Composition of American Food Materials — *Continued*

Food Materials	Number of Analyses	Refuse	Water	Protein N × 6.25	Protein By Difference	Fat	Total Carbo-hydrates	Ash	Fuel Value per Pound
Animal Food—*Continued*									
pork, fresh—*Continued*									
Shoulder—*Continued*		Per Cent	Per Cent	Per Cent	Per Cent	Per Cent	Per Cent	Per Cent	Cal-ories
As purchased —									
Average	19	12.4	44.9	12.0	*12.2*	29.8	——	0.7	1480
Side, lard and other fat included:									
Edible portion —									
Average	3	——	29.4	9.4	*8.5*	61.7	——	0.4	2780
As purchased —									
Average	3	11.2	26.1	8.3	*7.5*	54.8	——	0.4	2465
Side, not including lard and kidney:									
Edible portion [1] —									
Average	11	——	34.4	9.1	*9.8*	55.3	——	0.5	2505
As purchased —									
Average	11	11.5	30.4	8.0	*8.6*	49.0	——	0.5	2215
Clear backs:									
Edible portion [2] —									
Average	8	——	25.1	6.4	*6.9*	67.6	——	0.4	2970
As purchased —									
Average	8	5.7	23.7	6.0	*6.4*	63.8	——	0.4	2805
Clear bellies:									
Edible portion [3] —									
Average	8	——	31.4	6.9	*7.8*	60.4	——	0.4	2675
As purchased —									
Average	8	6.2	29.5	6.5	*7.3*	56.6	——	0.4	2510
Back fat, as purchased:									
Average	3	——	7.7	3.6	*2.3*	89.9	——	0.1	3860
Belly fat, as purchased:									
Average	3	——	13.8	5.2	*4.1*	81.9	——	0.2	3555

[1] Eight samples contained an average of lecithin 0.35, gelatinoids 1, and "flesh bases" 1.5 per cent.

[2] Eight samples contained an average of lecithin 0.21, gelatinoids 0.6, and "flesh bases" 0.8 per cent.

[3] Eight samples contained an average of lecithin 0.18. gelatinoids 0.6. and "flesh bases" 0.9 per cent.

CHEMICAL COMPOSITION OF AMERICAN FOOD MATERIALS — *Continued*

FOOD MATERIALS	NUMBER OF ANALYSES	REFUSE	WATER	PROTEIN N × 6.25	PROTEIN By Difference	FAT	TOTAL CARBOHYDRATES	ASH	FUEL VALUE PER POUND
ANIMAL FOOD—*Continued*									
PORK, FRESH—*Continued*		Per Cent	Per Cent	Per Cent	Per Cent	Per Cent	Per Cent	Per Cent	Cal-ories
Ham fat, as purchased:									
Average	3	—	9.1	3.5	*2.7*	88.0	—	0.2	3780
Jowl fat, as purchased:									
Average	3	—	16.0	5.9	*5.0*	78.8	—	0.2	3435
Feet:									
Edible portion [1] —									
Average	8	—	55.4	15.8	*17.5*	26.3	—	0.8	1405
As purchased —									
Average	8	74.1	14.3	4.1	*4.5*	6.9	—	0.2	365
Tails:									
Edible portion [2] —									
Average	8	—	17.4	4.8	*5.2*	77.1	—	0.3	3340
As purchased —									
Average	8	13.3	15.0	4.1	*4.5*	66.9	—	0.3	2900
Trimmings:									
Edible portion —									
Average	8	—	23.3	5.4	*6.2*	70.2	—	0.3	3060
As purchased —									
Average	8	7.4	21.6	5.0	*5.7*	65.0	—	0.3	2835
PORK ORGANS, ETC.									
Brains, as purchased	1	—	75.8	11.7	*12.3*	10.3	—	1.6	655
Heart, as purchased . .	1	—	75.6	17.1	*17.1*	6.3	—	1.0	585
Kidneys, as purchased:									
Average	2	—	77.8	15.5	*16.2*	4.8	—	1.2	490
Liver, as purchased . .	1	—	71.4	21.3	*21.3*	4.5	1.4	1.4	615
Lungs, as purchased . .	1	—	83.3	11.9	*11.8*	4.0	—	0.9	390
Marrow, as purchased:									
Average	6	—	14.6	2.3	*4.2*	81.2	—	[3]	3470
Skin, as purchased:									
Average	7	—	46.3	26.4	*30.4*	22.7	—	0.6	1450

[1] Eight samples contained an average of lecithin 0.32, gelatinoids 3.5, and "flesh bases" 2 per cent.

[2] Eight samples contained an average of lecithin 0.20, gelatinoids 0.6, and "flesh bases" 0.6 per cent.　　　　　　[3] Ash not determined.

Chemical Composition of American Food Materials — *Continued*

Food Materials	Number of Analyses	Refuse	Water	Protein N × 6.25	Protein By Difference	Fat	Total Carbohydrates	Ash	Fuel Value per Pound
ANIMAL FOOD—*Continued*									
PORK, PICKLED, SALTED, AND SMOKED									
Ham, smoked, lean:		Per Cent	Per Cent	Per Cent	Per Cent	Per Cent	Per Cent	Per Cent	Calories
Edible portion —									
Average	3	—	53.5	19.8	*20.2*	20.8	—	5.5	1245
As purchased —									
Average	3	11.5	47.2	17.5	*17.9*	18.5	—	4.9	1105
Ham, smoked, medium fat:									
Edible portion —									
Average	14	—	40.3	16.3	*16.1*	38.8	—	4.8	1940
As purchased —									
Average	14	13.6	34.8	14.2	*14.0*	33.4	—	4.2	1675
Ham, smoked, fat:									
Edible portion —									
Average	4	—	27.9	14.8	*16.1*	52.3	—	3.7	2485
As purchased —									
Average . . .	2	3.4	25.2	12.4	*14.2*	53.7	—	3.5	2495
Ham, smoked, all analyses.									
Edible portion . .	21	—	39.8	16.5	*16.7*	38.8	—	4.7	1945
As purchased .	19	12.2	35.8	14.5	*14.6*	33.2	—	4.2	1670
Ham skin, as purchased	1	—	27.2	15.4	*16.0*	53.7	—	3.1	2555
Ham, smoked, boiled, as purchased:									
Average	2	—	51.3	20.2	*20.2*	22.4	—	6.1	1320
Ham, smoked, fried, as purchased . .	1	—	36.6	22.2	*24.4*	33.2	—	5.8	1815
Ham, boneless, raw:									
Edible portion —									
Average	4	—	50.1	14.9	*15.4*	28.5	—	6.0	1480
As purchased —									
Average	4	3.3[1]	48.5	14.3	*14.9*	27.5	—	5.8	1425
Ham, luncheon, cooked:									
Edible portion —									
Average	2	—	49.2	22.5	*24.0*	21.0	—	5.8	1305

[1] Refuse, case.

CHEMICAL COMPOSITION OF AMERICAN FOOD MATERIALS — *Continued*

FOOD MATERIALS	NUMBER OF ANALYSES	REFUSE	WATER	PROTEIN N × 6.25	PROTEIN By Difference	FAT	TOTAL CARBO-HYDRATES	ASH	FUEL VALUE PER POUND
ANIMAL FOOD—*Continued* PORK, PICKLED, SALTED, AND SMOKED—*Continued*									
Ham, luncheon, cooked —*Continued* As purchased —		Per Cent	Per Cent	Per Cent	Per Cent	Per Cent	Per Cent	Per Cent	Cal-ories
Average	2	2.1¹	48.1	22.1	*23.5*	20.6	——	5.7	1280
Shoulder, smoked, medium fat: Edible portion —									
Average	3	——	45.0	15.9	*15.8*	32.5	——	6.7	1665
As purchased —									
Average	3	18.2	36.8	13.0	*12.9*	26.6	——	5.5	1365
Shoulder, smoked, fat: Edible portion —									
Average	2	——	26.5	15.1	*14.7*	53.6	——	5.2	2545
As purchased —									
Average	2	20.0	21.4	12.1	*11.8*	42.6	——	4.2	2020
Shoulder, smoked, all analyses:									
Edible portion . . .	5	——	37.6	15.5	*15.3*	41.0	——	6.1	2020
As purchased . . .	5	18.9	30.7	12.4	*12.4*	33.0	——	5.0	1625
Pigs' tongues, pickled: Edible portion —									
Average	2	——	58.6	17.7	*18.0*	19.8	——	3.6	1165
As purchased —									
Average	2	3.2	56.8	17.1	*17.5*	19.1	——	3.4	1125
Pigs' feet, pickled: Edible portion —									
Average	2	——	68.2	16.3	*16.1*	14.8	——	0.9	930
As purchased —									
Average	2	35.5	44.6	10.2	*10.0*	9.3	——	0.6	585
Dry-salted backs: Edible portion —									
Average	2	——	17.3	7.7	*7.2*	72.7	——	2.8	3210
As purchased —									
Average	2	8.1	15.9	7.1	*6.5*	66.8	——	2.7	2950

¹ Refuse, case.

CHEMICAL COMPOSITION OF AMERICAN FOOD MATERIALS —
Continued

FOOD MATERIALS	NUMBER OF ANALYSES	REFUSE	WATER	PROTEIN		FAT	TOTAL CARBO-HYDRATES	ASH	FUEL VALUE PER POUND
				N × 6.25	By Difference				
ANIMAL FOOD—*Continued*									
PORK, PICKLED, SALTED, AND SMOKED—*Continued*									
Dry-salted bellies:		Per Cent	Per Cent	Per Cent	Per Cent	Per Cent	Per Cent	Per Cent	Cal-ories
Edible portion —									
Average	2	—	17.7	8.4	*6.7*	72.2	—	3.4	3200
As purchased —									
Average	2	8.2	16.2	7.7	*6.2*	66.2	—	3.2	2935
Salt pork, clear fat, as purchased:									
Average	7	—	7.9	1.9	*2.0*	86.2	—	3.9	3670
Salt pork, lean ends:									
Edible portion —									
Average	4	—	19.9	8.4	*7.3*	67.1	—	5.7	2985
As purchased —									
Average	4	11.2	17.6	7.4	*6.5*	59.6	—	5.1	2655
Bacon, smoked, lean:									
Edible portion —									
Average	2	—	31.8	15.5	*14.6*	42.6	—	11.0	2085
As purchased —									
Average	2	17.0	26.5	13.0	*12.3*	35.5	—	8.7	1740
Bacon, smoked, medium fat:									
Edible portion —									
Average	17	—	18.8	9.9	*9.4*	67.4	—	4.4	3030
As purchased —									
Average	17	7.7	17.4	9.1	*8.6*	62.2	—	4.1	2795
Bacon, smoked, all analyses:									
Edible portion . .	19	—	20.2	10.5	*9.9*	64.8	—	5.1	2930
As purchased . .	19	8.7	18.4	9.5	*9.0*	59.4	—	4.5	2685
Ribs, cooked, as purchased	1	—	33.6	24.8	*26.6*	37.6	—	2.2	2050
Steak, cooked, as purchased	1	—	33.2	—	*19.9*	45.4	—	1.5	2285
PORK, CANNED									
Brawn, boars' brains, as purchased:									
Average	2	—	49.0	25.2	*23.4*	23.0	—	4.6	1440

CHEMICAL COMPOSITION OF AMERICAN FOOD MATERIALS — *Continued*

FOOD MATERIALS	NUMBER OF ANALYSES	REFUSE	WATER	PROTEIN N × 6.25	PROTEIN By Difference	FAT	TOTAL CARBO-HYDRATES	ASH	FUEL VALUE PER POUND
ANIMAL FOOD—*Continued* PORK, CANNED—*Continued*									
Boars' heads, as purchased:		Per Cent	Per Cent	Per Cent	Per Cent	Per Cent	Per Cent	Per Cent	Calories
Average	2	—	55.3	20.7	*19.2*	22.2	—	3.3	1320
Ham, deviled, as purchased:									
Average	6	—	44.1	19.0	*18.5*	34.1	—	3.3	1790
SAUSAGE [1]									
Arles:									
Edible portion . . .	1	—	17.2	26.8	*24.9*	50.6	—	7.3	2635
As purchased . . .	1	5.2	16.3	25.4	*23.6*	48.0	—	6.9	2495
Banquet:									
Edible portion . . .	1	—	62.7	18.3	*17.9*	15.7	—	3.7	1005
As purchased . . .	1	1.6	61.7	18.0	*17.7*	15.4	—	3.6	985
Bologna :.									
Edible portion —									
Average	8	—	60.0	18.7	*18.4*	17.6	0.3	3.7	1095
As purchased —									
Average	4	3.3	55.2	18.2	*18.0*	19.7	—	3.8	1170
Farmer:									
Edible portion . . .	1	—	23.2	29.0	*27.2*	42.0	—	7.6	2310
As purchased . . .	. 1	3.9	22.2	27.9	*26.2*	40.4	—	7.3	2225
Frankfort, as purchased:									
Average	8	—	57.2	19.6	*19.7*	18.6	1.1	3.4	1170
Holsteiner:									
Edible portion . . .	1	—	25.6	29.4	*29.4*	37.3	3.4	4.3	2220
As purchased . . .	1	2.2	25.1	28.7	*28.7*	36.5	3.3	4.2	2135
Lyons, pure ham:									
Edible portion . . .	1	—	32.5	32.3	*32.3*	27.2	——	8.0	1750
As purchased . . .	1	10.0	29.2	29.1	*29.1*	24.5	——	7.2	1575
Pork, as purchased:									
Average	11	—	39.8	13.0	*12.7*	44.2	1.1	2.2	2125

[1] In some cases the sum of the percentages of water, protein, fat, and ash in sausage does not make 100. In such cases the difference is estimated as carbohydrates. There are, however, no tests showing the presence of these, and it may be more nearly correct to give no value for carbohydrates.

CHEMICAL COMPOSITION OF AMERICAN FOOD MATERIALS —
Continued

FOOD MATERIALS	NUMBER OF ANALYSES	REFUSE	WATER	PROTEIN		FAT	TOTAL CARBO-HYDRATES	ASH	FUEL VALUE PER POUND
				N × 6.25	By Differ-ence				
ANIMAL FOOD—*Continued*									
SAUSAGE—*Continued*		Per Cent	Per Cent	Per Cent	Per Cent	Per Cent	Per Cent	Per Cent	Cal-ories
Pork sausage meat, as purchased . . .	1	——	46.2	17.4	*17.9*	32.5	——	3.4	1695
Pork and beef chopped together, as pur-chased	1	——	55.4	19.4	*19.5*	24.1	——	1.0	1380
Salmi :									
Edible portion —									
Average	2	——	**30.5**	**24.1**	*22.6*	**39.9**	——	**7.0**	**2130**
As purchased —									
Average	2	9.3	27.6	21.8	*20.5*	36.2	——	6.4	1935
Summer :									
Edible portion —									
Average	3	——	**23.2**	**26.0**	*24.6*	**44.5**	——	**7.7**	**2360**
As purchased —									
Average	2	7.0	20.9	24.5	*23.0*	42.1	——	7.0	2230
Tongue, as purchased .	1	——	46.4	20.1	*17.3*	33.1	——	3.2	1770
Wienerwurst, as pur-chased	1	——	43.9	28.0	——	22.1	1.6	4.4	1485
SAUSAGE, CANNED									
Beef, as purchased . .	1	——	59.6	17.9	*17.8*	20.6	——	2.0	1200
Bologna, Italian, as pur-chased	1	——	42.6	24.9	*23.2*	27.8	——	6.4	1635
Frankfort, as purchased	1	——	72.7	14.9	*14.6*	9.9	——	2.8	695
Oxford, as purchased .	1	——	28.9	9.9	*9.9*	58.5	0.6	2.1	2665
Pork :									
Edible portion . . .	1	——	56.6	16.6	*16.6*	24.8	——	2.0	1355
As purchased . . .	1	12.6[1]	49.5	14.5	*14.5*	21.6	——	1.8	1180
POULTRY AND GAME, FRESH									
Chicken, broilers :									
Edible portion —									
Average	3	——	**74.8**	**21.5**	*21.6*	**2.5**	——	**1.1**	**505**

[1] Refuse liquid.

CHEMICAL COMPOSITION OF AMERICAN FOOD MATERIALS —
Continued

FOOD MATERIALS	NUMBER OF ANALYSES	REFUSE	WATER	PROTEIN N × 6.25	PROTEIN By Difference	FAT	TOTAL CARBO-HYDRATES	ASH	FUEL VALUE PER POUND
ANIMAL FOOD—*Continued*									
POULTRY AND GAME, FRESH									
—*Continued*									
Chicken, broilers — *Continued*		Per Cent	Per Cent	Per Cent	Per Cent	Per Cent	Per Cent	Per Cent	Calories
As purchased —									
Average	3	41.6	43.7	12.8	*12.6*	1.4	——	0.7	295
Fowls :									
Edible portion —									
Average	26	——	63.7	19.3	*19.0*	16.3	——	1.0	1045
As purchased —									
Average	26	25.9	47.1	13.7	*14.0*	12.3	——	0.7	775
Goose, young :									
Edible portion . . .	1	——	46.7	16.3	*16.3*	36.2	——	0.8	1830
As purchased . . .	1	17.6	38.5	13.4	*13.4*	29.8	——	0.7	1505
Turkey :									
Edible portion —									
Average	3	——	55.5	21.1	*20.6*	22.9	——	1.0	1360
As purchased —									
Average	3	22.7	42.4	16.1	*15.7*	18.4	——	0.8	1075
Chicken gizzard, as purchased	1	——	72.5	24.7	*24.7*	1.4	——	1.4	520
Chicken heart, as purchased	1	——	72.0	20.7	*21.1*	5.5	——	1.4	615
Chicken liver, as purchased . . .	1	——	69.3	22.4	——	4.2	2.4	1.7	640
Goose gizzard	1	——	73.8	19.6	*19.4*	5.8	——	1.0	610
Goose liver, as purchased	1	——	62.6	16.6	——	15.9	3.7	1.2	1050
Turkey gizzard, as purchased	1	——	62.7	20.5	——	14.5	1.2	1.1	1015
Turkey heart, as purchased	1	——	68.6	16.8	*17.2*	13.2	——	1.0	870
Turkey liver, as purchased	1	——	69.6	22.9	——	5.2	0.6	1.7	655
POULTRY AND GAME, COOKED									
Capon :									
Edible portion . . .	1	——	59.9	27.0	*27.3*	11.5	——	1.3	985

2 c

CHEMICAL COMPOSITION OF AMERICAN FOOD MATERIALS — *Continued*

FOOD MATERIALS	NUMBER OF ANALYSES	REFUSE	WATER	PROTEIN N × 6.25	PROTEIN By Difference	FAT	TOTAL CARBOHYDRATES	ASH	FUEL VALUE PER POUND
ANIMAL FOOD—*Continued* POULTRY AND GAME, COOKED—*Continued*		Per Cent	Per Cent	Per Cent	Per Cent	Per Cent	Per Cent	Per Cent	Calories
Capon — *Continued*									
As purchased . . .	1	10.4	53.6	24.2	*24.5*	10.3	——	1.2	885
Capon, with stuffing:									
Edible portion . .	1	——	62.1	21.8	——	10.9	3.8	1.4	935
As purchased . . .	1	7.7	57.2	20.1	——	10.3	3.5	1.2	875
Chicken, fricasseed, edible portion . .	1	——	67.5	17.6	——	11.5	2.4	1.0	855
Turkey, roast, edible portion . . .	1	——	52.0	27.8	*28.4*	18.4	——	1.2	1295
Turkey, roast, light and dark meat and stuffing, edible portion	1	——	65.0	——	*17.1*	10.8	5.5	1.6	870
POULTRY AND GAME, CANNED									
Chicken, sandwich, as purchased . .	1	——	46.9	20.8	*20.5*	30.0	——	2.6	1655
Turkey. sandwich. as purchased . . .	1	——	47.4	20.7	*20.7*	29.2	——	2.7	1615
Plover, roast, as purchased	1	——	57.7	22.4	——	10.2	7.6	2.1	985
Quail, as purchased . .	1	——	66.9	21.8	——	8.0	1.7	1.6	775
FISH, FRESH [1]									
Alewife, whole: Edible portion — Average	2	——	*74.4*	*19.4*	*19.2*	*4.9*	——	*1.5*	*570*

[1] A considerable number of determinations of phosphorus, sulfur, and chlorine have been made in the flesh of fresh fish. These are recorded in the following table in terms of phosphoric anhydrid (P_2O_5), sulfuric anhydrid (SO_3), and chlorine (Cl), and in percentages of the total weight of "edible portion" or flesh;

CHEMICAL COMPOSITION OF AMERICAN FOOD MATERIALS —
Continued

PHOSPHORIC ANHYDRID, SULFURIC ANHYDRID, AND CHLORINE IN SAMPLES OF
FRESH FISH

KIND OF FISH	PHOSPHORIC ANHYDRID		SULFURIC ANHYDRID		CHLORINE	
	Number of Determinations	Average	Number of Determinations	Average	Number of Determinations	Average
		Per Cent		Per Cent		Per Cent
Alewife	1	0.50	—	—	—	—
Bass:						
Black	1	0.44	1	0.89	—	—
Striped . . .	2	0.48	1	0.47	—	—
Blackfish . . .	1	0.52	1	0.46	1	0.24
Bluefish	1	0.62	—	—	—	—
Cod	2	0.45	—	—	—	—
Eels, salt water .	1	0.51	—	—	—	—
Flounder . . .	2	0.40	2	0.42	—	—
Haddock . . .	2	0.47	1	0.41	—	—
Halibut	2	0.44	1	0.49	—	—
Herring	1	0.55	1	0.55	—	—
Mackerel . . .	4	0.56	2	0.47	—	—
Muskellunge . .	1	0.52	1	0.37	—	—
Perch:						
White	2	0.44	2	0.65	—	—
Pike	1	0.46	1	0.90	—	—
Porgy'	2	0.59	1	0.52	—	—
Red snapper . .	2	0.47	2	0.47	—	—
Salmon	2	0.57	1	0.61	—	—
Landlocked . .	2	0.51	2	0.40	—	—
California . .	1	0.69	1	0.43	—	—
Shad	2	0.60	1	0.52	—	—
Sheepshead . .	1	0.45	1	0.48	—	—
Smelt	1	0.81	1	0.55	—	—
Spanish mackerel	1	0.60	1	0.58	—	—
Trout, brook . .	1	0.61	1	0.48	—	—
Turbot	1	0.48	1	0.32	—	—
Whitefish . . .	1	0.71	1	0.41	—	—

CHEMICAL COMPOSITION OF AMERICAN FOOD MATERIALS —
Continued

Food Materials	Number of Analyses	Refuse	Water	Protein N × 6.25	Protein By Difference	Fat	Total Carbohydrates	Ash	Fuel Value per Pound
ANIMAL FOOD—*Continued*									
FISH, FRESH—*Continued*									
Alewife, whole — *Continued*		Per Cent	Per Cent	Per Cent	Per Cent	Per Cent	Per Cent	Per Cent	Calories
As purchased —									
Average . . .	—	49.5	37.6	9.8	9.7	2.4	——	0.8	285
Bass, black, whole:									
Edible portion —									
Average . . .	2	——	76.7	20.6	20.4	1.7	——	1.2	455
As purchased —									
Average . . .	2	54.8	34.6	9.3	9.3	0.8	——	0.5	205
Bass, red, whole:									
Edible portion . . .	1	——	81.6	16.9	16.7	0.5	——	1.2	335
As purchased . . .	1	63.5	29.8	6.2	6.1	0.2	——	0.4	125
Bass, sea, whole:									
Edible portion . . .	1	——	79.3	19.8	18.8	0.5	——	1.4	390
As purchased . . .	1	56.1	34.8	8.7	8.3	0.2	——	0.6	170
Bass, striped, whole:									
Edible portion —									
Average . . .	6	——	77.7	18.6	18.3	2.8	——	1.2	465
As purchased —									
Average . . .	5	55.0	35.1	8.4	8.3	1.1	——	0.5	200
Bass, striped, entrails removed, as purchased . . .	1	51.2	37.4	8.8	8.7	2.2	——	0.5	255
Blackfish, whole:									
Edible portion —									
Average . . .	4	——	79.1	18.7	18.5	1.3	——	1.1	405
As purchased —									
Average . . .	2	60.2	31.4	7.4	7.3	0.7	——	0.4	165
Blackfish, entrails removed, as purchased:									
Average . . .	2	55.7	35.0	8.4	8.3	0.5	——	0.5	175
Bluefish, entrails removed:									
Edible portion . . .	1	——	78.5	19.4	19.0	1.2	——	1.3	410

CHEMICAL COMPOSITION OF AMERICAN FOOD MATERIALS —
Continued

| FOOD MATERIALS | NUMBER OF ANALYSES | REFUSE | WATER | PROTEIN | | FAT | TOTAL CARBO-HYDRATES | ASH | FUEL VALUE PER POUND |
				N × 6.25	By Difference				
ANIMAL FOOD—*Continued*									
FISH, FRESH—*Continued*									
Bluefish, entrails removed — *Continued*		Per Cent	Per Cent	Per Cent	Per Cent	Per Cent	Per Cent	Per Cent	Calories
As purchased . . .	1	48.6	40.3	10.0	*9.8*	0.6	——	0.7	210
Buffalo fish, entrails removed :									
Edible portion . . .	1	——	78.6	18.0	*17.9*	2.3	——	1.2	430
As purchased . . .	1	52.5	37.3	8.5	*8.5*	1.1	——	0.6	205
Butter-fish, whole :									
Edible portion . . .	1	——	70.0	18.0	*17.8*	11.0	——	1.2	800
As purchased . . .	1	42.8	40.1	10.3	*10.2*	6.3	——	0.6	460
Catfish :									
Edible portion . . .	1	——	64.1	14.4	*14.4*	20.6	——	0.9	1135
As purchased . . .	1	19.4	51.7	11.6	*11.6*	16.6	——	0.7	915
Ciscoe, whole :									
Edible portion —									
Average	3	——	**74.0**	**18.5**	*18.1*	**6.8**	——	**1.1**	**630**
As purchased . . .	1	42.7	43.6	11.1	*11.0*	2.0	——	0.7	290
Ciscoe, entrails removed, as purchased :									
Average . .	2	**10.1**	**65.6**	**16.3**	*15.9*	**7.5**	——	**0.9**	**620**
Cod, whole :									
Edible portion —									
Average	5	——	**82.6**	**16.5**	*15.8*	**0.4**	——	**1.2**	**325**
As purchased —									
Average	2	**52.5**	**38.7**	**8.4**	*8.0*	**0.2**	——	**0.6**	**165**
Cod, dressed, as purchased :									
Average	3	**29.9**	**58.5**	**11.1**	*10.6*	**0.2**	——	**0.8**	**215**
Cod, sections, edible portion :									
Average	3	——	**82.5**	**16.7**	*16.3*	**0.3**	——	**0.9**	**325**
Cod, steaks :									
Edible portion . . .	1	——	79.7	18.7	*18.6*	0.5	——	1.2	370
As purchased . . .	1	9.2	72.4	17.0	*16.9*	0.5	——	1.0	335
Cusk, entrails removed :									
Edible portion . . .	1	——	82.0	17.0	*16.9*	0.2	——	0.9	325

CHEMICAL COMPOSITION OF AMERICAN FOOD MATERIALS —
Continued

Food Materials	Number of Analyses	Refuse	Water	Protein N × 6.25	Protein By Difference	Fat	Total Carbo-hydrates	Ash	Fuel Value per Pound
ANIMAL FOOD—*Continued*									
FISH, FRESH—*Continued*									
Cusk, entrails removed—*Continued*		Per Cent	Per Cent	Per Cent	Per Cent	Per Cent	Per Cent	Per Cent	Cal-ories
As purchased . . .	1	40.3	49.0	10.1	*10.1*	0.1	——	0.5	190
Eels, salt water, head, skin, and entrails removed:									
Edible portion — Average	2	——	71.6	18.6	*18.3*	9.1	——	1.0	730
As purchased — Average . . .	2	20.2	57.2	14.8	*14.6*	7.2	——	0.8	580
Flounder, whole:									
Edible portion — Average	3	——	84.2	14.2	*13.9*	0.6	——	1.3	290
As purchased — Average	2	61.5	32.6	5.4	*5.1*	0.3	——	0.5	115
Flounder, entrails removed, as purchased . . .	1	57.0	35.8	6.4	*6.3*	0.3	——	0.6	130
Haddock, entrails removed:									
Edible portion — Average	4	——	81.7	17.2	*16.8*	0.3	——	1.2	335
As purchased — Average	4	51.0	40.0	8.4	*8.2*	0.2	——	0.6	165
Hake, entrails removed:									
Edible portion . . .	1	——	83.1	15.4	*15.2*	0.7	——	1.0	315
As purchased . . .	1	52.5	39.5	7.3	*7.2*	0.3	——	0.5	150
Halibut, steaks or sections:									
Edible portion — Average	3	——	75.4	18.6	*18.4*	5.2	——	1.0	565
As purchased — Average	3	17.7	61.9	15.3	*15.1*	4.4	——	0.9	470
Herring, whole:									
Edible portion — Average	2	——	72.5	19.5	*18.9*	7.1	——	1.5	660

CHEMICAL COMPOSITION OF AMERICAN FOOD MATERIALS —
Continued

FOOD MATERIALS	NUMBER OF ANALYSES	REFUSE	WATER	PROTEIN N × 6.25	PROTEIN By Difference	FAT	TOTAL CARBO-HYDRATES	ASH	FUEL VALUE PER POUND
ANIMAL FOOD—*Continued*									
FISH, FRESH—*Continued*									
Herring, whole — *Continued*		Per Cent	Per Cent	Per Cent	Per Cent	Per Cent	Per Cent	Per Cent	Cal-ories
As purchased —									
Average	2	**42.6**	**41.7**	**11.2**	*10.9*	**3.9**	——	**0.9**	**375**
Kingfish, whole:									
Edible portion . . .	1	——	79.2	18.9	*18.7*	0.9	——	1.2	390
As purchased . . .	1	56.6	34.4	8.2	*8.1*	0.4	——	0.5	170
Lamprey, whole:									
Edible portion . . .	1	——	71.1	15.0	*14.9*	13.3	——	0.7	840
As purchased . . .	1	45.8	38.5	8.1	*8.1*	7.2	——	0.4	455
Mackerel, whole:									
Edible portion — ·									
Average	6	——	**73.4**	**18.7**	*18.3*	**7.1**	——	**1.2**	**645**
As purchased —									
Average	5	**44.7**	**40.4**	**10.2**	*10.0*	**4.2**	——	**0.7**	**365**
Mackerel, entrails removed, as purchased	1	40.7	43.7	11.6	*11.4*	3.5	——	0.7	365
Mullet, whole:									
Edible portion . . .	1	——	74.9	19.5	*19.3*	4.6	——	1.2	555
As purchased . . .	1	57.9	31.5	8.2	*8.1*	2.0	——	0.5	235
Muskellunge, whole:									
Edible portion . . .	1	——	76.3	20.2	*19.6*	2.5	——	1.6	480
As purchased . . .	1	29.2	38.7	10.2	*10.0*	1.3	——	0.8	245
Perch, white, whole:									
Edible portion —									
Average	2	——	**75.7**	**19.3**	*19.1*	**4.0**	——	**1.2**	**530**
As purchased —									
Average	2	**62.5**	**28.4**	**7.3**	*7.2*	**1.5**	——	**0.4**	**200**
Perch, pike (wall-eyed pike):									
Edible portion . . .	1	——	79.7	18.6	*18.4*	0.5	——	1.4	365
As purchased . . .	1	57.3	34.0	7.9	*7.9*	0.2	——	0.6	155
Perch, yellow, whole:									
Edible portion —									
Average	2	——	**79.3**	**18.7**	*18.7*	**0.8**	——	**1.2**	**380**

CHEMICAL COMPOSITION OF AMERICAN FOOD MATERIALS — *Continued*

FOOD MATERIALS	NUMBER OF ANALYSES	REFUSE	WATER	PROTEIN N × 6.25	PROTEIN By Difference	FAT	TOTAL CARBO-HYDRATES	ASH	FUEL VALUE PER POUND
ANIMAL FOOD—*Continued* FISH, FRESH—*Continued*		Per Cent	Per Cent	Per Cent	Per Cent	Per Cent	Per Cent	Per Cent	Cal-ories
Perch, yellow, whole — *Continued*									
As purchased . . .	1	62.7	30.0	6.6	*6.7*	0.2	——	0.4	130
Perch, yellow, dressed, as purchased . .	1	35.1	50.7	12.8	*12.6*	0.7	——	0.9	265
Pickerel, pike, whole: Edible portion —									
Average	3	——	79.8	18.7	*18.6*	**0.5**	——	**1.1**	**370**
As purchased —									
Average . . .	2	47.1	42.2	9.9	*9.9*	0.2	——	0.6	190
Pickerel, pike, entrails removed as purchased	1	42.7	45.7	10.7	*10.7*	0.3	——	0.6	210
Pike, gray, whole:									
Edible portion . . .	1	——	80.8	17.9	*17.3*	0.8	——	1.1	365
As purchased . . .	1	63.2	29.7	6.6	*6.4*	0.3	——	0.4	135
Pollock, dressed:									
Edible portion . . .	1	——	76.0	21.6	*21.7*	0.8	——	1.5	435
As purchased . . .	1	28.5	54.3	15.4	*15.5*	0.6	——	1.1	310
Pompano, whole: Edible portion —									
Average .	2	——	72.8	18.8	*18.7*	7.5	——	1.0	665
As purchased —									
Average	2	45.5	39.5	10.3	*10.2*	4.3	——	0.5	375
Porgy, whole: Edible portion —									
Average	3	——	75.0	18.6	*18.5*	5.1	——	1.4	560
As purchased —									
Average	3	60.0	29.9	7.4	*7.4*	2.1	——	0.6	225
Red grouper, entrails removed: Edible portion —									
Average . . .	2	——	79.5	19.3	*18.8*	0.6	——	1.1	385
As purchased —									
Average . . .	2	55.9	35.0	8.5	*8.4*	0.2	——	0.5	165
Red snapper, whole: Edible portion —									
Average	3	——	78.5	19.7	*19.2*	1.0	——	1.3	410

CHEMICAL COMPOSITION OF AMERICAN FOOD MATERIALS — *Continued*

FOOD MATERIALS	NUMBER OF ANALYSES	REFUSE	WATER	PROTEIN N × 6.25	PROTEIN By Difference	FAT	TOTAL CARBOHYDRATES	ASH	FUEL VALUE PER POUND
ANIMAL FOOD—*Continued*									
FISH, FRESH—*Continued*									
Red snapper, whole — *Continued*		Per Cent	Per Cent	Per Cent	Per Cent	Per Cent	Per Cent	Per Cent	Cal- ories
As purchased —									
Average	2	46.1	42.0	10.8	*10.6*	0.6	——	0.7	225
Red snapper, entrails and gills removed, as purchased . . .	1	45.3	43.7	10.6	*10.0*	0.3	——	0.7	210
Salmon, whole:									
Edible portion —									
Average	6	——	64.6	22.0	*21.2*	12.8	——	1.4	950
As purchased —									
Average	4	34.9	40.9	15.3	*14.4*	8.9	——	0.9	660
Salmon, entrails removed, as purchased:									
Average	2	29.5	48.1	13.8	*13.5*	8.1	——	0.8	600
Salmon, landlocked, whole, spent:									
Edible portion —									
Average	4	——	77.7	17.8	*17.8*	3.3	——	1.2	470
As purchased —									
Average	4	45.5	42.3	9.7	*9.8*	1.8	——	0.6	255
Salmon, California, anterior sections:									
Edible portion —									
Average	2	——	63.6	17.8	*17.5*	17.8	——	1.1	1080
As purchased . . .	1	10.3	57.9	16.7	*16.1*	14.8	——	0.9	935
Shad, whole:									
Edible portion —									
Average	7	——	70.6	18.8	*18.6*	9.5	——	1.3	750
As purchased —									
Average	7	50.1	35.2	9.4	*9.2*	4.8	——	0.7	380
Shad, roe, as purchased	1	——	71.2	20.9	——	3.8	2.6	1.5	600
Sheepshead, whole:									
Edible portion —									
Average	2	——	75.6	20.1	*19.5*	3.7	——	1.2	530
As purchased . . .	1	66.0	26.9	6.6	*6.4*	0.2	——	0.5	130
Sheepshead, entrails removed, as purchased	1	56.6	31.2	9.0	*8.8*	2.9	——	0.5	290

CHEMICAL COMPOSITION OF AMERICAN FOOD MATERIALS —
Continued

FOOD MATERIALS	NUMBER OF ANALYSES	REFUSE	WATER	PROTEIN N × 6.25	PROTEIN By Difference	FAT	TOTAL CARBO-HYDRATES	ASH	FUEL VALUE PER POUND
ANIMAL FOOD—*Continued*									
FISH, FRESH—*Continued*		Per Cent	Per Cent	Per Cent	Per Cent	Per Cent	Per Cent	Per Cent	Cal-ories
Skate, lobe of body:									
Edible portion . .	1	——	82.2	18.2	*15.3*	1.4	——	1.1	400
As purchased . .	1	51.0	40.2	8.9	*7.5*	0.7	——	0.6	195
Smelt, whole:									
Edible portion —									
Average . . .	2	——	79.2	17.6	*17.3*	1.8	——	1.7	405
As purchased —									
Average	2	41.9	46.1	10.1	*10.0*	1.0	——	1.0	230
Spanish mackerel, whole:									
Edible portion . . .	1	——	68.1	21.5	*21.0*	9.4	——	1.5	795
As purchased . .	1	34.6	44.5	14.1	*13.7*	6.2	——	1.0	525
Sturgeon, anterior sections:									
Edible portion . . .	1	——	78.7	18.1	*18.0*	1.9	——	1.4	415
As purchased . .	1	14.4	67.4	15.1	*15.4*	1.6	——	1.2	350
Tomcod, whole:									
Edible portion . . .	1	——	81.5	17.2	*17.1*	0.4	——	1.0	335
As purchased . . .	1	59.9	32.7	6.9	*6.8*	0.2	——	0.4	135
Trout, brook, whole:									
Edible portion —									
Average	3	——	77.8	19.2	*18.9*	2.1	——	1.2	445
As purchased —									
Average	3	48.1	40.4	9.9	*9.8*	1.1	——	0.6	230
Trout, salmon or lake:									
Edible portion —									
Average	2	——	70.8	17.8	*17.7*	10.3	——	1 2	765
As purchased —									
Average	2	48.5	36.6	9.1	*9.2*	5.1	——	0.6	385
Turbot:									
Edible portion . .	1	——	71.4	14.8	*12.9*	14.4	——	1.3	885
As purchased . . .	1	47.7	37.3	7.7	*6.8*	7.5	——	0.7	460
Weakfish, whole:									
Edible portion . . .	1	——	79.0	17.8	*17.4*	2.4	——	1.2	430
As purchased . .	1	51.9	38.0	8.6	*8.4*	1.1	——	0.6	205
Whitefish, whole:									
Edible portion . . .	1	——	69.8	22.9	*22.1*	6.5	——	1.6	700
As purchased . . .	1	53.5	32.5	10.6	*10.3*	3.0	——	0.7	325

CHEMICAL COMPOSITION OF AMERICAN FOOD MATERIALS — *Continued*

FOOD MATERIALS	NUMBER OF ANALYSES	REFUSE	WATER	N × 6.25	By Difference	FAT	TOTAL CARBOHYDRATES	ASH	FUEL VALUE PER POUND
				PROTEIN					
ANIMAL FOOD—*Continued*									
FISH, COOKED		Per	Per	Per	Per	Per	Per	Per	Cal-
Bluefish, cooked, edible		Cent	Cent	Cent	Cent	Cent	Cent	Cent	·ories
portion	1	—	68.2	25.9	*26.1*	4.5	—	1.2	670
Spanish mackerel, broiled									
Edible portion . .	1	—	68.9	23.7	*23.2*	6.5	—	1.4	715
As purchased . . .	1	7.9	63.5	21.8	*21.4*	5,9	—	1.3	655
FISH, PRESERVED AND CANNED [1]									
Cod, salt: [2]									
Edible portion —									
Average	2	—	**53.5**	**25.4**	*21.5*	**0.3**	—	**24.7** [3]	**410**

[1] A considerable number of determinations of phosphorus, sulfur, and chlorine have been made in the flesh of preserved and canned fish. These are recorded in the following table in terms of phosphoric anhydrid (P_2O_5), sulfuric anhydrid (SO_3) and chlorine (Cl), and in percentages of the total weight of "edible portion" or flesh:

PHOSPHORIC ANHYDRID, SULFURIC ANHYDRID, AND CHLORINE IN SAMPLES OF PRESERVED AND CANNED FISH

KIND OF FISH	Number of Determinations	Average	Number of Determinations	Average	Number of Determinations	Average
	PHOSPHORIC ANHYDRID		SULFURIC ANHYDRID		CHLORINE	
		Per Cent		Per Cent		Per Cent
Cod, salt . . .	2	0.25	2	0.74	2	11.92
Cod, salt, boneless	1	0.36	1	0.68	1	11.19
Halibut, smoked .	1	0.47	1	0.44	1	8.66
Herring, smoked .	1	0.84	1	1.24	1	7.21
Mackerel, salt . .	1	0.35	1	0.61	—	—
Salmon, canned .	1	0.61	1	0.44	—	—

[2] It is observable that in salt cod the proportion of protein by difference is much smaller than by factor. The former value is apparently more nearly correct, and has been used in estimating the fuel value per pound.

[3] Two samples averaged 23 per cent common salt.

CHEMICAL COMPOSITION OF AMERICAN FOOD MATERIALS —
Continued

Food Materials	Number of Analyses	Refuse	Water	Protein N × 6.25	Protein By Difference	Fat	Total Carbohydrates	Ash	Fuel Value per Pound
ANIMAL FOOD—*Continued*									
FISH, PRESERVED AND CANNED —*Continued*									
Cod, salt—*Continued*		Per Cent	Per Cent	Per Cent	Per Cent	Per Cent	Per Cent	Per Cent	Cal-ories
As purchased —									
Average	2	24.9	40.2	19.0	*16.0*	0.4	——	18.5	315
Cod, salt, "boneless":									
Edible portion —									
Average	2	——	55.0	27.3	*25.7*	0.3	——	19.0 [1]	490
As purchased	1	1.6	54.8	27.7	*28.6*	0.3	——	14.7	545
Haddock, smoked:									
Edible portion	1	——	72.5	23.3	*23.7*	0.2	——	3.6	440
As purchased	1	32.2	49.2	15.8	*16.1*	0.1	——	2.4	305
Haddock, smoked, cooked, canned, as purchased	1	——	68.7	22.3	*21.8*	2.3	——	7.2	510
Halibut, smoked:									
Edible portion —									
Average	2	——	49.4	20.7	*20.6*	15.0	——	15.0 [2]	1020
As purchased —									
Average	2	7.0	46.0	19.3	*19.1*	14.0	——	13.9	950
Herring, smoked:									
Edible portion	1	——	34.6	36.9	*36.4*	15.8	——	13.2 [3]	1355
As purchased	1	44.4	19.2	20.5	*20.2*	8.8	——	7.4	750
Lamprey, canned:									
Edible portion	1	——	63.3	16.9	——	12.2	3.6	4.0	895
As purchased	1	18.2 [4]	51.7	13.8	——	10.0	3.0	3.3	735
Mackerel, salt, entrails removed:									
Edible portion	1	——	42.2	21.1	*22.0*	22.6	——	13.2 [5]	1345
As purchased	1	22.9	32.5	16.3	*17.0*	17.4	——	10.2	1035
Mackerel, salt, canned, as purchased	1	——	68.2	19.6	*19.9*	8.7	——	3.2	730

[1] One sample contained 19.1 per cent common salt.
[2] One sample contained 12.1 per cent common salt.
[3] Contained 11.7 per cent common salt.
[4] Refuse, oil.   [5] Contained 9.2 per cent common salt.

CHEMICAL COMPOSITION OF AMERICAN FOOD MATERIALS — *Continued*

FOOD MATERIALS	NUMBER OF ANALYSES	REFUSE	WATER	PROTEIN N × 6.25	PROTEIN By Difference	FAT	TOTAL CARBOHYDRATES	ASH	FUEL VALUE PER POUND
ANIMAL FOOD—*Continued*									
FISH, PRESERVED AND CANNED—*Continued*									
Mackerel, salt, canned in oil:		Per Cent	Per Cent	Per Cent	Per Cent	Per Cent	Per Cent	Per Cent	Calories
Edible portion . . .	1	——	58.3	25.4	*23.5*	14.1	——	4.1	1065
As purchased . . .	1	31.5 [1]	39.9	17.4	*16.1*	9.7	——	2.8	735
Mackerel, salt, dressed:									
Edible portion —									
Average	2	——	**43.4**	**17.3**	*17.3*	**26.4**	——	**12.9** [2]	**1435**
As purchased —									
Average	2	**19.7**	**34.8**	**13.9**	*13.9*	**21.2**	——	**10.4**	**1155**
Minogy, pickled, canned:									
Edible portion . . .	1	——	56.5	22.0	*21.9*	18.6	——	3.0	1195
As purchased . . .	1	18.7 [3]	46.0	17.9	*17.8*	15.1	——	2.4	970
Pilchard in tomatoes, canned, Russia, as purchased . . .	1	——	52.7	27.9	*27.5*	15.8	——	4.0	1185
Salmon, canned:									
Edible portion —									
Average . . .	7	——	**63.5**	**21.8**	*21.8*	**12.1**	——	**2.6**	**915**
As purchased —									
Average . . .	3	**14.2**	**56.8**	**19.5**	*19.5*	**7.5**	——	**2.0**	**680**
Sardines, canned:									
Edible portion —									
Average	2	——	**52.3**	**23.0**	*22.4*	**19.7**	——	**5.6**	**1260**
As purchased . .	1	5.0 [1]	53.6	23.7	*24.0*	12.1	——	5.3	950
Sturgeon, dried, Russia:									
Edible portion . . .	1	——	50.6	31.8	*32.2*	9.6	——	7.6	995
As purchased . . .	1	12.7	44.1	27.8	*28.1*	8.4	——	6.7	870
Sturgeon, caviare, pressed Russian, as purchased	1	——	38.1	30.0	——	19.7	7.6	4.6	1530
Trout, brook:									
Edible portion . . .	1	——	68.4	22.3	*22.8*	6.1	——	3.7	670
As purchased . . .	1	3.5	66.1	21.5	*20.9*	5.9	——	3.6	650

[1] Refuse, oil.   [2] Contained 10.4 per cent common salt.

[3] Refuse, liquids.

CHEMICAL COMPOSITION OF AMERICAN FOOD MATERIALS —
Continued

| FOOD MATERIALS | NUMBER OF ANALYSES | REFUSE | WATER | PROTEIN | | FAT | TOTAL CARBOHYDRATES | ASH | FUEL VALUE PER POUND |
				N × 6.25	By Difference				
ANIMAL FOOD—*Continued*									
FISH, PRESERVED AND CANNED—*Continued*		Per Cent	Per Cent	Per Cent	Per Cent	Per Cent	Per Cent	Per Cent	Calories
Tunney, as purchased .	1	——	72.7	21.7	*21.5*	4.1	——	1.7	575
Tunney, canned in oil, Russia:									
Edible portion . . .	1	——	51.3	23.8	——	20.0	0.6	4.3	1300
As purchased . . .	1	16.7 [1]	42.7	20.3	——	16.7	——	3.6	1085
AMPHIBIA									
Frogs' legs:									
Edible portion —									
Average	2	——	83.7	**15.5**	*15.1*	**0.2**	——	**1.0**	**295**
As purchased —									
Average	**2**	32.0	56.9	**10.5**	*10.3*	**0.1**	——	**0.7**	**200**
SHELLFISH, ETC., FRESH [2]									
Clams, long, in shell:									
Edible portion —									
Average	4	——	85.8	8.6	——	**1.0**	2.0	2.6	240

[1] Refuse, oil.

[2] A considerable number of determinations of phosphorus and sulfur have been made in the flesh of shellfish. These are recorded in the following table in terms of phosphoric anhydrid (P_2O_5) and sulfuric anhydrid (SO_3) and in percentages of the total weight of "edible portion" or flesh:

PHOSPHORIC ANHYDRID AND SULFURIC ANHYDRID IN SAMPLES OF SHELLFISH

| KIND OF FISH | PHOSPHORIC ANHYDRID | | SULFURIC ANHYDRID | |
	Number of Determinations	Average	Number of Determinations	Average
		Per Cent		Per Cent
Clams, long	2	0.48	2	0.56
Clams, round	1	0.40	1	0.89
Crayfish	1	0.53	1	0.26
Lobster	3	0.38	3	0.42
Oysters .	14	0.30	14	0.68
Scallops	2	0.48	2	0.49
Lobster, canned . . .	1	0.23	1	0.48
Oysters, canned . . .	1	0.35	1	0.20

CHEMICAL COMPOSITION OF AMERICAN FOOD MATERIALS —
Continued

FOOD MATERIALS	NUMBER OF ANALYSES	REFUSE	WATER	PROTEIN N × 6.25	PROTEIN By Difference	FAT	TOTAL CARBOHYDRATES	ASH	FUEL VALUE PER POUND
ANIMAL FOOD—*Continued*									
SHELLFISH, ETC., FRESH—*Continued*									
Clams, long, in shell — *Continued*		Per Cent	Per Cent	Per Cent	Per Cent	Per Cent	Per Cent	Per Cent	Cal-ories
As purchased —									
Average	4	41.9	49.9	5.0	——	0.6	1.1	1.5	140
Clams, round, in shell:									
Edible portion . . .	1	——	86.2	6.5	——	0.4	4.2	2.7	215
As purchased . . .	1	67.5	28.0	2.1	——	0.1	1.4	0.9	70
Clams, round, removed from shell, as purchased	1	——	80.8	10.6	——	1.1	5.2	2.3	340
Crabs, hardshell, whole:									
Edible portion . . .	1	——	77.1	16.6	——	2.0	1.2	3.1	415
As purchased . . .	1	52.4	36.7	7.9	——	0.9	0.6	1.5	195
Crayfish, abdomen, whole									
Edible portion . .	1	——	81.2	16.0	——	0.5	1.0	1.3	340
As purchased . . .	1	86.6 [1]	10.9	2.1	——	0.1	0.1	0.2	45
Lobster, whole:									
Edible portion —									
Average	5	——	79.2	16.4	——	1.8	0.4	2.2	390
As purchased —									
Average . .	5	61.7	30.7	5.9	——	0.7	0.2	0.8	140
Mussels, in shell:									
Edible portion . . .	1	——	84.2	8.7	——	1.1	4.1	1.9	285
As purchased . . .	1	46.7	44.9	4.6	——	0.6	2.2	1.0	150
Oysters in shell:									
Edible portion —									
Average	34	——	86.9	6.2	——	1.2	3.7	2.0	235
As purchased —									
Average	34	81.4	16.1	1.2	——	0.2	0.7	0.4	45
Oysters, solids, as purchased:									
Average	9	——	88.3	6.0	——	1.3	3.3	1.1	230
Scallops, as purchased:									
Average	2	——	80.3	14.8	——	0.1	3.4	1.4	345

[1] Refuse of whole.

CHEMICAL COMPOSITION OF AMERICAN FOOD MATERIALS — *Continued*

FOOD MATERIALS	NUMBER OF ANALYSES	REFUSE	WATER	PROTEIN N × 6.25	PROTEIN By Difference	FAT	TOTAL CARBO-HYDRATES	ASH	FUEL VALUE PER POUND
ANIMAL FOOD—*Continued*									
SHELLFISH, ETC., FRESH—*Continued*		Per Cent	Per Cent	Per Cent	Per Cent	Per Cent	Per Cent	Per Cent	Cal-ories
Terrapin:									
Edible portion . . .	1	—	74.5	21.2	*21.0*	3.5	—	1.0	545
As purchased . . .	1	75.4	18.3	5.2	*5.2*	0.9	—	0.2	135
Turtle, green, whole:									
Edible portion . . .	1	—	79.8	19.8	*18.5*	0.5	—	1.2	390
As purchased . . .	1	76.0	19.2	4.7	*4.4*	0.1	—	0.3	90
SHELLFISH, ETC., CANNED									
Clams, long, as purchased	1	—	84.5	9.0	—	1.3	2.9	2.3	275
Clams, round, as purchased	1	—	82.9	10.5	—	0.8	3.0	2.8	285
Crabs, as purchased:									
Average	2	—	80.0	15.8	—	1.5	0.7	2.0	370
Lobster, as purchased:									
Average	2	—	77.8	18.1	—	1.1	0.5	2.5	390
Oysters, as purchased:									
Average	4	—	83.4	8.8	—	2.4	3.9	1.5	335
Shrimp, as purchased .	1	—	70.8	25.4	—	1.0	0.2	2.6	520
EGGS									
Hens, uncooked: [1]									
Edible portion —									
Average	60	—	73.7	13.4	*14.8*	10.5	—	1.0	720
As purchased . . .	—	11.2 [2]	65.5	11.9	*13.1*	9.3	—	0.9	635
Hens', boiled:									
Edible portion —									
Average	19	—	73.2	13.2	*14.0*	12.0	—	0.8	765
As purchased . . .	—	11.2 [2]	65.0	11.7	*12.4*	10.7	—	0.7	680

[1] Eggs are difficult of analysis, and the discrepancy between the protein by factor and by difference may be due in part to incomplete determination of nitrogen and fat. It is also probable that the factor 6.25 is not correct for eggs. The value of protein by difference is perhaps the more nearly correct and has been used in the computation of the fuel value per pound.

[2] Average percentage refuse (shell) in 34 samples.

CHEMICAL COMPOSITION OF AMERICAN FOOD MATERIALS — *Continued*

FOOD MATERIALS	NUMBER OF ANALYSES	REFUSE	WATER	PROTEIN' N × 6.25	PROTEIN' By Difference	FAT	TOTAL CARBO-HYDRATES	ASH	FUEL VALUE PER POUND
ANIMAL FOOD—*Continued*									
EGGS — *Continued*									
Hens', boiled whites:		Per Cent	Per Cent	Per Cent	Per Cent	Per Cent	Per Cent	Per Cent	Cal-ories
Edible portion [1] —									
Average	11	—	86.2	12.3	*13.0*	0.2	—	0.6	250
Hens', boiled yolks:									
Edible portion [2] —									
Average	11	—	49.5	15.7	*16.1*	33.3	—	1.1	1705
DAIRY PRODUCTS, ETC.									
Butter, as purchased [3] .	—	—	11.0	1.0	—	85.0	—	3.0	3605
Buttermilk, as purchased	—	—	91.0	3.0	—	0.5	4.8	0.7	165
Cheese, American, pale, as purchased [4] .	1	—	31.6	28.8	—	35.9	0.3 [5]	3.4	2055
Cheese, American, red, as purchased [6] .	1	—	28.6	—	*29.6*	38.3	—	3.5	2165
Cheese, Boudon, as pur-chased [7] . . .	1	—	55.2	15.4	—	20.8	1.6 [8]	7.0	1195
Cheese, California flat, as purchased . .	4	—	34.0	24.3	—	33.4	4.5	3.8	1945
Cheese, Cheddar. as pur-chased [9] . . .	6	—	27.4	27.7	—	36.8	4.1	4.0	2145
Cheese, Cheshire, as pur-chased [10] . . .	1	—	37.1	26.9	—	30.7	0.9 [5]	4.4	1810
Cheese, cottage, as pur-chased:									
Average	2	—	72.0	20.9	—	1.0	4.3	1.8	510

[1] The ash of the whites of 73 eggs contained 3.3 per cent phosphoric anhydrid.
[2] The ash of the yolks of 73 eggs contained 57.2 per cent phosphoric anhydrid.
[3] The averages given for butter, buttermilk, cream, skimmed milk, and whole milk are assumed from the most reliable data available, but are not averages of all analyses.   [4] Contained 0.82 per cent common salt.
[5] Lactic acid.   [6] Contained 0.72 per cent common salt.
[7] Contained 3.16 per cent common salt.
[8] Milk sugar 0.7 per cent; lactic acid 0.9 per cent.
[9] One sample contained 0.45 per cent lactic acid and 1.43 per cent common salt.
[10] Contained 1.69 per cent common salt.

2 D

CHEMICAL COMPOSITION OF AMERICAN FOOD MATERIALS — *Continued*

FOOD MATERIALS	NUMBER OF ANALYSES	REFUSE	WATER	PROTEIN N × 6.25	PROTEIN By Difference	FAT	TOTAL CARBOHYDRATES	ASH	FUEL VALUE PER POUND
ANIMAL FOOD—*Continued* DAIRY PRODUCTS — *Continued*									
Cheese, Crown brand cream, as purchased [1] . . .	1	Per Cent —	Per Cent 31.4	Per Cent 5.2	Per Cent —	Per Cent 58.0	Per Cent 2.2	Per Cent 3.2	Calories 2585
Cheese, Dutch, as purchased: Average	2	—	35.2	.	37.1	17.7	—	10.0	1435
Cheese, Fromage de Brie, as purchased [2] .	1	—	60.2	15.9	—	21.0	1.4	1.5	1210
Cheese, full cream, as purchased: [3] Average . . .	25	—	34.2	25.9	—	33.7	2.4	3.8	1950
Cheese, imitation full cream, Ohio, as purchased . . .	1	—	37.9	—	25.9	31.7	—	4.5	1820
Cheese, imitation old English, as purchased [4] . . .	1	—	20.7	30.1	—	42.7	1.3	5.2	2385
Cheese, Limburger, as purchased [5] . .	1	—	42.1	23.0	—	29.4	0.4	5.1	1675
Cheese, Neuchatel, as purchased: [6] Average	2	—	50.0	18.7	.	27.4	1.5	2.4	1530

[1] Contained 2.72 per cent common salt.
[2] Contained 0.40 per cent common salt.
[3] Four cheeses were analyzed when 1, 3, and 5 weeks old. The average composition is as follows: When 7 days old, water 35.4, protein 21.6, fat 35.8, carbohydrates 3.9, and ash 3.3 per cent; when 21 days old, water 34.7, protein 22.7, fat 36.6, carbohydrates 2.1, and ash 3.9 per cent; when 35 days old, water 34.9, protein 23.3, fat 36.7, carbohydrates 0.7, and ash 4.4 per cent. The average of 20 analyses in which protein and carbohydrates were determined by difference gives: Water 28.3, protein and carbohydrates 38, fat 32.7, and ash 4 per cent. The average of 78 analyses in which the carbohydrates and ash were determined by difference gives: Water 24.9, protein 38, fat 32.7, carbohydrates and ash 4.4 per cent. The average of 148 analyses of green cheese in which the carbohydrates and ash were determined by difference gives: Water 33, protein 28.6, fat 33.7, carbohydrates and ash 4.7 per cent.
[4] Contained 1.47 per cent common salt.
[5] Contained 3.51 per cent common salt.
[6] The average of 10 analyses in which protein and sugar were not determined

CHEMICAL COMPOSITION OF AMERICAN FOOD MATERIALS — *Continued*

FOOD MATERIALS	NUMBER OF ANALYSES	REFUSE	WATER	N × 6.25	By Difference	FAT	TOTAL CARBO-HYDRATES	ASH	FUEL VALUE PER POUND
				PROTEIN					
ANIMAL FOOD—*Continued*									
DAIRY PRODUCTS, ETC.— *Continued*									
Cheese, partly skimmed milk, as purchased : [1]		Per Cent	Per Cent	Per Cent	Per Cent	Per Cent	Per Cent	Per Cent	Calories
Average	3	——	38.2	25.4	——	29.5	3.6	3.3	1785
Cheese, pineapple, as purchased : [2]									
Average	5	——	23.0	29.9	——	38.9	2.6	5.6	2245
Cheese, Roquefort, as purchased [3] . .	1	——	39.3	22.6	——	29.5	1.8	6.8	1700
Cheese, skimmed milk, as purchased : [4]									
Average	9	——	45.7	31.5	——	16.4	2.2	4.2	1320
Cheese, Swiss, as purchased : [5]									
Average	2	——	31.4	27.6	——	34.9	1.3	4.8	2010
Cheese, whole milk. (*See* Full cream cheese.)									
Cream, as purchased [6] .	—	——	74.0	2.5	——	18.5	4.5	0.5	910
Koumiss, as purchased : [7]									
Average	8	——	89.3	2.8	——	2.1	5.4	0.4	240

gives: Water 53.6, protein and sugar (by difference) 18.9, fat 27.7, lactic acid 1.2, and ash 2.6 per cent (including 1.4 per cent common salt).

[1] Three cheeses were analyzed when 1, 3, and 5 weeks old. The average composition is as follows: When 1 week old, water 38.4, protein 25, fat 30, carbohydrates 3.3, and ash 3.3 per cent; when 3 weeks old, water 38.4, protein 25.3, fat 29, carbohydrates 4, and ash 3.3 per cent; when 5 weeks old, water 37.7, protein 26, fat 29.7, carbohydrates 3.2, and ash 3.4 per cent.

[2] Four samples contained an average of 2.13 per cent common salt.

[3] Contained 5.3 per cent common salt.

[4] Two samples contained an average of 1.5 per cent common salt.

[5] Contained 1.9 per cent common salt.

[6] The averages given for butter, buttermilk, cream, skim milk, and whole milk are assumed from the most reliable data available, but are not averages of all analyses.

[7] Contained, on the average, 4.4 per cent cane sugar and 0.76 per cent alcohol Ash not reported, but assumed from European analyses.

CHEMICAL COMPOSITION OF AMERICAN FOOD MATERIALS —
Continued

FOOD MATERIALS	NUMBER OF ANALYSES	REFUSE	WATER	PROTEIN N × 6.25	PROTEIN By Difference	FAT	TOTAL CARBO-HYDRATES	ASH	FUEL VALUE PER POUND
ANIMAL FOOD—*Continued*									
DAIRY PRODUCTS, ETC.—*Continued*									
Milk, condensed, sweetened, as purchased:[1]		Per Cent	Per Cent	Per Cent	Per Cent	Per Cent	Per Cent	Per Cent	Calories
Average	24	—	26.9	8.8	—	8.3	54.1	1.9	1520
Milk, condensed, unsweetened, "evaporated cream," as purchased:									
Average . . .	6	—	68.2	9.6	—	9.3	11.2	1.7	780
Milk, skimmed, as purchased [2]	—	—	90.5	3.4	—	0.3	5.1	0.7	170
Milk, whole, as purchased[2]	—	—	87.0	3.3	—	4.0	5.0	0.7 [3]	325
Whey, as purchased .	—	—	93.0	1.0	—	0.3	5.0	0.7	125
MISCELLANEOUS									
Gelatin, as purchased:									
Average	6	—	13.6	91.4	*84.2*	0.1	—	2.1	1705
Calf's-foot jelly, as purchased . . .	1	—	77.6	4.3	—	—	17.4	0.7	405
Isinglass, sturgeon, as purchased . . .	1	—	19.0	89.3	*77.4*	1.6	—	2.0	1730
Spinal column, sturgeon, as purchased . .	1	—	17.7	59.8	—	17.1	0.8	4.6	1850
Lard, refined, as purchased . . .	1	—	—	—	—	100.0	—	—	4220
Lard, unrefined, as purchased:									
Average	3	—	4.8	2.2	*1.1*	94.0	—	0.1	4010
Tallow, refined, as purchased . . .	1	—	—	—	—	100.0	—	—	4220
Cottolene, as purchased .	1	—	—	—	—	100.0	—	—	4220
Oleomargarine, as purchased . . .	41	—	9.5	1.2	—	83.0	—	6.3	3525
Beef juice, as purchased	1	—	93.0	4.9	—	0.6	—	1.5	115

[1] Sixteen samples contained, on the average, 43.6 per cent cane sugar.

[2] The averages given for butter, buttermilk, cream, skim milk, and whole milk are assumed from the most reliable data available, but are not averages of all analyses.

[3] According to Farrington and Woll the ash of cow's milk contains, on the average, K_2O 25.6, Na_2O 12.5, CaO 24.6, P_2O_5 21.2, and Cl 16.3 per cent.

CHEMICAL COMPOSITION OF AMERICAN FOOD MATERIALS —
Continued

FOOD MATERIALS	NUMBER OF ANALYSES	REFUSE	WATER	PROTEIN	FAT	TOTAL CARBOHY-DRATES (Including Fiber)	FIBER (Number of Determinations in Parentheses)	ASH	FUEL VALUE PER POUND
VEGETABLE FOOD FLOURS, MEALS, ETC.		Per Cent	Per Cent	Per Cent	Per Cent	Per Cent	Per Cent	Per Cent	Cal-ories
Barley, granulated . .	1	—	10.9	7.5	0.9	79.8	*0.7*	0.9	1660
Barley meal and flour:									
Average	3	—	11.9	10.5	2.2	72.8	(3)*6.5*	2.6	1640
Barley, pearled:									
Average	3	—	11.5	8.5	1.1	77.8	(1)*0.3*	1.1	1650
Buckwheat flour:									
Average	17	—	13.6	6.4	1.2	77.9	(8)*0.4*	0.9	1620
Buckwheat preparations:									
Farina and groats —									
Average	2	—	10.9	4.1	0.4	84.1	*0.2*	0.5	1660
Seif-raising —									
Average	14	—	11.6	8.2	1.2	73.4	(1)*0.4*	5.6	1570
Corn flour: [1]									
Average	3	—	12.6	7.1	1.3	78.4	*0.9*	0.6	1645
Corn meal, granular: [2]									
Average	19	—	12.5	9.2	1.9	75.4	(1)*1.0*	1.0	1655
Corn meal, unbolted:									
Edible portion —									
Average . . .	7	—	11.6	8.4	4.7	74.0	—	1.3	1730
As purchased —									
Average	7	10.9	10.3	7.5	4.2	65.9	—	1.2	1545
Pop corn:									
Average	2	—	4.3	10.7	5.0	78.7	*1.4*	1.3	1875
Corn preparations:									
Cerealine [3] —									
Average	5	—	10.3	9.6	1.1	78.3	(4)*0.4*	0.7	1680
Hominy —									
Average . . .	17	—	11.8	8.3	0.6	79.0	(12)*0.9*	0.3	1650
Hominy, cooked . .	1	—	79.3	2.2	0.2	17.8	—	0.5	380
Parched —									
Average	2	—	5.2	11.5	8.4	72.3	—	2.6	1915

[1] Average of 77 analyses of corn meal used for fodder gives water 15, protein 8.2, fat 3.8, carbohydrates 68.7, fiber 1.9, and ash 1.4 per cent; and fuel value 1610 calories.

[2] The ash of 1 sample contained 0.185 per cent phosphorus.

[3] The ash of 1 sample contained 0.192 per cent phosphorus.

CHEMICAL COMPOSITION OF AMERICAN FOOD MATERIALS — *Continued*

FOOD MATERIALS	NUMBER OF ANALYSES	REFUSE	WATER	PROTEIN	FAT	TOTAL CARBOHYDRATES (including Fiber)	FIBER (Number of Determinations in Parentheses)	ASH	FUEL VALUE PER POUND
VEGETABLE FOOD—*Continued*									
FLOURS, MEALS, ETC.—*Continued*		Per Cent	Per Cent	Per Cent	Per Cent	Per Cent	Per Cent	Per Cent	Calories
Kafir corn	1	——	16.8	6.6	3.8	70.6	*1.1*	2.2	1595
Oatmeal: [1]									
Average	16	——	7.3	16.1	7.2	67.5	([9])*0.9*	1.9	1860
Oatmeal, boiled . . .	1	——	84.5	2.8	0.5	11.5	——	0.7	285
Oatmeal gruel:									
Average	2	——	91.6	1.2	0.4	6.3	——	0.5	155
Oatmeal water:									
Average	2	——	96.0	0.7	0.1	2.9	——	0.3	70
Oats, other preparations:[2]									
Rolled oats —									
Average . .	20	——	7.7	16.7	7.3	66.2	([2])*1.3*	2.1	1850
Miscellaneous —									
Average	26	——	7.9	16.3	7.3	66.8	([20])*0.9*	1.7	1855
All analyses, average[3]	46	——	7.8	16.5	7.3	66.5	([22])*1.0*	1.9	1850
Rice:									
Average	21	——	12.3	8.0	0.3	79.0	([13])*0.2*	0.4	1630
Rice, boiled:									
Average	3	——	72.5	2.8	0.1	24.4	——	0.2	510
Rice, flaked:									
Average	2	——	9.5	7.9	0.4	81.9	*0.2*	0.3	1685
Rice flour: [4]									
Average	4	——	8.5	8.6	6.1	68.0	*16.1*	8.8	1680
Rye flour:									
Average	8	——	12.9	6.8	0.9	78.7	([4])*0.4*	0.7	1630
Rye meal	1	——	11.4	13.6	2.0	71.5	*1.8*	1.5	1665

[1] The ash of 1 sample contained 0.414 per cent phosphorus.

[2] The preparations analyzed include a considerable number of brands, each of which varies in composition only slightly from the average.

[3] The ash of 5 samples contained an average of 0.418 per cent phosphorus.

[4] Rice flour is used mainly as a fodder, and varies considerably in composition. The ash of 2 samples contained an average of P_2O_5 29.1, K_2O 12.6, CaO 1, MgO 7.6, and SO_3 0.3 per cent. Two samples contained an average of protein (N×6.25) 11.8, and proteids 11.6 per cent.

CHEMICAL COMPOSITION OF AMERICAN FOOD MATERIALS —
Continued

FOOD MATERIALS	NUMBER OF ANALYSES	REFUSE	WATER	PROTEIN	FAT	TOTAL CARBOHYDRATES (including Fiber)	FIBER (Number of Determinations in Parentheses)	ASH	FUEL VALUE PER POUND
VEGETABLE FOOD— *Continued*									
FLOURS, MEALS, ETC.— *Continued*									
Wheat flour, California fine : [1]		Per Cent	Per Cent	Per Cent	Per Cent	Per Cent	Per Cent	Per Cent	Calories
Average	3	—	13.8	7.9	1.4	76.4	—	0.5	1625
Wheat flour, entire wheat :									
Average	9	—	11.4	13.8	1.9	71.9	(3)*0.9*	1.0	1675
Wheat flour, gluten :									
Average	5	—	12.0	14.2	1.8	71.1	(1)*0.6*	0.9	1665
Wheat flour, Graham :									
Average	13	—	11.3	13.3	2.2	71.4	(3)*1.9*	1.8	1670
Wheat flour, prepared (self-raising) : [2]									
Average	29	—	10.8	10.2	1.2	73.0	(3)*0.4*	4.8	1600
Wheat flour, patent roller process, bakers' grade :									
Average . . .	14	—	11.9	13.3	1.5	72.7	(6)*0.7*	0.6	1665
Wheat flour, patent roller process, family and straight grade :									
Spring wheat —									
Average	3	—	11.9	10.9	1.1	75.6	(1)*0.1*	0.5	1655
Winter wheat [3] —									
Average	6	—	13.1	12.3	1.1	73.0	(4)*0.3*	0.5	1635
Undesignated —									
Average	19	—	12.9	10.4	1.0	75.2	(1)*0.1*	0.5	1635
All analyses, average .	28	—	12.8	10.8	1.1	74.8	(6)*0.2*	0.5	1640

[1] The ash of 3 complete samples contained an average of 49.3 per cent P_2O_5.

[2] The flours analyzed included 18 varieties or brands. The variation between different samples of the same brand is as wide as that between the averages of the different brands. The widest variation is in the ash, which of course depends upon the mineral matters added for raising.

[3] The ash of 1 sample contained K_2O 36.3. CaO 5.7, MgO 6.4, and P_2O_5 49.3 per cent. In 1 sample protein (N × 6.25) 11.4 and proteids 10.8 per cent.

CHEMICAL COMPOSITION OF AMERICAN FOOD MATERIALS — *Continued*

FOOD MATERIALS	NUMBER OF ANALYSES	REFUSE	WATER	PROTEIN	FAT	TOTAL CARBOHYDRATES (including Fiber)	FIBER (Number of Determinations in Parentheses)	ASH	FUEL VALUE PER POUND
VEGETABLE FOOD— *Continued* **FLOURS, MEALS, ETC.** *Continued*									
Wheat flour, patent roller process, grade not indicated:		Per Cent	Per Cent	Per Cent	Per Cent	Per Cent	Per Cent	Per Cent	Calories
Average	111	——	11.5	11.4	1.0	75.6	(15)0.2	0.5	1660
Wheat flour, patent roller process, high grade Spring wheat —									
Average	23	——	12.3	11.7	1.1	74.5	(7)0.1	0.4	1650
Winter wheat [1] —									
Average	6	——	13.3	11.0	0.9	74.4	0.3	0.4	1625
Undesignated —									
Average	28	——	12.5	10.8	1.0	75.2	(1)0.1	0.5	1640
All analyses, average .	57	——	12.4	11.2	1.0	74.9	(14)0.2	0.5	1645
Average of all analyses of high and medium grades and grade not indicated . . .	210	——	12.0	11.4	1.0	75.1	(41)0.3	0.5	1650
Wheat flour, patent roller process, low grade[2]									
Average	13	——	12.0	14.0	1.9	71.2	(7)0.8	0.9	1665
Wheat flour, unclassified process, grade not indicated: Spring wheat [3] —									
Average	4	——	12.4	10.5	1.0	75.4	(3)0.5	0.7	1640

[1] The ash of 1 sample contained K₂O 38.5, CaO 5.6, MO 4.4, P₂O₅ 48.1, and SO₃ 0.2 per cent.   In 1 sample protein (N + 6.25) 10.6 and proteids 10.3 per cent.

[2] The ash of 1 sample contained K₂O 32.3, CaO 4.5, MgO 9.3, and P₂O₅ 53.1 per cent.   In 1 sample protein (N × 6.25) 14.1 and proteids 13.8 per cent.

[3] Three samples contained an average of starch 70.8, dextrin 1.5, and sugar, etc., 1.8 per cent.

CHEMICAL COMPOSITION OF AMERICAN FOOD MATERIALS —
Continued

FOOD MATERIALS	NUMBER OF ANALYSES	REFUSE	WATER	PROTEIN	FAT	TOTAL CARBOHY-DRATES (including Fiber)	FIBER (Number of Determinations in Parentheses)	ASH	FUEL VALUE PER POUND
VEGETABLE FOOD— *Continued*									
FLOURS, MEALS, ETC. — *Continued*									
Wheat flour, unclassified process, grade not indicated: — *Continued*		Per Cent	Per Cent	Per Cent	Per Cent	Per Cent	Per Cent	Per Cent	Calories
Winter wheat [1] —									
Average	21	——	11.9	10.7	1.0	75.8	([5])*0.4*	0.6	1650
Undesignated [2] —									
Average	8	——	9.4	10.4	1.2	78.4	([3])*0.9*	0.6	1700
All analyses, average .	33	——	11.4	10.6	1.1	76.3	([10])*0.2*	0.6	1665
Wheat preparations, breakfast foods: [3]									
Cracked and crushed[4]—									
Average	11	——	10.1	11.1	1.7	75.5	([7])*1.7*	1.6	1685
Farina [5] —									
Average	9	——	10.9	11.0	1.4	76.3	([7])*0.4*	0.4	1685
Flaked [6] —									
Average	7	——	8.7	13.4	1.4	74.3	*1.8*	2.2	1690
Germs [6] —									
Average	10	——	10.4	10.5	2.0	76.0	([8])*0.9*	1.1	1695
Glutens [7] —									
Average	3	——	8.9	13.6	1.7	74.6	*1.3*	1.2	1715

[1] Four samples contained an average of starch 71.9, dextrin 2.3, and sugar, etc., 1.6 per cent.

[2] Three samples contained an average of starch 71.8, dextrin 2, and sugar, etc., 1.7 per cent.

[3] The different groups of wheat breakfast foods contain various brands, which have been arranged as far as possible according to similarity in method of preparation. The varieties under each group differ only slightly from the average in percentage composition.

[4] The ash of 2 samples contained an average of 0.282 per cent of phosphorus.

[5] The ash of 1 sample contained 0.153 per cent of phosphorus.

[6] The ash of 2 samples contained an average of 0.247 per cent of phosphorus.

[7] The ash of 1 sample contained 0.251 per cent of phosphorus.

CHEMICAL COMPOSITION OF AMERICAN FOOD MATERIALS —
Continued

Food Materials	Number of Analyses	Refuse	Water	Protein	Fat	Total Carbohydrates (including Fiber)	Fiber (Number of Determinations in Parentheses)	Ash	Fuel Value per Pound
VEGETABLE FOOD— *Continued*									
FLOURS, MEALS, ETC.— *Continued*									
Wheat preparations, breakfast foods [1] —*Continued*		Per Cent	Per Cent	Per Cent	Per Cent	Per Cent	Per Cent	Per Cent	Cal-ories
Miscellaneous [2] — Average	22	——	9.4	13.1	2.1	74.1	(16)*0.9*	1.3	1710
Parched and toasted [3]— Average	6	——	8.6	13.6	2.4	74.5	*0.8*	0.9	1740
Shredded — Average	6	——	8.1	10.5	1.4	77.9	(3)*1.7*	2.1	1700
All analyses, average .	74	——	9.6	12.1	1.8	75.2	*1.0*	1.3	1700
Wheat preparations: Macaroni — Average	11	——	10.3	13.4	0.9	74.1	——	1.3	1665
Macaroni, cooked . .	1	——	78.4	3.0	1.5	15.8	——	1.3	415
Noodles — Average	2	——	10.7	11.7	1.0	75.6	*0.4*	1.0	1665
Spaghetti — Average	3	——	10.6	12.1	0.4	76.3	(2)*0.4*	0.6	1660
Vermicelli — Average	15	——	11.0	10.9	2.0	72.0	——	4.1	1625
BREAD, CRACKERS, PASTRY, ETC.									
Bread, brown, as purchased — Average	2	——	43.6	5.4	1.8	47.1	——	2.1	1050

[1] The different groups of wheat breakfast foods contain various brands, which have been arranged as far as possible according to similarity in method of preparation. The varieties under each group differ only slightly from the average in percentage composition.

[2] The ash of 4 samples contained an average of 0.35 per cent of phosphorus.

[3] The ash of 1 sample contained 0.288 per cent of phosphorus.

CHEMICAL COMPOSITION OF AMERICAN FOOD MATERIALS — *Continued*

FOOD MATERIALS	NUMBER OF ANALYSES	REFUSE	WATER	PROTEIN	FAT	TOTAL CARBOHYDRATES (including Fiber)	FIBER (Number of Determinations in Parentheses)	ASH	FUEL VALUE PER POUND
VEGETABLE FOOD— *Continued*									
BREAD, CRACKERS, PASTRY, ETC.—*Continued*			Per Cent	Per Cent	Per Cent	Per Cent	Per Cent	Per Cent	Per Cent	Calories
Bread, cassava, as purchased	1	—	10.5	9.1	0.3	79.0	—	1.1	1650
Bread, corn (johnnycake) as purchased : [1]									
Average	5	—	38.9	7.9	4.7	46.3	—	2.2	1205
Bread, rye, as purchased :									
Average	21	—	35.7	9.0	0.6	53.2	(9)0.5	1.5	1180
Bread, rye, black, as purchased	1	—	36.9	9.6	0.6	48.9	—	4.0	1115
Bread, rye, whole, as purchased —									
Average	2	—	50.7	11.9	0.6	35.9	1.2	0.9	915
Bread, rye and wheat, as purchased . . .	1	—	35.3	11.9	0.3	51.5	—	1.0	1190
Bread, wheat :									
Buns, as purchased .	1	—	29.0	6.3	6.5	57.3	0.4	0.9	1455
Buns, cinnamon, as purchased . . .	1	—	23.6	9.4	7.2	59.1	—	0.7	1575
Buns, currant, as purchased	1	—	27.5	6.7	7.6	57.6	1.1	0.6	1515
Buns, hot cross, as purchased	1	—	36.7	7.9	4.8	49.7	—	0.9	1275
Buns, sugar, as purchased [2] —									
Average	3	—	29.6	8.1	6.9	54.2	(1)0.3	1.2	1450
Gluten bread, as purchased —									
Average . . .	6	—	38.2	9.3	1.4	49.8	—	1.3	1160

[1] Corn bread (johnnycake), made of Indian meal mixed with sour milk or buttermilk.

[2] One sample contained sugar 7.9, dextrin 3.2, and starch 47 per cent.

CHEMICAL COMPOSITION OF AMERICAN FOOD MATERIALS —
Continued

Food Materials	Number of Analyses	Refuse	Water	Protein	Fat	Total Carbohydrates (including Fiber)	Fiber (Number of Determinations in Parentheses)	Ash	Fuel Value per Pound
VEGETABLE FOOD— *Continued*									
BREAD, CRACKERS, PASTRY, ETC.—*Continued*									
Bread, wheat—*Continued* Graham bread, as purchased [1] —		Per Cent	Per Cent	Per Cent	Per Cent	Per Cent	Per Cent	Per Cent	Calories
Average	27	——	35.7	8.9	1.8	52.1	(11)1.1	1.5	1210
Biscuit, homemade, as purchased [2] —									
Average	3	——	32.9	8.7	2.6	55.3	(2)0.7	0.5	1300
Biscuit, Maryland, as purchased [3] —									
Average	2	——	24.6	8.4	5.6	60.1	1.3	1.3	1510
Biscuit, soda, as purchased . . .	1	——	22.9	9.3	13.7	52.6	——	1.5	1730
Rolls, French, as purchased [4]									
Average . . .	2	——	32.0	8.5	2.5	55.7	0.6	1.3	1300
Rolls, plain as purchased —									
Average	5	——	25.2	9.7	4.2	59.9	(2)0.3	1.0	1470
Rolls, Vienna, as purchased . . .	1	——	31.7	8.5	2.2	56.5	0.4	1.1	1300
Rolls, water, as purchased —									
Average	2	——	32.6	9.0	3.0	54.2	——	1.2	1300
Rolls, all analyses, as purchased . . .	20	——	29.2	8.9	4.1	56.7	(12)0.6	1.1	1395
Rolls, large, cheap, as purchased . . .	1	——	29.4	9.4	0.8	59.4	——	1.0	1315

[1] Two samples contained an average of sugar 3.2, dextrin 3.1, and starch 40.8 per cent.

[2] Two samples contained an average of sugar 2.7, dextrin 5.5, and starch 41.5 per cent.

[3] One sample contained sugar 3.9, dextrin 2.8, and starch 52.2 per cent.

[4] One sample contained sugar 2.9, dextrin 2.8, and starch 48.6 per cent.

CHEMICAL COMPOSITION OF AMERICAN FOOD MATERIALS —
Continued

FOOD MATERIALS	NUMBER OF ANALYSES	REFUSE	WATER	PROTEIN	FAT	TOTAL CARBOHY-DRATES (including Fiber)	FIBER (Number of Determinations in Parentheses)	ASH	FUEL VALUE PER POUND
VEGETABLE FOOD— *Continued*									
BREAD, CRACKERS, PASTRY, ETC.—*Continued*									
Bread, wheat—*Continued* Toasted bread, as purchased —		Per Cent	Per Cent	Per Cent	Per Cent	Per Cent	Per Cent	Per Cent	Calories
Average	5	—	24.0	11.5	1.6	61.2	—	1.7	1420
White bread, biscuit, as purchased —									
Average	3	—	35.2	8.0	1.4	54.3	(²)*0.3*	1.1	1220
White bread, butter, as purchased —	1	—	32.2	7.9	1.1	57.7	0.4	1.1	1265
White bread, cheap grade, as purchased —									
Average	6	—	33.2	10.9	1.3	53.6	—	1.0	1255
White bread, cream, as purchased —									
Average	6	—	33.2	9.8	0.9	55.0	(¹)*0.2*	1.1	1245
White bread, homemade, as purchased —									
Average	38	—	35.0	9.1	1.6	53.3	(²)*0.2*	1.0	1225
White bread, milk, as purchased —									
Average . . . ,	8	—	36.5	9.6	1.4	51.1	—	1.4	1190
White bread, miscellaneous, as purchased : ¹									
Average	103	—	35.6	9.3	1.2	52.7	(⁸)*0.5*	1.2	1205
White bread, New England, as purchased :									
Average	7	—	36.6	9.1	1.2	52.1	—	1.0	1190
White bread, Quaker, as purchased —									
Average	4	—	35.8	8.3	1.1	53.7	(³)*0.3*	1.1	1200

ᴸ Four samples contained an average of sugar 2.3, dextrin 4.2, and starch 48.2 per cent.

CHEMICAL COMPOSITION OF AMERICAN FOOD MATERIALS —
Continued

FOOD MATERIALS	NUMBER OF ANALYSES	REFUSE	WATER	PROTEIN	FAT	TOTAL CARBOHYDRATES (including Fiber)	FIBER (Number of Determinations in Parentheses)	ASH	FUEL VALUE PER POUND
VEGETABLE FOOD — *Continued* BREAD, CRACKERS, PASTRY, ETC. — *Continued* Bread, wheat—*Continued* White bread, split. as purchased —		Per Cent	Per Cent	Per Cent	Per Cent	Per Cent	Per Cent	Per Cent	Calories
Average	3	——	34.6	9.3	1.0	54.1	(¹)0.2	1.0	1220
White bread, Vienna, as purchased —									
Average	25	——	34.2	9.4	1.2	54.1	(⁹)0.5	1.1	1230
White bread, all analyses, as purchased, average [1]	198	——	35.3	9.2	1.3	53.1	(²⁷)0.5	1.1	1215
Whole wheat bread, as purchased —									
Average	12	——	38.4	9.7	0.9	49.7	(¹)1.2	1.3	1140
Zwieback, as purchased —									
Average	4	——	5.8	9.8	9.9	73.5	——	1.0	1970

[1] Analyses of similar bread made from different grades of flour, from high to low grade :

	WATER	PROTEIN	FAT	CARBOHYDRATES	FIBER	ASH	FUEL VALUE PER POUND
	Per Cent	Per Cent	Per Cent	Per Cent	Per Cent	Per Cent	Calories
White bread from high-grade patent flour	32.9	8.7	1.4	56.5	——	0.5	1270
White bread from regular patent flour	34.1	9.0	1.3	54.9	——	0.7	1245
White bread from baker's flour . .	39.1	10.6	1.2	48.3	——	0.9	1145
White bread from low-grade flour .	40.7	12.6	1.1	44.3	——	1.3	1105

CHEMICAL COMPOSITION OF AMERICAN FOOD MATERIALS —
Continued

FOOD MATERIALS	NUMBER OF ANALYSES	REFUSE	WATER	PROTEIN	FAT	TOTAL CARBOHY-DRATES (including Fiber)	FIBER (Number of Determinations in Parentheses)	ASH	FUEL VALUE PER POUND
VEGETABLE FOOD — *Continued* BREAD, CRACKERS, PASTRY, ETC.— *Continued*									
Crackers:									
Boston (split) crackers, as purchased —		Per Cent	Per Cent	Per Cent	Per Cent	Per Cent	Per Cent	Per Cent	Calories
Average	2	—	7.5	11.0,	8.5	71.1	(¹)0.8	1.9	1885
Butter crackers, as purchased :									
Average . . .	3	—	7.2	9.6	10.1	71.6	(²)0.4	1.5	1935
Cream crackers, as purchased —									
Average	9	—	6.8	9.7	12.1	69.7	(⁵)0.6	1.7	1990
Egg crackers, as purchased —									
Average	2	—	5.8	12.6	14.0	66.6	0.4	1.0	2060
Flatbread, as purchased :									
Average	3	—	9.8	14.9	0.5	73.6	—	1.2	1665
Graham crackers, as purchased —									
Average	4	—	5.4	10.0	9.4	73.8	(²)1.5	1.4	1955
Miscellaneous, as purchased —									
Average	21	—	7.1	10.2	8.8	72.4	(¹⁷)0.4	1.5	1905
Oatmeal crackers, as purchased —									
Average	2	—	6.3	11.8	11.1	69.0	(¹)1.9	1.8	1970
Oyster crackers, as purchased —									
Average	7	—	4.8	11.3	10.5	70.5	(¹)0.2	2.9	1965
Pilot bread, as purchased :									
Average . . .	3	—	8.7	11.1	5.0	74.2	(²)0.3	1.0	1800
Pretzels, as purchased :									
Average . . .	2	—	9.6	9.7	3.9	72.8	(²)0.5	4.0	1700
Saltines, as purchased :									
Average . .	2	—	5.6	10.6	12.7	68.5	0.5	2.6	2005

CHEMICAL COMPOSITION OF AMERICAN FOOD MATERIALS —
Continued

FOOD MATERIALS	NUMBER OF ANALYSES	REFUSE	WATER	PROTEIN	FAT	TOTAL CARBOHYDRATES (including Fiber)	FIBER (Number of Determinations in Parentheses)	ASH	FUEL VALUE PER POUND
VEGETABLE FOOD — *Continued* BREAD, CRACKERS, PASTRY, ETC.— *Continued*									
Crackers — *Continued* Soda crackers, as purchased —		Per Cent	Per Cent	Per Cent	Per Cent	Per Cent	Per Cent	Per Cent	Calories
Average	5	——	5.9	9.8	9.1	73.1	(¹)0.3	2.1	1925
Water crackers, as purchased —									
Average	6	——	6.4	11.7	5.0	75.7	0.4	1.2	1835
All analyses, as purchased, average .	71	——	6.8	10.7	8.8	71.9	(45)0.5	1.8	1905
Cracker meal, as purchased —									
Average	2	——	9.2	10.9	6.0	72.9	0.2	1.0	1810
Cake: Baker's cake, as purchased —									
Average	2	——	31.4	6.3	4.6	56.9	——	0.8	1370
Chocolate layer cake, as purchased .	1	——	20.5	6.2	8.1	64.1	——	1.1	1650
Coffee cake, as purchased —									
Average	5	——	21.3	7.1	7.5	63.2	(⁴)0.4	0.9	1625
Cup cake, as purchased: Average	2	——	15.6	5.9	9.0	68.5	(¹)0.3	1.0	1765
Drop cake, as purchased	1	——	16.6	7.6	14.7	60.3	0.1	0.8	1885
Frosted cake, as purchased —									
Average	7	——	18.2	5.9	9.0	64.8	——	2.1	1695
Fruit cake, as purchased —									
Average	4	——	17.3	5.9	10.9	64.1	——	1.8	1760
Gingerbread, as purchased —									
Average	2	——	18.8	5.8	9.0	63.5	(¹)0.9	2.9	1670

CHEMICAL COMPOSITION OF AMERICAN FOOD MATERIALS — *Continued*

FOOD MATERIALS	NUMBER OF ANALYSES	REFUSE	WATER	PROTEIN	FAT	TOTAL CARBOHY-DRATES (including Fiber)	FIBER (Number of Determinations in Parentheses)	ASH	FUEL VALUE PER POUND
VEGETABLE FOOD — *Continued*									
BREAD, CRACKERS, PASTRY, ETC. — *Continued*									
Cake — *Continued*									
Miscellaneous, as purchased —		Per Cent	Per Cent	Per Cent	Per Cent	Per Cent	Per Cent	Per Cent	Calories
Average	4	—	21.9	5.9	10.6	60.1	—	1.5	1675
Sponge cake, as purchased —									
Average	3	—	15.3	6.3	10.7	65.9	—	1.8	1795
All analyses, except fruit, as purchased, average .	27	—	19.9	6.3	9.0	63.3	(7)0.4	1.5	1675
Cookies, cakes, etc.:									
Molasses cookies, as purchased [1] —									
Average	6	—	6.2	7.2	8.7	75.7	—	2.2	1910
Miscellaneous cookies, as purchased —									
Average . . .	5	—	10.3	6.7	9.6	72.4	1.2	1.0	1875
Sugar cookies. as purchased [2] —									
Average	9	—	8.3	7.0	10.2	73.2	(3)1.1	1.3	1920
All analyses, as purchased, average .	20	—	8.1	7.0	9.7	73.7	0.5	1.5	1910
Fig biscuits or bars, as purchased . . .	1	—	17.9	4.6	6.6	69.8	1.7	1.1	1660
Ginger snaps, as purchased —									
Average	7	—	6.3	6.5	8.6	76.0	(5)0.7	2.6	1895
Lady fingers, as purchased —									
Average	3	—	15.0	8.8	5.0	70.6	(2)0.2	0.6	1685

[1] One sample contained sugar 32.4, dextrin 3.2, and starch 40.6 per cent.
[2] One sample contained sugar 25.2, dextrin 1.8, and starch 42.7 per cent.

2 E

CHEMICAL COMPOSITION OF AMERICAN FOOD MATERIALS — *Continued*

FOOD MATERIALS	NUMBER OF ANALYSES	REFUSE	WATER	PROTEIN	FAT	TOTAL CARBOHYDRATES (including Fiber)	FIBER (Number of Determinations in Parentheses)	ASH	FUEL VALUE PER POUND
VEGETABLE FOOD— *Continued* BREAD, CRACKERS, PASTRY, ETC. — *Continued* Cookies, cakes, etc.— *Continued* Macaroons, as purchased —		Per Cent	Per Cent	Per Cent	Per Cent	Per Cent	Per Cent	Per Cent	Calories
Average	4	——	12.3	6.5	15.2	65.2	*1.1*	0.8	1975
Wafers, miscellaneous, as purchased — Average	5	——	6.6	8.7	8.6	74.5	*0.4*	1.6	1910
Wafers, vanilla, as purchased — Average	6	——	6.7	6.6	14.0	71.6	(5)*0.3*	1.1	2045
Wafers, all analyses, as purchased, average	11	——	6.6	7.6	11.6	72.9	(10)*0.3*	1.3	1985
Miscellaneous cakes, as purchased — Average . . .	17	——	8.2	7.6	9.0	74.0	(16)*0.3*	1.2	1900
Doughnuts, as purchased Average	9	——	18.3	6.7	21.0	53.1	(2)*0.7*	0.9	2000
Jumbles, as purchased: Average	4	——	14.3	7.4	13.5	63.7	(3)*0.5*	1.1	1890
Pie, apple, as purchased: Average . . .	4	——	42.5	3.1	9.8	42.8	——	1.8	1270
Pie, cream, as purchased: Average	3	——	32.0	4.4	11.4	51.2	——	1.0	1515
Pie, custard, as purchased:	1	——	62.4	4.2	6.3	26.1	——	1.0	830
Pie, lemon, as purchased:	1	——	47.4	3.6	10.1	37.4	——	1.5	1190
Pie, mince, as purchased: Average	3	——	41.3	5.8	12.3	38.1	——	2.5	1335
Pie, raisin, as purchased:	1	——	37.0	3.0	11.3	47.2	——	1.5	1410
Pie, squash, as purchased:	1	——	64.2	4.4	8.4	21.7	——	1.3	840
Pudding, Indian meal, as purchased . .	1	——	60.7	5.5	4.8	27.5	——	1.5	815
Pudding, rice custard, as purchased . .	1	——	59.4	4.0	4.6	31.4	——	0.6	825

CHEMICAL COMPOSITION OF AMERICAN FOOD MATERIALS —
Continued

FOOD MATERIALS	NUMBER OF ANALYSES	REFUSE	WATER	PROTEIN	FAT	TOTAL CARBOHY-DRATES (including Fiber)	FIBER (Number of Determinations in Parentheses)	ASH	FUEL VALUE PER POUND
VEGETABLE FOOD— *Continued* BREAD, CRACKERS, PASTRY, ETC. — *Continued*									
Pudding, tapioca, as purchased—		Per Cent	Per Cent	Per Cent	Per Cent	Per Cent	Per Cent	Per Cent	Calories
Average	3	—	64.5	3.3	3.2	28.2	—	0.8	720
Pudding, tapioca, with apples, as purchased	1	—	70.1	0.3	0.1	29.3	—	0.2	575
SUGARS, STARCHES, ETC.									
Candy, as purchased: [1]	—	—	—	—	—	96.0	—	—	1785

[1] AVERAGE COMPOSITION OF SOME COMMON CANDIES

	NUMBER OF ANALYSES	WATER	SUCROSE	INVERT SUGAR	ASH	INSOLUBLE IN COLD WATER	REMARKS
		Per Cent	Per Cent	Per Cent	Per Cent	Per Cent	
Broken candy .	8	4.6	75.3	14.0	2.7	0.9 in one sample.	
Cream candy . .	20	5.3	77.1	8.7	0.1	0.2 in one sample.	
Marshmallows .	3	5.6	33.3	24.1	1.1	27.0	One sample contained 44.8 per cent insoluble matter (starch and flour).
Caramels . . .	3	3.3	37.5	15.2	1.4	32.2	One sample contained 66.3 per cent insoluble matter (starch and flour).
Chocolate creams	1	3.8	58.3	13.8	0.5	15.4	

CHEMICAL COMPOSITION OF AMERICAN FOOD MATERIALS — *Continued*

FOOD MATERIALS	NUMBER OF ANALYSES	REFUSE	WATER	PROTEIN	FAT	TOTAL CARBOHYDRATES (including Fiber)	FIBER (Number of Determinations in Parentheses)	ASH	FUEL VALUE PER POUND
VEGETABLE FOOD— *Continued*									
SUGARS, STARCHES, ETC.— *Continued*		Per Cent	Per Cent	Per Cent	Per Cent	Per Cent	Per Cent	Per Cent	Cal-ories
Honey, as purchased: [1]									
Average	17	——	18.2	0.4	——	81.2	——	0.2	1520
Molasses, cane, as purchased:									
Average	15	——	25.1	2.4	——	69.3	——	3.2	1290
Starch, arrowroot, as purchased	1	——	2.3	——	——	97.5	——	0.2	1815
Starch, cornstarch, as purchased	—	——	——	——	——	90.0	——	——	1675
Starch, manioca, as purchased	1	——	10.5	0.5	0.1	88.8	——	0.1	1665
Starch, sago, as purchased	1	——	12.2	9.0	0.4	78.1	——	0.3	1635
Starch, tapioca, as purchased:									
Average	7	——	11.4	0.4	0.1	88.0	(5)0.1	0.1	1650
Sugar, coffee or brown sugar, as purchased	328	——	——	——	——	95.0	——	——	1765
Sugar, granulated sugar, as purchased	—	——	——	——	——	100.0	——	——	1860
Sugar, maple, as purchased:									
Average	17	——	——	——	——	82.8	——	——	1540
Sugar, powdered, as purchased	—	——	——	——	——	100.0	——	——	1860
Syrup, maple, as purchased:									
Average	50	——	——	——	——	71.4	——	——	1330

[1] Contained an average of cane sugar 2.8 and reducing sugar 71.1 per cent. The reducing sugar was composed of about equal amounts of glucose (dextrose) and fruit sugar (levulose).

CHEMICAL COMPOSITION OF AMERICAN FOOD MATERIALS —
Continued

FOOD MATERIALS	NUMBER OF ANALYSES	REFUSE	WATER	PROTEIN	FAT	TOTAL CARBOHYDRATES (including Fiber)	FIBER (Number of Determinations in Parentheses)	ASH	FUEL VALUE PER POUND
VEGETABLE FOOD— *Continued*									
VEGETABLES [1]		Per Cent	Per Cent	Per Cent	Per Cent	Per Cent	Per Cent	Per Cent	Calories
Artichokes, as purchased :[2]									
Average	2	——	79.5	2.6	0.2	16.7	*0.8*	1.0	365
Asparagus, fresh, as purchased : [3]									
Average	3	——	94.0	1.8	0.2	3.3	*0.8*	0.7	105
Asparagus, cooked, as purchased . . .	1	——	91.6	2.1	3.3	2.2	——	0.8	220
Beans, butter, green :									
Edible portion . . .	1	——	58.9	9.4	0.6	29.1	——	2.0	740
As purchased . . .	1	50.0	29.4	4.7	0.3	14.6	——	1.0	370
Beans, dried, as purchased :									
Average	11	——	12.6	22.5	1.8	59.6	[4] *4.4*	3.5	1605
Beans, frijoles (New Mexico), as purchased :									
Average	4	——	7.5	21.9	1.3	65.1	——	4.2	1675
Beans, lima, dried, as purchased :									
Average	4	——	10.4	18.1	1.5	65.9	——	4.1	1625
Beans, lima, fresh : [4]									
Edible portion . . .	1	——	68.5	7.1	0.7	22.0	*1.7*	1.7	570
As purchased . .	—	55.0	30.8	3.2	0.3	9.9	*0.8*	0.8	255
Beans, mesquite, dry, as purchased . .	1	——	4.8	12.2	2.5	77.1	——	3.4	1765

[1] Such vegetables as potatoes, squash, beets, etc., have a certain amount of inedible material, skin, seeds, etc. The amount varies with the method of preparing the vegetables, and cannot be accurately estimated. The figures given for refuse of vegetables, fruits, etc., are assumed to represent approximately the amount of refuse in these foods as ordinarily prepared.

[2] In 1 sample, protein (N×6.25) 2.2 and proteids 1.2 per cent contained an average protein (N×6.25) 1.83 and proteids 0.94 per cent.

[3] Two samples contained an average of 0.23 per cent free acid. Three samples contained an average protein (N × 6.25) 1.83 and proteids 0.94 per cent.

[4] Contained protein (N×6.25) 7.1 and proteids 5.7 per cent.

CHEMICAL COMPOSITION OF AMERICAN FOOD MATERIALS — *Continued*

FOOD MATERIALS	NUMBER OF ANALYSES	REFUSE	WATER	PROTEIN	FAT	TOTAL CARBOHYDRATES (including Fiber)	FIBER (Number of Determinations in Parentheses)	ASH	FUEL VALUE PER POUND
VEGETABLE FOOD—*Continued*									
VEGETABLES—*Continued*		Per Cent	Per Cent	Per Cent	Per Cent	Per Cent	Per Cent	Per Cent	Calories
Beans, string, cooked, edible portion	1	——	95.3	0.8	1.1	1.9	——	0.9	95
Beans, string, fresh: [1]									
Edible portion —									
Average	5	——	89.2	2.3	0.3	7.4	[2]*1.9*	0.8	**195**
As purchased	—	7.0	83.0	2.1	0.3	6.9	*1.8*	0.7	180
Beets, cooked, edible portion	1	——	88.6	2.3	0.1	7.4	——	1.6	185
Beets, fresh: [2]									
Edible portion —									
Average	24	——	87.5	1.6	0.1	9.7	[18]*0.9*	1.1	**215**
As purchased	—	20.0	70.0	1.3	0.1	7.7	——	0.9	170
Cabbage: [3]									
Edible portion —									
Average	16	——	91.5	1.6	0.3	5.6	[8]*1.1*	1.0	**145**
As purchased	—	15.0	77.7	1.4	0.2	4.8	——	0.9	125
Cabbage, curly, as purchased	1	——	87.3	4.1	0.6	6.2	——	1.8	215
Cabbage sprouts:									
Edible portion	1	——	88.2	4.7	1.1	4.3	——	1.7	215
As purchased	1	61.8	33.7	1.8	0.4	1.7	——	0.6	80
Carrots, fresh: [4]									
Edible portion —									
Average	18	——	88.2	1.1	0.4	9.3	[15]*1.1*	1.0	**210**
As purchased	—	20.0	70.6	0.9	0.2	7.4	——	0.9	160

[1] One sample contained free acid 0.49, protein (N × 6.25)1.7, and proteids 0.87 per cent.

[2] The ash of 8 samples contained an average of CaO 6.2, K_2O 44, MgO 3.1, P_2O_5 9.4, Na_2O 10.3, and Fe_2O_3 0.3 per cent. Seven samples contained an average of protein (N×6.25) 1.6, and proteids 0.55 per cent.

[3] The ash of 2 samples contained an average of CaO 4.7, MgO 1.9, P_2O_5 5.5, Na_2O 6.3, and K_2O 61.5 per cent. Five samples contained an average of protein (N×6.25) 2.4 and proteids 1.4 per cent.

[4] The ash of 1 sample contained CaO 7.3, K_2O 53.7, MgO 2.8, P_2O_5 9.8, Na_2O 1.4,

CHEMICAL COMPOSITION OF AMERICAN FOOD MATERIALS —
Continued

FOOD MATERIALS	NUMBER OF ANALYSES	REFUSE	WATER	PROTEIN	FAT	TOTAL CARBOHYDRATES (including Fiber)	FIBER (Number of Determinations in Parentheses)	ASH	FUEL VALUE PER POUND
VEGETABLE FOOD— *Continued*		Per Cent	Per Cent	Per Cent	Per Cent	Per Cent	Per Cent	Per Cent	Calories
VEGETABLES—*Continued*									
Carrots, cooked, edible portion	1	—	3.5	7.7	3.6	80.3		4.9	1790
Cauliflower, as purchased:[1]									
Average	2	—	92.3	1.8	0.5	4.7	(1)1.0	0.7	140
Celery:									
Edible portion —									
Average	5	—	94.5	1.1	0.1	3.3		1.0	85
As purchased . . .	—	20.0	75.6	0.9	0.1	2.6		0.8	70
Collards:[2]									
Edible portion —									
Average	2	—	87.1	4.5	0.6	6.3		1.5	225
As purchased . . .	1	55.3	39.5	1.5	0.2	2.9		0.6	90
Corn, green:[3]									
Edible portion —									
Average	3	—	75.4	3.1	1.1	19.7	(1)0.5	0.7	470
As purchased . . .	—	61.0	29.4	1.2	0.4	7.7		0.3	180
Cucumbers:[4]									
Edible portion —									
Average	4	—	95.4	0.8	0.2	3.1	(2)0.7	0.5	80
As purchased . . .	—	15.0	81.1	0.7	0.2	2.6		0.4	70
Eggplant, edible portion [5]	1	—	92.9	1.2	0.3	5.1	0.8	0.5	130
Greens, beet, cooked, as purchased . . .	1	—	89.5	2.2	3.4	3.2		1.7	245

and Fe_2O_2 0.8 per cent. One sample contained protein (N × 6.25) 1 and proteids 0.5 per cent. One sample contained cane sugar 3.6 and fruit sugar 3 per cent.

[1] One sample contained free acid 0.6. protein (N × 6.25) 1.6, and proteids 1 per cent.

[2] One sample contained protein (N × 6.25) 5.7 and proteids 2.9 per cent.

[3] One sample contained free acid 0.01, protein (N × 6.25) 2.8, and proteids 2.2 per cent.

[4] One sample contained 0.02 per cent free acid. Two samples contained an average of protein (N × 6.25), 0.8, and proteids 0.4 per cent.

[5] Contained free acid 0.01, protein (N × 6.25) 1.2, and proteids 0.6 per cent,

CHEMICAL COMPOSITION OF AMERICAN FOOD MATERIALS —
Continued

Food Materials	Number of Analyses	Refuse	Water	Protein	Fat	Total Carbohydrates (including Fiber)	Fiber (Number of Determinations in Parentheses)	Ash	Fuel Value per Pound
VEGETABLE FOOD—*Continued* VEGETABLES—*Continued*		Per Cent	Per Cent	Per Cent	Per Cent	Per Cent	Per Cent	Per Cent	Calories
Greens, dandelion, as purchased . . .	1	—	81.4	2.4	1.0	10.6	—	4.6	285
Greens, turnip-salad, as purchased :									
Average	2	—	86.7	4.2	0.6	6.3	—	2.2	220
Kohl-rabi, edible portion : [1]									
Average	2	—	91.1	2.0	0.1	5.5	1.3	1.3	145
Leeks :									
Edible portion . . .	1	—	91.8	1.2	0.5	5.8	—	0.7	150
As purchased . . .	1	15.0	78.0	1.0	0.4	5.0	0.6	0.6	130
Lentils, dried, as purchased :									
Average	3	—	8.4	25.7	1.0	59.2	—	5.7	1620
Lettuce : [2]									
Edible portion —									
Average	8	—	94.7	1.2	0.3	2.9	(7)0.7	0.9	90
As purchased . . .	—	15.0	80.5	1.0	0.2	2.5	—	0.8	75
Mushrooms, as purchased : [3]									
Average	11	—	88.1	3.5	0.4	6.8	(8)0.8	1.2	210
Okra :									
Edible portion —									
Average	2	—	90.2	1.6	0.2	7.4	(1)3.4	0.6	175
As purchased . . .	—	12.5	78.9	1.4	0.2	6.5	—	0.5	155

[1] Two samples contained an average of protein (N × 6.25) 2 and proteids 0.5 per cent.

[2] The ash of 2 samples contained an average of CaO 5.1, K₂O 46.6, MgO 0.8, P₂O₅ 5.3, and Na₂O 3.3 per cent. Five samples contained an average of protein (N × 6.25)1.4 and proteins 0.8 per cent.

[3] Eight samples contained an average of 3.1 protein (N × 6.25) and 2.2 per cent proteids.

CHEMICAL COMPOSITION OF AMERICAN FOOD MATERIALS —
Continued

FOOD MATERIALS	NUMBER OF ANALYSES	REFUSE	WATER	PROTEIN	FAT	TOTAL CARBOHY-DRATES (including Fiber)	FIBER (Number of Determinations in Parentheses)	ASH	FUEL VALUE PER POUND
VEGETABLE FOOD— *Continued* VEGETABLES—*Continued*									
Onions, fresh: [1] Edible portion —			Per Cent	Per Cent	Per Cent	Per Cent	Per Cent	Per Cent	Calories
Average	15	—	87.6	1.6	0.3	9.9	(7)*0.8*	0.6	225
As purchased . . .	—	10.0	78.9	1.4	0.3	8.9	—	0.5	205
Onions, cooked, prepared as purchased . .	1	—	91.2	1.2	1.8	4.9	—	0.9	190
Onions, green, (New Mexico) : Edible portion —									
Average	2	—	87.1	1.0	0.1	11.2	—	0.6	230
As purchased . . .	—	51.0	42.6	0.5	0.1	5.5	—	0.3	115
Parsnips : [2] Edible portion —									
Average	3	—	83.0	1.6	0.5	13.5	(1)*2.5*	1.4	300
As purchased . . .	—	20.0	66.4	1.3	0.4	10.8	—	1.1	240
Peas, dried, as purchased : Average	8	—	9.5	24.6	1.0	62.0	(2)*4.5*	2.9	1655
Peas, green : [3] Edible portion —									
Average	5	—	74.6	7.0	0.5	16.9	(1)*1.7*	1.0	465
As purchased . . .	—	45.0 [4]	40.8	3.6	0.2	9.8	—	0.6	255
Peas, green, cooked, as purchased . . .	1	—	73.8	6.7	3.4	14.6	—	1.5	540
Peas, sugar, green, edible portion	1	—	81.8	3.4	0.4	13.7	*1.6*	0.7	335

[1] The ash of 1 sample contained CaO 6.4, K₂O 30.2, MgO 2.9, and P₂O₅ 12.4 per cent. Four samples contained an average of protein (N × 6.25) 1.3 and proteids 0.6 per cent.

[2] One sample contained CaO 6, K₂O 42.2, MgO 3.1, P₂O₅ 12.8, Na₂O 0.4, and Fe₂O₃ 0.3 per cent.

[3] One sample contained protein (N × 6.25) 4.4, and proteids 4.3 per cent.

[4] Refuse, pods.

CHEMICAL COMPOSITION OF AMERICAN FOOD MATERIALS —
Continued

FOOD MATERIALS	NUMBER OF ANALYSES	REFUSE	WATER	PROTEIN	FAT	TOTAL CARBOHYDRATES (including Fiber)	FIBER (Number of Determinations in Parentheses)	ASH	FUEL VALUE PER POUND
VEGETABLE FOOD — *Continued* VEGETABLES—*Continued*									
Cowpeas. dried. as purchased:		Per Cent	Per Cent	Per Cent	Per Cent	Per Cent	Per Cent	Per Cent	Calories
Average	13	——	13.0	21.4	1.4	60.8	*4.1*	3.4	1590
Cowpeas, green, edible portion	1	——	65.9	9.4	0.6	22.7	——	1.4	620
Potatoes, raw or fresh : [1] Edible portion —									
Average	136	——	78.3	2.2	0.1	18.4	(53)*0.4*	1.0	385
As purchased . . .	—	20.0	62.6	1.8	0.1	14.7	——	0.8	310
Potatoes, evaporated, as purchased:									
Average	3	——	7.1	8.5	0.4	80.9	——	3.1	1680
Potatoes, cooked, boiled, as purchased : [2]									
Average	11	——	75.5	2.5	0.1	20.9	(1)*0.6*	1.0	440
Potatoes, cooked, chips, as purchased:									
Average	2	——	2.2	6.8	39.8	46.7	——	4.5	2675
Potatoes, cooked, mashed, and creamed, as purchased:									
Average . . .	4	——	75.1	2.6	3.0	17.8	——	1.5	505
Potatoes, sweet. raw, or fresh : [3] Edible portion —									
Average	95	——	69.0	1.8	0.7	27.4	(88)*1.3*	1.1	570
As purchased . . .	—	20.0	55.2	1.4	0.6	21.9	——	0.9	460

[1] One sample contained 0.02 per cent free acid.   In 4 samples the average amount of proteid nitrogen was 57 per cent of the total nitrogen.   Twenty samples contained an average of 0.8 per cent malic acid, pectose substances, etc.   The ash of 40 samples contained an average of CaO 1, K_2O 59.2, MgO 4.5, P_2O_5 13.8, Na_2O 4, and SO_2 6.5 per cent.

[2] One sample contained cane sugar 0.2, glucose 0.2, and starch 17.4 per cent.

[3] The edible portion of 26 samples contained an average of cane sugar 2.5 and

CHEMICAL COMPOSITION OF AMERICAN FOOD MATERIALS — *Continued*

Food Materials	Number of Analyses	Refuse	Water	Protein	Fat	Total Carbohydrates (including Fiber)	Fiber (Number of Determinations in Parentheses)	Ash	Fuel Value per Pound
VEGETABLE FOOD — *Continued* VEGETABLES — *Continued*									
Potatoes, sweet, cooked, and prepared, as purchased . . .	1	Per Cent —	Per Cent 51.9	Per Cent 3.0	Per Cent 2.1	Per Cent 42.1	Per Cent	Per Cent 0.9	Cal-ories 925
Pumpkins: Edible portion —									
Average	3	—	93.1	1.0	0.1	5.2	*1.2*	0.6	120
As purchased . . .	—	50.0	46.5	0.5	0.1	2.6	—	0.3	60
Radishes: Edible portion —									
Average . . .	4	—	91.8	1.3	0.1	5.8	(2)0.7	1.0	135
As purchased . . .	—	30.0	64.3	0.9	0.1	4.0	—	0.7	95
Rhubarb:[1] Edible portion —									
Average	2	—	94.4	0.6	0.7	3.6	(1)1.1	0.7	105
As purchased . . .	—	40.0	56.6	0.4	0.4	2.2	—	0.4	65
Ruta-bagas:[2] Edible portion —									
Average	5	—	88.9	1.3	0.2	8.5	*1.2*	1.1	190
As purchased . . .	—	30.0	62.2	0.9	0.1	6.0	—	0.8	135
Sauerkraut, as purchased: Average	2	—	88.8	1.7	0.5	3.8	,—	5.2	125
Spinach, fresh, as purchased:[3] Average	3	—	92.3	2.1	0.3	3.2	*0.9*	2.1	110
Spinach, cooked, as purchased	1	—	89.8	2.1	4.1	2.6	—	1.4	260

invert sugar 3.4 per cent. Two samples contained, in the edible portion, an average of protein (N × 6.25) 1.8 and proteids 1.3 per cent.

[1] The edible portion of 1 sample contained free acid 0.5, protein (N × 6.25) 0.7, and proteids 0.4 per cent.

[2] The ash of the edible portion of 3 samples contained an average of CaO 9.4, K_2O 43.6, MgO 2.8, P_2O_5 11.7, Na_2O 10.2, and Fe_2O_3 0.5 per cent. One sample contained protein (N × 6.25) 2 and proteids 0.9 per cent.

[3] The ash of 2 samples contained an average of CaO 2 6, K_2O 39.9, MgO 2.2

Chemical Composition of American Food Materials — *Continued*

Food Materials	Number of Analyses	Refuse	Water	Protein	Fat	Total Carbohydrates (including Fiber)	Fiber (Number of Determinations in Parentheses)	Ash	Fuel Value per Pound
Vegetable Food — *Continued*									
Vegetables — *Continued*									
Squash: [1]			Per Cent	Per Cent	Per Cent	Per Cent	Per Cent	Per Cent	Per Cent	Cal-ories
Edible portion —									
Average	10	——	88.3	1.4	0.5	9.0	(5)0.8	0.8	215
As purchased . . .	—	50.0	44.2	0.7	0.2	4.5	——	0.4	105
Tomatoes, fresh, as purchased: [2]									
Average	27	——	94.3	0.9	0.4	3.9	(22)0.6	0.5	105
Tomatoes, dried, as purchased	1	——	7.3	12.9	8.1	62.3	——	9.4	1740
Turnips: [3]									
Edible portion —									
Average	19	——	89.6	1.3	0.2	8.1	(9)1.3	0.8	185
As purchased . . .	—	30.0	62.7	0.9	0.1	5.7	——	0.6	125
Vegetables, Canned									
Artichokes, as purchased:									
Average	3	——	92.5	0.8	——	5.0	0.6	1.7	110
Asparagus, as purchased:									
Average	14	——	94.4	1.5	0.1	2.8	0.5	1.2	85
Beans, baked, as purchased:									
Average	21	——	68.9	6.9	2.5	19.6	(12)2.5	2.1	600

P_2O_5 2.2, and Na_2O 9.4 per cent. One sample contained 0.01 per cent free acid. One sample contained protein ($N \times 6.25$) 2.1 and proteids 1.3 per cent.

[1] The edible portion of 2 samples contained an average of protein ($N \times 6.25$) 0.6 and proteids 0.5 per cent.

[2] The ash of 1 sample contained CaO 5.8, K_2O 68.1, MgO 3.7, and P_2O_5, 8.7 per cent. Six samples contained an average of protein ($N \times 6.25$) 0.8 and proteids 0.5 per cent.

[3] The ash of the edible portion of 4 samples contained an average of CaO 8.8, K_2O 43, MgO 2.7, P_2O_5 11.4, and Na_2O 8.3 per cent. One sample contained protein ($N \times 6.25$) 0.8 and proteids 0.2 per cent. One sample contained 4.4 per cent sugar.

CHEMICAL COMPOSITION OF AMERICAN FOOD MATERIALS —
Continued

FOOD MATERIALS	NUMBER OF ANALYSES	REFUSE	WATER	PROTEIN	FAT	TOTAL CARBOHY-DRATES (including Fiber)	FIBER (Number of Determinations in Parentheses)	ASH	FUEL VALUE PER POUND
VEGETABLE FOOD — *Continued* VEGETABLES, CANNED — *Continued*									
Beans, string, as purchased:		Per Cent	Per Cent	Per Cent	Per Cent	Per Cent	Per Cent	Per Cent	Cal-ories
Average	29	—	93.7	1.1	0.1	3.8	(18)*0.5*	1.3	95
Beans, little green, as purchased . . .	1	—	93.8	1.2	0.1	3.4	*0.6*	1.5	90
Beans, wax, as purchased	1	—	94.6	1.0	0.1	3.1	*0.6*	1.2	80
Beans, haricots verts, as purchased:									
Average	7	—	95.2	1.1	0.1	2.5	*0.5*	1.1	70
Beans, haricots flageolets, as purchased:									
Average	3	—	81.6	4.6	0.1	12.5	*1.0*	1.2	320
Beans, haricots panaches, as purchased . .	1	—	86.1	3.7	—	9.2	*1.0*	1.0	240
Beans, Lima, as purchased:									
Average	16	—	79.5	4.0	0.3	14.6	(15)*1.2*	1.6	360
Beans, red kidney, as purchased [1] . .	1	—	72.7	7.0	0.2	18.5	*1.2*	1.6	480
Brussels sprouts, as purchased	1	—	93.7	1.5	0.1	3.4	*0.5*	1.3	95
Corn, green, as purchased: [2]									
Average	52	—	76.1	2.8	1.2	19.0	(43)*0.8*	0.9	455
Corn and tomatoes, as purchased:									
Average	2	—	87.6	1.6	0.4	9.6	*0.5*	0.8	225
Macedoine (mixed vegetables), as purchased:									
Average	5	—	93.1	1.4	—	4.5	*0.6*	1.0	110

[1] Shelled.
[2] Thirty-two samples contained an average of 0.4 per cent NaCl.

CHEMICAL COMPOSITION OF AMERICAN FOOD MATERIALS —
Continued

FOOD MATERIALS	NUMBER OF ANALYSES	REFUSE	WATER	PROTEIN	FAT	TOTAL CARBOHYDRATES (including Fiber)	FIBER (Number of Determinations in Parentheses)	ASH	FUEL VALUE PER POUND
VEGETABLE FOOD — *Continued*									
VEGETABLES, CANNED — *Continued*		Per Cent	Per Cent	Per Cent	Per Cent	Per Cent	Per Cent	Per Cent	Calories
Okra, as purchased: [1]									
Average	4	——	94.4	0.7	0.1	3.6	*0.7*	1.2	85
Okra and tomatoes, as purchased: [2]									
Average	3	——	91.8	1.1	0.3	5.2	*0.5*	1.6	130
Peas, green, as purchased: [3]									
Average	88	——	85.3	3.6	0.2	9.8	(83)*1.2*	1.1	255
Potatoes, sweet, as purchased:									
Average	2	——	55.2	1.9	0.4	41.4	(1)*0.8*	1.1	820
Pumpkins, as purchased:									
Average	7	——	91.6	0.8	0.2	6.7	(5)*1.1*	0.7	150
Squash, as purchased:									
Average	5	——	87.6	0.9	0.5	10.5	(2)*0.7*	0.5	235
Succotash, as purchased:									
Average	12	——	75.9	3.6	1.0	18.6	(10)*0.9*	0.9	455
Tomatoes, as purchased: [4]									
Average	19	——	94.0	1.2	0.2	4.0	(11)*0.5*	0.6	105
PICKLES, CONDIMENTS, ETC.									
Catsup, tomato, as purchased:									
Average	2	——	82.8	1.5	0.2	12.3	——	3.2	265
Horse-radish, as purchased:									
Average	2	——	86.4	1.4	0.2	10.5	——	1.5	230
Horse-radish, evaporated, as purchased . .	1	——	4.3	11.0	0.8	77.7	——	6.2	1685

[1] Three samples contained an average of 1.1 per cent NaCl.
[2] Three samples contained an average of 1 per cent NaCl.
[3] Eighty samples contained an average of 0.7 per cent NaCl.
[4] Seven samples contained an average of 0.1 per cent NaCl.

CHEMICAL COMPOSITION OF AMERICAN FOOD MATERIALS — *Continued*

FOOD MATERIALS	NUMBER OF ANALYSES	REFUSE	WATER	PROTEIN	FAT	TOTAL CARBOHYDRATES (including Fiber)	FIBER (Number of Determinations in Parentheses)	ASH	FUEL VALUE PER POUND
VEGETABLE FOOD — *Continued*									
PICKLES, CONDIMENTS, ETC. — *Continued*		Per Cent	Per Cent	Per Cent	Per Cent	Per Cent	Per Cent	Per Cent	Calories
Olives, green:									
Edible portion . . .	1	——	58.0	1.1	27.6	11.6	——	1.7	1400
As purchased . . .	1	27.0	42.3	0.8	20.2	8.5	——	1.2	1025
Olives, ripe:									
Edible portion . . .	1	——	64.7	1.7	25.9	4.3	——	3.4	1205
As purchased . . .	1	19.0	52.4	1.4	21.0	3.5	——	2.7	975
Peppers (paprika), green, dried, as purchased	1	——	5.0	15.5	8.5	63.0	——	8.0	1820
Peppers, red chili, as purchased: [1]									
Average	5	——	5.3	9.4	7.7	70.0	——	7.6	1800
Pickles, cucumber, as purchased:									
Average	3	——	92.9	0.5	0.3	2.7	——	3.6	70
Pickles, mixed, as purchased . . .	1	——	93.8	1.1	0.4	4.0	——	0.7	110
Pickles, spiced, as purchased	1	——	77.1	0.4	0.1	20.7	——	1.7	395
FRUITS, BERRIES, ETC., FRESH [2]									
Apples: [3]									
Edible portion — Average	29	——	84.6	0.4	0.5	14.2	(7)1.2	0.3	290
As purchased. . . .	—	25.0	63.3	0.3	0.3	10.8	——	0.3	220

[1] Refuse, seeds and stem.

[2] Fruits contain a certain proportion of inedible materials, as skin, seeds, etc., which are properly classed as refuse. In some fruits, as oranges and prunes, the amount rejected in eating is practically the same as the refuse. In others, as apples and pears, more or less of the edible material is ordinarily rejected with the skin and seeds and other inedible portions. The edible material which is thus thrown away, and should properly be classed with the waste, is here classed with the refuse. The figures for refuse here given represent, as nearly as can be ascertained, the quantities ordinarily rejected.

[3] The edible portion of 1 sample contained glucose 6.4, cane sugar 6, and starch

CHEMICAL COMPOSITION OF AMERICAN FOOD MATERIALS — *Continued*

FOOD MATERIALS	NUMBER OF ANALYSES	REFUSE	WATER	PROTEIN	FAT	TOTAL CARBOHY-DRATES (including Fiber)	FIBER (Number of Determinations in Parentheses)	ASH	FUEL VALUE PER POUND
VEGETABLE FOOD — *Continued*									
FRUITS, BERRIES, ETC., FRESH—*Continued*									
Apricots: [1]			Per Cent	Per Cent	Per Cent	Per Cent	Per Cent	Per Cent	Cal-ories
Edible portion —									
Average	11	—	85.0	1.1	—	13.4		0.5	270
As purchased . .	—	6.0	79.9	1.0	—	12.6		0.5	255
Bananas, yellow: [2]									
Edible portion —									
Average	6	—	75.3	1.3	0.6	22.0	(1)1.0	0.8	460
As purchased .	—	35.0	48.9	0.8	0.4	14.3		0.6	300
Blackberries, as purchased: [3]									
Average	9	—	86.3	1.3	1.0	10.9	(1)2.5	0.5	270
Cherries: [4]									
Edible portion —									
Average	16	—	80.9	1.0	0.8	16.7	(1)0.2	0.6	365
As purchased . . .	—	5.0	76.8	0.9	0.8	15.9		0.6	345
Cranberries, as purchased:									
Average . . .	3	—	88.9	0.4	0.6	9.9	(2)1.5	0.2	215
Currants, as purchased .	1	—	85.0	1.5	—	12.8		0.7	265
Figs, fresh, as purchased:									
Average [5]	28	—	79.1	1.5	—	18.8		0.6	380

acids, etc., 12 per cent. The edible portion of 1 sample contained protein (N×6.25) 0.6 and proteids 0.4 per cent.

[1] The edible portion of 1 sample contained 11.9 per cent sugar. The fat was not determined.

[2] The edible portion of 1 sample contained protein (N × 6.25) 1.4 and proteids 1.2 per cent. The edible portion of 1 sample contained 0.1 per cent free acid.

[3] One sample contained protein (N × 6.25) 0.9 and proteids 0.7 per cent.

[4] The ash of 1 sample contained CaO 4.2, K₂O 57.7, MgO 5.5, P₂O₅ 15.1, Na₂O 6.8, and SO₃ 5.8 per cent. The edible portion of 1 sample contained protein (N × 6.25) 1.1 and proteids 0.4 per cent. The edible portion of 1 sample contained 0.1 per cent free acid. Six samples contained an average of 11 per cent sugar.

[5] The ash of 3 samples contained an average of CaO 2.4, K₂O 55.8, MgO 5.6, P₂O₅ 12.4, and SO₃ 3.9 per cent. Fat not determined.

CHEMICAL COMPOSITION OF AMERICAN FOOD MATERIALS — *Continued*

Food Materials	Number of Analyses	Refuse	Water	Protein	Fat	Total Carbohydrates (including Fiber)	Fiber (Number of Determinations in Parentheses)	Ash	Fuel Value per Pound
VEGETABLE FOOD — *Continued*									
FRUITS, BERRIES, ETC., FRESH — *Continued*									
Grapes:[1]		Per Cent	Per Cent	Per Cent	Per Cent	Per Cent	Per Cent	Per Cent	Calories
Edible portion —									
Average	5	—	77.4	1.3	1.6	19 2	(1)4.3	0.5	450
As purchased	—	25.0	58.0	1.0	1.2	14.4	—	0.4	335
Huckleberries, edible portion	1	—	81.9	0.6	0.6	16.6	—	0.3	345
Lemons:[2]									
Edible portion —									
Average	4	—	89.3	1.0	0.7	8.5	(2)1.1	0.5	205
As purchased	—	30.0	62.5	0.7	0.5	5.9	—	0.4	145
Lemon juice	22	—	—	—	—	9.8 3	—	—	180
Muskmelons:									
Edible portion	1	—	89.5	0.6	—	9.3	2.1	0.6	185
As purchased	1	50.0	44.8	0.3	—	4.6	—	0.3	90
Nectarines:[4]									
Edible portion	1	—	82.9	0.6	—	15.9	—	0.6	305
As purchased	1	6.6	77.4	0.6	—	14.8	—	0.6	285
Oranges:[5]									
Edible portion —									
Average	23	—	86.9	0.8	0.2	11.6	—	0.5	240
As purchased	—	27.0	63.4	0.6	0.1	8.5	—	0.4	170

[1] The ash of 5 samples contained an average of CaO 5, K_2O 50.9, MgO 3, P_2O_5 21.2, and SO_3 4.3 per cent.

[2] The ash of 2 samples contained an average of CaO 29.9, K_2O 48.3, MgO 4.4, P_2O_5 11.1, and SO^3 2.8 per cent. Two samples contained an average of protein (N × 6.25) 0.9 and proteids 0.5 per cent.

[3] Sugar 2.3, citric acid 7.5 per cent.

[4] Fat not determined.

[5] The ash of 9 samples contained an average of CaO 22.7, K_2O 48.9, MgO 5.4, P_2O_5 12.4, and SO_3 5.2 per cent. Fat determined in 8 samples, the mean of these assumed to be an average. Eight samples contained an average of 9 per cent sugar.

2 F

CHEMICAL COMPOSITION OF AMERICAN FOOD MATERIALS — *Continued*

Food Materials	Number of Analyses	Refuse	Water	Protein	Fat	Total Carbohydrates (including Fiber)	Fiber (Number of Determinations in Parentheses)	Ash	Fuel Value per Pound
VEGETABLE FOOD— *Continued* FRUITS, BERRIES, ETC., FRESH—*Continued*									
Pears: [1] Edible portion —			Per Cent	Per Cent	Per Cent	Per Cent	Per Cent	Per Cent	Calories
Average	2	—	84.4	0.6	0.5	14.1	(1)2.7	0.4	295
As purchased	—	10.0	76.0	0.5	0.4	12.7	—	0.4	260
Persimmons, edible portion [2]	1	—	66.1	0.8	0.7	31.5	1.8	0.9	630
Pineapple, edible portion [3]	1	—	89.3	0.4	0.3	9.7	0.4	0.3	200
Plums: [4] Edible portion, average	3	—	78.4	1.0	—	20.1	—	0.5	395
As purchased	—	5.0	74.5	0.9	—	19.1	—	0.5	370
Pomegranates, edible portion: [5] Average	2	—	76.8	1.5	1.6	19.5	2.7	0.6	460
Prunes: [6] Edible portion, average	24	—	79.6	0.9	—	18.9	—	0.6	370
As purchased	20	5.8	75.6	0.7	—	17.4	—	0.5	335
Raspberries, red, as purchased [7]	1	—	85.8	1.0	—	12.6	2.9	0.6	255
Raspberries, black, edible portion: Average	3	—	84.1	1.7	1.0	12.6	—	0.6	310

[1] One sample contained protein (N × 6.25) 0.6 and proteids 0.3 per cent.
[2] Contained glucose 13.5, cane sugar 1 per cent.
[3] Contained protein (N × 6.25) 0.4 and proteids 0.1 per cent.
[4] The edible portion contained 13.2 per cent sugar Fat not determined
[5] Two samples contained an average of glucose 11, of cane sugar 0.7 per cent.
[6] The ash of the edible portion of 3 samples contained an average of CaO 4.7, K_2O 63.8, MgO 5.5, P_2O_5 14.1, and SO_3 2.7 per cent. Edible portion of 20 samples contained an average of 16.1 per cent sugar. Fat was not determined.
[7] Fat not determined.

CHEMICAL COMPOSITION OF AMERICAN FOOD MATERIALS —
Continued

FOOD MATERIALS	NUMBER OF ANALYSES	REFUSE	WATER	PROTEIN	FAT	TOTAL CARBOHY-DRATES (including Fiber)	FIBER (Number of Determinations in Parentheses)	ASH	FUEL VALUE PER POUND
VEGETABLE FOOD— *Continued* FRUITS, BERRIES, ETC., FRESH—*Continued*		Per Cent	Per Cent	Per Cent	Per Cent	Per Cent	Per Cent	Per Cent	Cal- ories
Raspberry juice, edible portion	1	—	49.3	0.5	—	49.9 [1]	—	0.3	935
Strawberries: [2] Edible portion —									
Average	22	—	90.4	1.0	0.6	7.4	(19) *1.4*	0.6	180
As purchased . . .	—	5.0	85.9	0.9	0.6	7.0	—	0.6	175
Watermelons: [3] Edible portion —									
Average	2	—	92.4	0.4	0.2	6.7	—	0.3	140
As purchased . . .	—	59.4	37.5	0.2	0.1	2.7	—	0.1	60
Whortleberries, as pur- chased [4] . . .	1	—	82.4	0.7	3.0	13.5	*3.2*	0.4	390
FRUITS, ETC., DRIED									
Apples, as purchased: [5] Average	3	—	28.1	1.6	2.2	66.1	—	2.0	1350
Apricots, as purchased: [6] Average	2	—	29.4	4.7	1.0	62.5	—	2.4	1290
Citron, as purchased: Average	2	—	19.0	0.5	1.5	78.1	—	0.9	1525

[1] Probably sweetened.
[2] Four samples contained an average of protein (N × 6.25) 0.7 and proteids 0.5 per cent. Fifteen samples contained an average of glucose 5.5 and free acid, calculated as malic acid, 1.4 per cent.
[3] In one melon the rind was 55.8 of the whole, the pulp 6.9, the seeds 2.2, and the juice 35.1 per cent. The edible portion of 1 sample contained protein (N × 6.25) 0.9 and proteids 0.3 per cent.
[4] Contained protein (N × 6.25) 0.7 and proteids 0.5 per cent.
[5] One sample contained 2 per cent free acid calculated as sulfuric acid.
[6] One sample contained 1.5 per cent free acid calculated as sulfuric acid.

CHEMICAL COMPOSITION OF AMERICAN FOOD MATERIALS — *Continued*

FOOD MATERIALS	NUMBER OF ANALYSES	REFUSE	WATER	PROTEIN	FAT	TOTAL CARBOHYDRATES (including Fiber)	FIBER (Number of Determinations in Parentheses)	ASH	FUEL VALUE PER POUND
VEGETABLE FOOD— *Continued* FRUITS, ETC., DRIED— *Continued*									
Currants, Zante, as purchased:		Per Cent	Per Cent	Per Cent	Per Cent	Per Cent	Per Cent	Per Cent	Calories
Average	4	——	17.2	2.4	1.7	74.2	——	4.5	1495
Dates:									
Edible portion —									
Average	2	——	15.4	2.1	2.8	78.4	——	1.3	1615
As purchased . . .	—	10.0	13.8	1.9	2.5	70.6	——	1.2	1450
Figs, as purchased : [1]									
Average	3	——	18.8	4.3	0.3	74.2	——	2.4	1475
Grapes, ground, as purchased [2] . . .	1	——	34.8	2.8	0.6	60.5	3.7	1.2	1205
Pears, as purchased . .	1	——	16.5	2.8	5.4 [3]	72.9	——	2.4	1635
Prunes: [4]									
Edible portion —									
Average	15	——	22.3	2.1	——	73.3	——	2.3	1400
As purchased . . .	—	15.0	19.0	1.8	——	62.2	——	2.0	1190
Raisins:									
Edible portion —									
Average . . .	3	——	14.6	2.6	3.3	76.1	——	3.4	1605
As purchased . . .	—	10.0	13.1	2.3	3.0	68.5	——	3.1	1445
Raspberries, as purchased	1	——	8.1	7.3	1.8	80.2	——	2.6	1705
FRUITS, ETC., CANNED ; AND JELLIES, PRESERVES, ETC.									
Apples, crab, as purchased	1	——	42.4	0.3	2.4	54.4	——	0.5	1120
Apple sauce, as purchased	1	——	61.1	0.2	0.8	37.2	——	0.7	730

[1] One sample contained 0.4 per cent free acid calculated as sulfuric acid.

[2] Contained 0.8 per cent free acid calculated as sulfuric acid and 1.3 per cent tannin.

[3] The percentage of fat given is evidently too high.

[4] Twelve samples contained an average of sugar 25.4 and free acid 0.3 per cent, calculated as sulfuric acid. Fat not determined.

CHEMICAL COMPOSITION OF AMERICAN FOOD MATERIALS —
Continued

FOOD MATERIALS	NUMBER OF ANALYSES	REFUSE	WATER	PROTEIN	FAT	TOTAL CARBOHYDRATES (including Fiber)	FIBER (Number of Determinations in Parentheses)	ASH	FUEL VALUE PER POUND
VEGETABLE FOOD— *Continued*									
FRUITS, ETC., CANNED; AND JELLIES, PRESERVES, ETC.— *Continued*		Per Cent	Per Cent	Per Cent	Per Cent	Per Cent	Per Cent	Per Cent	Calories
Apricots, as purchased	1	—	81.4	0.9	—	17.3	—	0.4	340
Apricot sauce, as purchased . .	1	—	45.2	1.9	1.3	48.8	—	2.8	1000
Blackberries, as purchased . . .	1	—	40.0	0.8	2.1	56.4	—	0.7	1150
Blueberries, as purchased Average	3	—	85.6	0.6	0.6	12.8	—	0.4	275
Cherries, as purchased .	1	—	77.2	1.1	0.1	21.1	—	0.5	415
Cherry jelly: 1st quality, as purchased . . .	1	—	21.0	1.1	—	77.2	—	0.7	1455
2d quality, as purchased . . .	1	—	38.4	1.2	—	59.8	—	0.6	1135
Figs, stewed, as purchased . . .	1	—	56.5	1.2	0.3	40.9	—	1.1	785
Grape butter, as purchased . . .	1	—	36.7	1.2	0.1	58.5	—	3.5	1115
Marmalade (orange peel), as purchased [1] .	1	—	14.5	0.6	0.1	84.5	—	0.3	1585
Peaches, as purchased: Average	3	—	88.1	0.7	0.1	10.8	—	0.3	220
Pears, as purchased: Average	4	—	81.1	0.3	0.3	18.0	—	0.3	355
Pineapples, as purchased	1	—	61.8	0.4	0.7	36.4	—	0.7	715
Prune sauce, as purchased	1	—	76.6	0.5	0.1	22.3	—	0.5	430
Strawberries, stewed, as purchased . . .	1	—	74.8	0.7	—	24.0	—	0.5	460

[1] Fifteen samples of marmalade contain an average of water 30.8, sugar 32.8, invert sugar 32.3, glucose 14.2, acid 0.5, and undetermined 3.6 per cent.

CHEMICAL COMPOSITION OF AMERICAN FOOD MATERIALS —
Continued

FOOD MATERIALS	NUMBER OF ANALYSES	REFUSE	WATER	PROTEIN	FAT	TOTAL CARBOHYDRATES (including Fiber)	FIBER (Number of Determinations in Parentheses)	ASH	FUEL VALUE PER POUND
VEGETABLE FOOD — *Continued* FRUITS, ETC., CANNED; AND JELLIES, PRESERVES, ETC. — *Continued*		Per Cent	Per Cent	Per Cent	Per Cent	Per Cent	Per Cent	Per Cent	Calories
Tomato preserves, as purchased . . .	1	——	40.9	0.7	0.1	57.6	——	0.7	1090
NUTS									
Almonds: [1]									
Edible portion — Average	11	——	4.8	21.0	54.9	17.3	2.0	2.0	3030
As purchased . . .	—	45.0	2.7	11.5	30.2	9.5	——	1.1	1660
Beechnuts:									
Edible portion . . .	1	——	4.0	21.9	57.4	13.2	——	3.5	3075
As purchased . . .	1	40.8	2.3	13.0	34.0	7.0	——	2.1	1820
"Biotes" (acorns), (*Quercus emoryi*):									
Edible portion . . .	1	——	4.1	8.1	37.4	48.0	——	2.4	2620
As purchased . . .	1	35.6	2.6	5.2	24.1	30.9	——	1.6	1690
Brazil nuts (*Bertholletia excelsa*):									
Edible portion . . .	1	——	5.3	17.0	66.8	7.0	——	3.9	3265
As purchased . . .	1	49.6	2.6	8.6	33.7	3.5	·——	2.0	1655
Butternuts (*Juglans cinerea*):									
Edible portion . . .	1	——	4.4	27.9	61.2	3.5	——	2.9	3165
As purchased . . .	1	86.4	0.6	3.8	8.3	0.5	——	0.4	430
Chestnuts, fresh: [2]									
Edible portion — Average . .	9	——	45.0	6.2	5.4	42.1	1.8	1.3	1125

[1] Fresh almonds contain from 40 to 42 per cent water. The ash of the kernel contains CaO 14.5, MgO 18.3, Na₂O 1.8, K₂O 11, MnO₂ 0.3, Fe₂O₃ + Al₂O₃ 0.8, P₂O₅ 48.1, SO₃ 4.6, SiO₂ 0.2, and Cl 0.3 per cent.

[2] The ash of 2 samples contained an average of CaO 4.6, MgO 8, Na₃O₂ 1.2,

CHEMICAL COMPOSITION OF AMERICAN FOOD MATERIALS —
Continued

FOOD MATERIALS	NUMBER OF ANALYSES	REFUSE	WATER	PROTEIN	FAT	TOTAL CARBOHY-DRATES (including Fiber)	FIBER (Number of Determinations in Parentheses)	Ash	FUEL VALUE PER POUND
VEGETABLE FOOD — *Continued* NUTS — *Continued*									
Chestnuts, fresh — *Continued*		Per Cent	Per Cent	Per Cent	Per Cent	Per Cent	Per Cent	Per Cent	Cal-ories
As purchased . . .	9	16.0	37.8	5.2	4.5	35.4	—	1.1	945
Chestnuts, dried:									
Edible portion —									
Average	8	—	5.9	10.7	7.0	74.2	2.7	2.2	1875
As purchased . . .	8	24.0	4.5	8.1	5.3	56.4	—	1.7	1425
Coconuts:									
Edible portion . . .	1	—	14.1	5.7	50.6	27.9	—	1.7	2760
As purchased . . .	1	48.8 [1]	7.2	2.9	25.9	14.3	—	0.9	1413
Coconut without milk, as purchased . .	1	37.3 [2]	8.9	3.6	31.7	17.5	—	1.0	1730
Coconut milk, as purchased	1	—	92.7	0.4	1.5	4.6	—	0.8	155
Coconut, prepared, as purchased:									
Average	2	—	3.5	6.3	57.4	31.5	—	1.3	3125
Filberts:									
Edible portion . . .	1	—	3.7	15.6	65.3	13.0	—	2.4	3290
As purchased . . .	1	52.1	1.8	7.5	31.3	6.2	—	1.1	1575
Hickory nuts:									
Edible portion . . .	1	—	3.7	15.4	67.4	11.4	—	2.1	3345
As purchased . . .	1	62.2	1.4	5.8	25.5	4.3	—	0.8	1265
Lichi nuts:									
Edible portion . . .	1	—	17.9	2.9	0.2	77.5	—	1.5	1505
As purchased . . .	1	41.6	10.5	1.7	0.1	45.2	—	0.9	875
Peanuts:									
Edible portion —									
Average	4	—	9.2	25.8	38.6	24.4	2.5	2.0	2560
As purchased . . .	—	24.5	6.9	19.5	29.1	18.5	—	1.5	1935

K₂O 48.7, MnO₂ 0.2, Fe₂O + Al₂₃O₃ 0.4, P₂O₅ 23.5, S₂O 12.8, SiO₂ 0.2, and Cl 0.3 per cent.

[1] Milk and shell.   [2] Shell only.

CHEMICAL COMPOSITION OF AMERICAN FOOD MATERIALS — *Continued*

FOOD MATERIALS	NUMBER OF ANALYSES	REFUSE	WATER	PROTEIN	FAT	TOTAL CARBOHYDRATES (including Fiber)	FIBER (Number of Determinations in Parentheses)	ASH	FUEL VALUE PER POUND
VEGETABLE FOOD — *Continued* NUTS — *Continued*		Per Cent	Per Cent	Per Cent	Per Cent	Per Cent	Per Cent	Per Cent	Calories
Peanut butter, as purchased	2	—	2.1	29.3	46.5	17.1	—	5.0 [1]	2825
Pecans, polished:									
Edible portion . . .	1	—	3.0	11.0	71.2	13.3	—	1.5	3455
As purchased . . .	1	53.2	1.4	5.2	33.3	6.2	—	0.7	1620
Pecans, unpolished:									
Edible portion . .	1	—	2.7	9.6	70.5	15.3	—	1.9	3435
As purchased . . .	1	46.3	1.5	5.1	37.9	8.2	—	1.0	1846
Pine nuts:									
Pignolias, edible portion	1	—	6.4	33.9	49.4	6.9	—	3.4	2845
Piniones (*Pinus monophylla*) —									
Edible portion . .	1	—	3.8	6.5	60.7	26.2	—	2.8	3170
As purchased . .	1	41.7	2.2	3.8	35.4	15.3	—	1.6	1850
Pinon (*Pinus edulis*) —									
Edible portion . .	1	—	3.4	14.6	61.9	17.3	—	2.8	3205
As purchased . .	1	40.6	2.0	8.7	36.8	10.2	—	1.7	1905
Sabine pine nut (*Pinus sabiniana*) —									
Edible portion . .	1	—	5.1	28.1	53.7	8.4	—	4.7	2945
As purchased . .	1	77.0	1.2	6.5	12.3	1.9	—	1.1	675
Pistachios:									
First quality, shelled, edible portion .	1	—	4.2	22.3	54.0	16.3	—	3.2	2995
Second quality, shelled, edible portion .	1	—	4.3	22.8	54.9	14.9	—	3.0	3020
Walnuts, California: [2]									
Edible portion . . .	1	—	2.5	18.4	64.4	13.0	*1.4*	1.7	3300
As purchased . . .	1	73.1	0.7	4.9	17.3	3.5	—	0.5	885

[1] 1 per cent salt.
[2] Fresh walnuts contain from 20 to 27 per cent water. The ash of 7 samples of kernel contained an average of CaO 5.6, MgO 16.6, Na_2O 1, K_2O 12.7, MnO_2 0.3, $Fe_2O_3 + Al_2O_3$ 3.2, P_2O_5 57.8, SO_3 1.3, SiO_2 0.7, and Cl 0.7 per cent.

CHEMICAL COMPOSITION OF AMERICAN FOOD MATERIALS —
Continued

FOOD MATERIALS	NUMBER OF ANALYSES	REFUSE	WATER	PROTEIN	FAT	TOTAL CARBOHYDRATES (including Fiber)	FIBER (Number of Determinations in Parentheses)	ASH	FUEL VALUE PER POUND
VEGETABLE FOOD — *Continued* NUTS — *Continued*									
Walnuts, California, black: Edible portion —		Per Cent	Per Cent	Per Cent	Per Cent	Per Cent	Per Cent	Per Cent	Cal- ories
Average	2	—	2.5	27.6	56.3	11.7	*1.7*	1.9	3105
As purchased . . .	—	74.1	0.6	7.2	14.6	3.0	—	0.5	805
Walnuts, California, soft shell: Edible portion —									
Average	4	—	2.5	16.6	63.4	16.1	*2.6*	1.4	3285
As purchased . . .	—	58.1	1.0	6.9	26.6	6.8	—	0.6	1375
"Malted nuts," as pur-chased	1	—	2.6	23.7	27.6	43.9	—	2.2	2240
MISCELLANEOUS									
Chocolate, as purchased: Average	2	—	5.9	12.9	48.7	30.3	—	2.2	2860
Cocoa, as purchased: Average	3	—	4.6	21.6	28.9	37.7	—	7.2	2320
Cereal coffee infusion (1 part boiled in 20 parts water) [1] .	5	—	98.2	0.2	—	1.4	—	0.2	30
Yeast, compressed, as purchased . . .	1	—	65.1	11.7	0.4	21.0	—	1.8	625

[1] The average of five analyses of cereal coffee grain is: Water 6.2, protein 13.3, fat 3.4, carbohydrates 72.6, and ash 4.5 per cent. Only a portion of the nutrients however, enter into the infusion. The average in the table represents the available nutrients in the cereal coffee infusion. Infusions of genuine coffee and of tea contain practically no nutrients.

CHEMICAL COMPOSITION OF AMERICAN FOOD MATERIALS —
Continued

FOOD MATERIALS	NUMBER OF ANALYSES	REFUSE	WATER	PROTEIN N × 6.25	PROTEIN By Difference	FAT	TOTAL CARBO-HYDRATES	ASH	FUEL VALUE PER POUND
UNCLASSIFIED FOOD MATERIALS									
ANIMAL AND VEGETABLE									
Soups, home-made.		Per Cent	Per Cent	Per Cent	Per Cent	Per Cent	Per Cent	Per Cent	Cal-ories
Beef soup, as purchased:									
Average	2	——	92.9	4.4	——	0.4	1.1	1.2	120
Bean soup, as purchased:	1	——	84.3	10.5	——	1.4	9.4	1.7	295
Chicken soup, as purchased	1	——	84.3	10.5	——	0.8	2.4	2.0	275
Clam chowder, as purchased:									
Average . . .	2	——	88.7	1.8	——	0.8	6.7	2.0	195
Meat stew, as purchased:									
Average	5	——	84.5	4.6	——	4.3	5.5	1.1	370
Soups, canned.									
Asparagus, cream of, as purchased . . .	1	——	87.4	2.5	——	3.2	5.5	1.4	285
Bouillon, as purchased:									
Average	3	——	96.6	2.2	——	0.1	0.2	0.9	50
Celery, cream of, as purchased	1	——	88.6	2.1	——	2.8	5.0	1.5	250
Chicken gumbo, as purchased:									
Average	2	——	89.2	3.8	——	0.9	4.7	1.4	195
Chicken soup, as purchased:									
Average	2	——	93.8	3.6	——	0.1	1.5	1.0	100
Consommé, as purchased	1	——	96.0	2.5	——	——	0.4	1.1	55
Cream, corn of, as purchased	1	——	86.8	2.5	——	1.9	7.8	1.0	270
Julienne, as purchased .	1	——	95.9	2.7	——	——	0.5	0.9	60
Mock turtle, as purchased:									
Average	2	——	89.8	5.2	——	0.9	2.8	1.3	185
Mulligatawny, as purchased:									
Average	2	——	89.3	3.7	——	0.1	5.7	1.2	180

CHEMICAL COMPOSITION OF AMERICAN FOOD MATERIALS —
Continued

FOOD MATERIALS	NUMBER OF ANALYSES	REFUSE	WATER	PROTEIN N × 6.25	PROTEIN By Difference	FAT	TOTAL CARBOHYDRATES	ASH	FUEL VALUE PER POUND
UNCLASSIFIED FOOD MATERIALS—*Continued* ANIMAL AND VEGETABLE — *Continued*									
Soups, canned—Continued									
Oxtail: Edible portion —			Per Cent	Per Cent	Per Cent	Per Cent	Per Cent	Per Cent	Calories
Average	2	—	88.8	4.0	—	1.3	4.3	1.6	210
As purchased . . .	1	1.8	87.8	3.8	—	0.5	4.2	1.9	170
Pea soup, as purchased:									
Average	4	—	86.9	3.6	—	0.7	7.6	1.2	235
Pea, cream of green, as purchased . . .	1	—	87.7	2.6	—	2.7	5.7	1.3	270
Tomato soup, as purchased:									
Average	2	—	90.0	1.8	—	1.1	5.6	1.5	185
Turtle, green, as purchased	1	—	86.6	6.1	—	1.9	3.9	1.5	265
Vegetable, as purchased	1	—	95.7	2.9	—	—	0.5	0.9	65
Miscellaneous									
Hash, as purchased . .	1	—	80.3	6.0	—	1.9	9.4	2.4	365
"Infants' and invalids' foods," as purchased: [1]									
Average	22	—	6.0	12.7	—	3.3	76.2	1.8	1795
Mincemeat, commercial, as purchased:									
Average	3	—	27.7	6.7	—	1.4	60.2	4.0	1305
Mincemeat, home-made, as purchased:									
Average	3	—	54.4	4.8	—	6.7	32.1	2.0	970
Salad, ham, as purchased	1	—	69.4	15.4	—	7.6	5.6	2.0	710
Sandwich, egg, as purchased	1	—	41.4	9.6	—	12.7	34.5	1.8	1355
Sandwich, chicken, as purchased . . .	1	—	48.5	12.3	—	5.4	32.1	1.7	1055

[1] This includes malted milk, infants' foods. and similar preparations which are sold under various trade names, but are similar in composition.

INDEX

Histones, 53.
Hordein, 52.
Hydrogen, relation to living organisms, 10; sources, 10,

Ice, disease germs in, 333; relation to health, 332.
Indol, 106.
Infant, effect of medicines on, 276; feeding, precautions in, 277.
Infants, artificial feeding of, 278; foods for, 289.
Inosite, 74.
Insects, depredations on foods, 347.
Intestinal juices, 105.
Intestines, bacteria in, 250; digestion in, 101.
Invertase, 92.
Iron, compounds of, 14; demand for, 14.

Lactase, 92.
Lactation, period of, 269.
Lacteals, function in absorption, 109.
Lactose, 70.
Lecithins, 82.
Leucocytes, 129.
Levulans, 74.
Levulose, 68.
Liver, the, 139; function of, 139.
Living, cost of, 237; examples of simple, 242.
Lunches, comparison of, 211.
Lungs, the, 133.

Maltose, 70.
Man, efficiency as a machine, 221.
Mannans, 74.
Mastication, 92.
Matter, classes of, 20; combustible, non-combustible, 21; organic, inorganic, 22.
Maysin, 50.
Meals, cheap, 231; elaborate, 241; costly, 231.

Measurements, physiological, 144; physiological, how made, 145.
Meat, baking, losses from, 316; boiling, losses from, 316; eating of, 256; extract, 301; extracts, commercial, 302; frying, losses from, 316; roasting, losses from, 316; toxins, 338; tubercular, 335; unhealthy, 334; juices, 301.
Meats, cuts of, 348; losses from cooking, 315.
Medicines, effects on child, 276.
Milk, abnormal, 273; adulteration of, 323; cow's, care of, 328; cow's, compared with human, 278; cow's, curdling of, 282; cow's, effect of food on, 275; cow's, disease germs in, 326; cow's, germ life in, 325; cow's, how modified, 322; cow's, humanizing, 283; cow's, infection of, 327; cow's, modifying of, 284; cow's, pasteurization of, 329; cow's, physical condition, 282; cow's, sanitation of, 321; goat's, as infant food, 287; human, 266; human, analyses of, 267; human, compared with cow's, 278; human, compounds in, 280; human, curdling of, 282; human, effect of individuality, 270; human, physical condition, 282; mother's, 266; mother's, conditions affecting, 269; normal, 322; products of, toxic, 338; secretion, demands on food, 270; secretion, effect of food, 272; secretion, insufficient diet, 272; secretion, necessary dietary, 272; solids, removal of, 325; standards, 324.
Milk fats, 81.
Milling, influences on ash constituents, 37.
Mineral compounds, elimination of, 138; foods supplying, 151; functions of, 149.

2 G

Printed in the United States of America.

Printed in the United States
80482LV00004B/40

9 781417 962969